Stroke Prevention, Treatment, and Rehabilitation

Notice

Medicine is an ever-changing science. As new research and clinical experience broaden our knowledge, changes in treatment and drug therapy are required. The authors and the publisher of this work have checked with sources believed to be reliable in their efforts to provide information that is complete and generally in accord with the standards accepted at the time of publication. However, in view of the possibility of human error or changes in medical sciences, neither the authors nor the publisher nor any other party who has been involved in the preparation or publication of this work warrants that the information contained herein is in every respect accurate or complete, and they disclaim all responsibility for any errors or omissions or for the results obtained from use of the information contained in this work. Readers are encouraged to confirm the information contained herein with other sources. For example and in particular, readers are advised to check the product information sheet included in the package of each drug they plan to administer to be certain that the information contained in this work is accurate and that changes have not been made in the recommended dose or in the contraindications for administration. This recommendation is of particular importance in connection with new or infrequently used drugs.

Stroke Prevention, Treatment, and Rehabilitation

J. David Spence, BA, MBA, MD, FRCPC, FCaHS
Professor of Neurology and Clinical Pharmacology
Stroke Prevention & Atherosclerosis Research Centre
Robarts Research Institute
Western University
London, Canada

Henry J. M. Barnett, MD, FRCPC, OC
Professor Emeritus of Clinical Neurological Sciences
Western University
Toronto, Canada

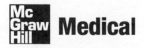
Medical

New York   Chicago   San Francisco   Lisbon   London   Madrid   Mexico City
New Delhi   San Juan   Seoul   Singapore   Sydney   Toronto

Stroke Prevention, Treatment, and Rehabilitation

1 2 3 4 5 6 7 8 9 0   DOC/DOC   17 16 15 14 13 12

ISBN 978-0-07-176235-9
MHID 0-07-176235-3

This book was set in Adobe Garamond by Cenveo Publisher Services.
The editors were Anne Sydor and Regina Y. Brown.
The production supervisor was Jeffrey Herzich.
Project management was provided by Manisha Singh, Cenveo Publisher Services.
The cover was designed by LaShae V. Ortiz.
RR Donnelley was printer and binder.

This book is printed on acid-free paper.

Cataloging-in Publication Data is on file with the Library of Congress.

McGraw-Hill books are available at special quantity discounts to use as premiums and sales promotions, or for use in corporate training programs. To contact a representative please e-mail us at bulksales@mcgraw-hill.com

Contents

Contributors

Francesco Arba, MD
Resident in Neurology
Department of Neurological and
Psychiatric Sciences
University of Florence
Florence, Italy

Eitan Auriel, MD, MSc
Department of Neurology
Tel-Aviv Sourasky Medical Center
Tel-Aviv University
Tel-Aviv, Israel

Joyce S. Balami, MD, MSc, MRCP
Stroke Physician and Geriatrician
Acute Stroke Programme
Department of Medicine and
Clinical Geratology
John Radcliffe Hospital
Oxford, United Kingdom

Henry J. M. Barnett, OC, MD, FRCP(C)
Professor Emeritus of Clinical
Neurological Sciences
Western University
Toronto, Canada

Natan M. Bornstein, MD
Professor of Neurology and Head of
Stroke Unit
Stourasky Medical Centre
Tel-Aviv Sourasky Medical Center
Tel-Aviv University
Tel-Aviv, Israel

**Alastair M. Buchan, DSc, LLD (Hon),
FMedSci, FRCP**
Head of Medical Sciences Division
Professor in Stroke Medicine
University of Oxford
Oxford, United Kingdom

Aurauma Chutinet, MD
Research Fellow
J. Philip Kistler MGH Stroke
Research Center
Boston, Massachusetts

Ross Feldman, MD
RW Gunton Professor of Therapeutics
Robarts Research Institute
Western University
London, Canada

Karen L. Furie, MD
Associate Professor of Neurology and
Director of Stroke Service
J. Philip Kistler MGH Stroke
Research Center
Boston, Massachusetts

Philip B. Gorelick, MD, MPH
Medical Director
Hauenstein Neuroscience Center
Michigan State University
St. Mary's Hospital
Grand Rapids, Michigan

Hen Hallevi, MD
Stroke Neurologist
Tel-Aviv Sourasky Medical Center
Tel-Aviv University
Tel-Aviv, Israel

**Marilyn MacKay-Lyons, BScPT,
MScPT, PhD**
Associate Professor
School of Physiotherapy
Dalhousie University
Halifax, Canada

Yongchai Nilanont, MD
Assistant Professor of Neurology
Director of Stroke Program
Division of Neurology
Siriraj Hospital
Mahidol University
Bangkok, Thailand

Niphon Poungvarin, MD, FRCP, FRI
Division of Neurology
Department of Medicine
Faculty of Medicine Siriraj Hospital
Mahidol University
Bangkok, Thailand

**Andrew Pipe, CM, MD, LLD (Hon),
DSc (Hon), OC**
Professor of Medicine and Chief
Division of Prevention and Rehabilitation
University of Ottawa Heart Institute
Ottawa, Canada

**John David Spence, BA, MBA, MD,
FRCPC, FCAHS**
Professor of Neurology and Clinical
    Pharmacology
Stroke Prevention & Atherosclerosis
    Research Centre
Robarts Research Institute
Western University
London, Canada

**Neville Suskin, MBChB, MSc, FRCPC,
FACC**
Associate Professor of Cardiology and
    Director of Cardiac Rehabilitation
University Hospital
London, Canada

Robert Teasell, MD, FRCPC
Chair of Rehabilitation Medicine
Parkwood Hospital
London, Canada

Fernando D. Testai, MD, PhD
Assistant Professor of Neurology
University of Illinois at Chicago
    Medical Center
Department of Neurology and Rehabilitation
Chicago, Illinois

Preface

More than 65 years ago when I was a medical student, I was taught that there were two kinds of stroke, namely cerebral thrombosis and cerebral haemorrhage. It was also recognized that sometimes cerebral infarction could result from embolism, when a blood clot, usually from the heart, flew off into a carotid artery and blocked one of the major cerebral vessels. Cerebral haemorrhage, we knew then, was largely the result of hypertension, though there was some neuropathological evidence to suggest that the presence of microaneurysms within the brain substance might be a factor. Even as a young trainee neurologist I was taught that relatively little could be done to treat a stroke apart from rehabilitative methods once the episode had terminated, and as for prevention, very little effective management was available, save for the treatment of hypertension.

How the position has changed over the last half century; one of the editors of this notable volume, Henry Barnett, has been acknowledged as a world leader in the field and as someone who has made seminal contributions to the diagnosis, management, and prevention of strokes of all types. In this excellent book, co-edited by him with Dr. J. David Spence, many effective measures for stroke prevention have been carefully and precisely detailed and analyzed. Very properly, the book begins with a consideration of epidemiology and highlights the urgency of treatment, a matter which has come increasingly to the fore in recent years, since it became recognized that early admission to hospital, with scanning to differentiate infarction from haemorrhage, followed by the use of thrombolytic drugs in the therapeutic window of three hours in those with infarcts, has had a major beneficial effect upon outcome. Subsequent chapters deal effectively with economics, nutrition, the crucial role of giving up smoking, the value of exercise, and the importance of treating hypertension. Barnett was one of the first to characterize fully transient ischaemic attacks, sometimes presaging major stroke, and was also one of the first to demonstrate the value of aspirin in treating such premonitory episodes as an important preventative tool. Appropriately, the book deals in detail with antiplatelet therapy, anticoagulation, and the role of lipid-lowering drugs, not forgetting the importance of treating diabetes and insulin resistance, which are sometimes a major factor in the aetiology of stroke. Additionally, of course, since the importance of carotid plaques in causing transient ischaemic attacks came to the fore, much work has been done on endarterectomy and stenting. The book concludes with a number of fascinating and in a sense provocative chapters, dealing specifically with finding the cause of TIAs and strokes, while Henry Barnett, perhaps with tongue in cheek, writes interestingly on the hazards of relying on publications, and while David Spence is keen to advise upon how one can minimize the adverse effects of cardiovascular therapy.

Without question, this publication must be regarded as an outstanding contribution to the cause of stroke prevention, and I believe it will be welcomed and avidly consulted by everyone with an interest in cardiovascular, but particularly cerebrovascular, disease.

John Walton (Lord Walton of Detchant)
Kt TD MA MD DSc FRCP FMedSci
Belford, Northumberland, UK

Section 1

Importance of Stroke and Stroke Prevention

Epidemiology of Stroke Prevention and Urgency of Treatment

1

Alastair M. Buchan
Joyce S. Balami
Francesco Arba

TOPICS

INTRODUCTION

Annually about 16 million first-ever strokes occur in the world, causing a total of 5.7 million deaths.[1] The burden of stroke is expected to increase to 18 million first-ever strokes and 6.5 million deaths in 2015.[2] According to World Health Organization (WHO) estimates, figures are predicted to increase further to 23 million first-time strokes, 77 million stroke survivors, 61 million disability-adjusted life years (DALYs), and 7.8 million deaths by 2030.[3,4] With an incidence of approximately 250 to 400 in 100,000 and a mortality of around 30%, stroke remains the third largest killer after heart disease and cancer in the developed world, and the most common cause of adult disability.[5] It has even been suggested that stroke can be ranked as the second most common single cause of death in the world population after ischemic heart disease, the third only if neoplastic diseases are considered as a group.[6] A review[7] has shown a statistically significant trend in stroke incidence rates over the past four decades, with a 42% decrease in stroke incidence in high-income countries and a greater than 100% increase in low- to middle-income countries. Nonetheless, stroke is a global epidemic and by no means a problem limited to developed or developing countries, thus making stroke and its consequences a worldwide health care problem.

2

INCIDENCE AND PREVALENCE

It has been difficult to assess the global incidence and prevalence of stroke, despite the large number of published epidemiological studies, due to lack of reliable data, particularly from developing countries. Several factors such as age, sex, race/ethnicity, population groups, socioeconomic status, and subtype of stroke determine the incidence and prevalence of stroke. Some studies repeated over successive time-points using the same methodology[8-13] have reported a significant decline in the incidence of stroke from the 1970s to the 1990s in the developed world, with more modest declines recently. Other studies have reported no change[14,15] or an increase in stroke incidence.[16-18]

The decline in stroke incidence has been suggested to be attributable to improvements in the primary prevention of stroke. For example, the Oxford Vascular Study in Oxfordshire, United Kingdom, reported a 29% decline in the incidence rate of stroke over a 20-year period that was attributed to the significant decrease in systolic and diastolic blood pressure, cholesterol levels, and prevalence of smoking.[8]

On the other hand, the increased stroke incidence, lack of change, or the modest decline shown in recent studies may reflect the aging demographic of the population and the fact that other risk factors such as obesity and diabetes mellitus may be on the rise, even though aggressive approaches to reducing hypertension, hypercholesterolemia, and smoking have been shown to play a role in the reduction of stroke incidence.[11]

In the United States about 795,000 people per year have stroke, of which 610,000 are first strokes and 185,000 are recurrent strokes.[19] It has been projected that the incidence will increase to 1 million by the year 2050.[20]

There is higher regional incidence and prevalence of stroke in the southeastern United States (referred to as the "stroke belt") than the northeast of the country.[21-23] The reason for this reported difference of nearly three times the number of strokes in the stroke belt region, consisting of 11 states, compared with that of the remaining 39 states in the northeast region is unclear; however, the reported higher prevalence of hypertension in the stroke belt may be partly responsible for the difference.

The number of stroke events in Europe is expected to increase from 1.1 million per year in 2000 to more than 1.5 million per year in 2025.[24] There is a considerable difference in total stroke incidence across Europe with reported lower rates in western and higher rates in eastern European countries.[25,26]

Data from the WHO MONICA Project (which is the first and to date the only multinational study reported on geographical stroke incidence using uniform criteria) showed a high incidence in Russia and Lithuania, and the lowest incidence in Italy.[27,28] Similarly, data from other studies have shown significantly higher stroke incidence rates in Ukraine,[29] and Russia,[30] and lower in Dijon, France.[31] For example, the incidence rates adjusted to the European population aged 45 to 84 years ranged from 238 per 100,000 people in Dijon to 938 per 100,000 people per year in the Ukraine.[29,31]

The East-West differences in stroke incidence rates have been attributed to higher levels of hypertension, smoking, and other risk factors in the Eastern countries as compared with the West.[27,28,32-34] Every year 110,000 people in England and Wales have their first stroke, and 30,000 of these people go on to have another one.[35]

Stroke can affect individuals of any age, but it primarily affects the elderly with the incidence as well as the prevalence increasing sharply with age.[36,37] For each successive 10 years after the age of 55, the stroke rate doubles in both men and women.[38] Around 75% to 89% of strokes occur after the age of 65, 50% in people who are aged 70 years or older and nearly 25% in individuals who are older than 85 years of age.[39,10] The age-specific incidence of stroke has been shown to rise from between 10 to 30 per 100,000 person-years in those aged less than 45 years, to 1200 to 2000 per 100,000 person-years in those 75 to 84 years of age.[16] The American Heart Association estimates that the prevalence of stroke in Americans older than 20 years is 6.4 million, with an overall prevalence of 2.9%. The prevalence of silent cerebral infarcts is age dependent and rises to about 11% for those aged 55 to 64 and to 43% for those aged 85.[19]

The older population is expected to increase in the future. By the year 2025 the global population older than 60 years is estimated to rise to 1.2 billion, and by 2050 the global number of old people (those aged >65) will exceed the number of young people (those aged <65).[40] Therefore, as the proportion of older people increases, stroke incidence is expected to rise, presenting a massive epidemic in the forthcoming years.

The incidence of pediatric stroke is estimated to be around two to three, to 13 per 100,000 children, with a higher incidence in boys than girls.[41] There is a higher incidence of ischemic stroke in men than women in patients under 80,[42,43] with a 25% to 33% higher rate in men than women.[44-46] In contrast, women comprised a larger proportion of the very old stroke patients (>80 years),[47-49] probably due to survival effects or women at risk of having their stroke later in life than men.[42]

A meta-analysis of the world population age-adjusted sex incidence rate ratios for 44 different populations showed a pooled age-adjusted rate ratio of 1.33 (95% confidence interval [CI], 1.30-1.37), suggesting a 33% greater stroke incidence in men than in women. The pooled age-adjusted rate was found to be 1.45 (95% CI, 1.39-1.51) for America and Australia populations (20 studies, 10,304 cases) and 1.24 (95% CI, 1.20-1.29) for European populations involving 24 studies with 11,687 cases.[49]

Although the analysis confirmed that stroke is more common among men than women, the difference tends to decrease with age, with women having their first stroke about four and a half years later than men.

In the United States the male-to-female incidence ratio is 1.25 in those aged 55 to 64 years, 1.50 in those aged 65 to 75, 1.07 for those aged 75 to 84, and falls to 0.76 in those aged 85 and older.[19]

European stroke incidence rates have been shown to vary from 141.3 per 100,000 in men to 94.6 per 100,000 in women.[25] There is also a regional variation, ranging in men from 101.2 per 100,000 (95% CI, 82.5-123.0) in Sesto Fiorentino, Italy, to 239.3 per 100,000 (95% CI, 209.9-271.6) in Kaunas, Lithuania. In women it ranged from 63.0 per 100,000 (95% CI, 48.5-80.7) in Sesto Fiorentino to 158.7 per 100,000 (95% CI, 135.0-185.4) in Kaunas.[25]

There is a racial disparity in the incidence of stroke as reported by numerous epidemiological studies.[50-53] Overall there are higher incidence rates of ischemic stroke among black patients, Asians, Hispanics, and other minority groups.

In the United States blacks and Hispanics have an increased incidence of stroke compared to whites. Blacks have been found to have a risk of first-ever stroke almost twice that of whites.[19] The age-adjusted incidence rate in people aged 45 to 84 years is 6.6 per 1000 in black men and 3.6 per 1000 in white men. In the Northern Manhattan study, the age-adjusted incidence of first ischemic stroke among whites, Hispanics, and blacks were 88, 149, and 191 per 100,000, respectively.[53] Also, Mexican Americans have been found to have an increased incidence of stroke compared to non-Hispanic whites.[54] Similarly, the prevalence of stroke in the United States has been reported to be higher for blacks than whites. The stroke prevalence rates (for those aged 18 and older) for whites, blacks, and Asians were 2.2%, 3.7%, and 2.6%, respectively.[19,55]

BURDEN OF STROKE

Mortality/Morbidity

Stroke exerts a substantial societal burden as the leading cause of adult long-term disability and is a major cause of mortality worldwide. Despite recent advances in the diagnosis and treatment of acute stroke in the past two decades, the mortality poststroke is still high. Although fatality from stroke has decreased in most populations, stroke remains a leading cause of death and disability in many developed countries. Declining stroke mortality rates were seen in the United States, Switzerland, Canada, Australia, and Western European countries like France,[56-58] and most Eastern European countries and Portugal, along with Yugoslavia in Southern Europe, have had an increase in stroke mortality.[7,56] The other parts of the world with high stroke mortality include North Asia, Central Africa, and the South Pacific regions.[7]

In the United States, age-adjusted mortality rates were reported to have stabilized in the 1990s, but started to decline from 1995 to 2005. During these years, there was a fall from 29.7% to 13.5% in stroke mortality.[59] Similarly, between 1996 and 2006 the death rate for stroke fell by 33.5%, with the total number of stroke deaths declining by 18.4%.[19] A similar trend of a 28.2% fall in the rate of stroke mortality between 1994 and 2004 was reported in a Canadian study as well as a 27.2% decrease in hospital admissions for stroke.[60]

It has been suggested that much of the observed decrease in stroke fatality is likely to be due to a decrease in case fatality rather than decreasing event rates.[61] This has been partly attributed to significant advances in the management of acute stroke care over the last decade, especially the advent of thrombolytic therapy,[62] which has revolutionized stroke care. This is in addition to endovascular treatments,[63,64] the use of aspirin,[65] and the introduction of stroke units[66] as well as decompressive surgery for supratentorial malignant hemispheric cerebral infarction.[67,68] (Hemicraniectomy is discussed in Chapter 17.) Other possible reasons for the decrease in stroke mortality may be improved detection and treatment of hypertension and increased public awareness.[59]

Numerous studies have shown the 30-day mortality after a first-ever stroke to be between 10% and 28%.[29,69-71] The three-month mortality varies between 18% and 33%,[70,72] and the six-month mortality between 20% and 30%.[73-75] Similarly, the one-year mortality has been reported to vary between 23.6% and 67.8%,[71,76,77] with a more than 50% risk of death during the subsequent five years and a more than 70% risk of death during the 10-year period poststroke.[69,78,79] A meta-analysis of the world population has shown how strokes are more severe in women, and case fatality at one month is higher among women.[46] Overall, about 10% of patients with first-ever strokes die in a month, 30% within three months, and 20% within six months, and about 30% or more are dependent on others for activities of daily living.[80,81] Stroke is also a leading cause of functional impairments; among stroke survivors 50% to 70% of patients regain functional independence, 15% to 30% are permanently disabled, and 20% require institutional care.[82]

In the United States about 134,000 people die yearly from stroke,[19] with a higher age-adjusted stroke mortality in the stroke belt than the rest of the country.[22,23,83] The total number of deaths from stroke in the 48 European countries was estimated at 1,239,000 per year.[84] Like the difference in the incidence and prevalence of stroke between the West and East, there is also a large disparity in mortality between the two European regions. The WHO MONICA Project reported a variation in the 28-day mortality within Europe, with higher mortality rates in some eastern countries.[85,86] The inequality in stroke mortality was partly attributable to the difference in hospitalization rates and level of care between the regions. Also accounting for the high mortality is the higher proportion of patients suffering from more severe strokes and therefore also having a higher case fatality rate.[32-34] Based on the data from the WHO MONICA Project and from other regional studies it has been concluded that the differences in early mortality of stroke are at least partly caused by the variation in quality and quantity of stroke throughout Europe.[34]

There are about 53,000 deaths from stroke every year in the United Kingdom, with a north–south variation with around 50% higher rates in the north compared to the south.[87] Stroke contributed to 1.5 and 3.5 million deaths in low- and middle-income countries, respectively.[4] About 87% of all stroke deaths are registered in low- and middle-income countries, which also account for 87% of total losses due to stroke in terms of DALYs.[88]

There is a relationship between race/ethnicity and stroke mortality. Several studies have shown increased mortality rates among blacks and other minority groups. Overall, blacks are more than twice as likely as whites to die of stroke.[89] This is probably due to socioeconomic and environmental factors, although much of the increase in mortality among blacks remains unexplained.[90] Spence has suggested that much of the excess stroke among blacks may be due to resistant hypertension from undiagnosed primary aldosteronism and Liddle syndrome variants.[91]

Cost

In addition to the relatively high mortality from stroke, the long-term needs of patients left disabled following stroke place an ongoing commitment of resources on the health care system. An international comparison of stroke cost studies showed that, on average, 0.27% of gross domestic product (GDP) was spent on stroke by national health systems, and stroke care accounted for approximately 3% of total health care expenditures.[92]

In the United States the total direct and indirect cost of stroke was estimated at $73.7 billion in 2010,[19] an increase from $68.9 billion in 2009[59] and $65.5 billion in 2008.[82] In the United States stroke is ranked among the most expensive chronic diseases, such as cancer, diabetes, and depression.[93] In European Union countries the total annual cost of stroke is estimated at 27 billion.[84] In the United Kingdom the cost for treatment and productivity loss arising from stroke has been estimated at £8.9 billion a year,[94] an increase from £4.5 billion in 2006-2007.[88]

The economic burden of stroke will also be a major challenge for developing countries, where stroke accounts for 87% of total losses in terms of DALYs.[87] Additionally, as the proportion of elderly stroke patients increases, the cost of stroke-related health care will continue to escalate and exert a major impact on medical resources, as well as an increasing toll on individuals and society,[95,96] especially in developed countries where the proportion of elderly people reaching advanced age is expected to increase substantially in the coming years. Individuals aged 80 years or older are the fastest growing age group in many industrialized countries.[97]

TYPES OF STROKE/CLASSIFICATION

Stroke has three distinct subtypes, each with different incidence rates, risk factors, and outcome profiles. The frequency of stroke subtypes also depends on age and racial differences. Overall, ischemic stroke (IS) is the most common subtype of stroke, accounting for approximately 67% to 80% of all strokes, followed by intracerebral hemorrhage (ICH), accounting for 7% to 20%, and subarachnoid hemorrhage (SAH), which accounts for between 1% and 13% of all strokes.[16] In the United States 87% of strokes are ischemic, 10% are primary intracerebral hemorrhage, and 3% are subarachnoid hemorrhage (SAH). Spontaneous intracerebral hemorrhage is more common in younger patients.[98] In the North Manhattan Stroke Study the stroke subtype in younger patients was 45% infarct, 31% intracerebral hemorrhage, and 24% subarachnoid hemorrhage.[99] On the other hand, due to the increasing prevalence of atherosclerosis and cardiovascular pathologies with aging, ischemic stroke accounts for most of the stroke subtypes in older patients. Furthermore, stroke has been classified using different classification systems: the Trial of Org 10172 in ACUTE Stroke Treatment (TOAST) criteria,[100] the Oxfordshire Community Stroke Project (OCSP) classification,[101] and the Atherothrombotic, Small vessel

Table 1–1. Stroke Classification

OCSP Classification	TOAST Classification	ASCO Classification
Lacunar infarcts (LACI): one of the 4 classic lacunar syndromes	**Large-artery athero-sclerosis** (embolus/thrombosis)	**Atherothrombosis** • Grade 1 • Grade 2 • Grade 3
Total anterior circulation infarcts (TACI): higher cerebral dysfunction + homonymous visual field defect + ipsilateral motor or sensory deficit of at least 2 areas of the face, arm, and leg	**Cardioembolism** (high-risk/medium risk)	**Small-vessel disease** • Grade 1 • Grade 2 • Grade 3
Partial anterior circulation infarcts (PACI): only 2 of the 3 components of the TACI syndrome	**Small-vessel occlusion** (lacune)	**Cardioembolism** • Grade 1 • Grade 2 • Grade 3
Posterior circulation infarcts (POCI): any of the following: • Ipsilateral cranial nerve palsy with contralateral motor and/or sensory deficit • Bilateral motor and/or sensory deficit • Disorder of conjugate eye movement • Cerebellar dysfunction without ipsilateral long tract deficit (ie, ataxic hemiparesis) • Isolated homonymous visual field defect	**Stroke of other deter-mined etiology**	**Other causes** • Grade 1 • Grade 2 • Grade 3
	Stroke of undeter-mined etiology • Two or more causes • Negative evaluation (cryptogenic) • Incomplete evaluation	

OCSP: Clinical pattern (signs and symptoms) at the time of the maximum deficit from first cerebrovascular event. It gives important information about the outcome and prognosis of stroke.

TOAST: Every category has a possible or probable subgroup on the basis of the examinations.

ASCO: Grade 1, 2, or 3 refers to the likelihood of pathology on the results of examinations:
    Grade 1: definitely a potential cause of index stroke
    Grade 2: causality uncertain
    Grade 3: unlikely a direct cause of the index stroke (but disease is present)

disease, Cardioembolic, Other Causes (ASCO) classification (Table 1–1).[102] The various classifications of the stroke subtypes have different purposes ranging from clinical decision making for therapy and stroke prevention, and predicting prognosis or clinical outcome, to selecting patients for epidemiological studies.

STROKE PATHOLOGY

Ischemic Stroke

Over 80% of strokes are ischemic and result from vascular occlusion, leading to reduced cerebral perfusion. Comprising only 2% of body weight, the brain utilizes nearly 20% of oxygen and glucose and is highly vulnerable to ischemia. The lack of adequate oxygen and energy supply during ischemia leads to depletion of adenosine triphosphate (ATP) and phosphocreatinine with subsequent reduction in ion transporter activity.[103] In the first 3 to 10 minutes after onset of ischemia, there is a progressive and marked reduction of neuronal membrane potential.[104] The tissue begins to accumulate lactate and hydrogen ions, resulting in a fall in pH and causing lactic acidosis.[105] Intracellular acidosis leads to disturbances in calcium sequestration in mitochondria and endoplasmic reticulum due to competitive relations with hydrogen ions and calcium for binding sites, and to accumulation of free calcium ions.[106] Calcium is overloaded in the cells resulting in swelling of the organelles, for example, mitochondria,[107] leading to necrotic neuronal cell death (necrosis), the predominant mechanism of cell death that follows acute permanent vascular occlusion.[108] Calcium accumulation further deteriorates ion dyshomeostasis via the calmodulin-dependent activation of neuronal nitric oxide synthase (nNOS).[109,110] Nitric oxide (NO) will then couple with ischemia-associated cytosolic and/or mitochondrial-derived superoxide to form toxic peroxynitrite, which leads to apoptosis, the main cause of cell death in milder injury, particularly within the ischemic penumbra.[111,112] The extent of apoptosis versus that of necrosis under specific conditions and in relation to regional changes in arterial perfusion remains uncertain.[113] Increased intracellular Na^+ and Cl^- results in osmotic movement of water[114] causing cytotoxic edema (the translocation of interstitial water into the intracellular compartment).[103] The brain microvasculature forming the blood-brain barrier (BBB) generates free radicals earlier than neurons,[115] and BBB disruption is observed 6 hours after the ischemia, while neuronal death becomes evident one to three days postischemia.[116,117] BBB disruption lets substances in the blood such as ions and serum proteins enter into the brain parenchyma, causing vasogenic edema (water movement from vascular to extravascular spaces).[118] Irreversible damage occurs in an ischemic core of severe hypoperfusion, surrounded by the *penumbra* and *oligemia*.[119] Tissue within the penumbra may be salvageable and is a key target for therapeutic intervention,[120,121] unlike the oligemic compartment, which is already infarcted and cannot be salvaged.[122]

The main pathophysiological mechanisms causing ischemic strokes are (1) thrombosis (the clot forms in a cerebral blood vessel most commonly by clot formation affecting the middle cerebral artery), (2) embolism (the clot forms in another part of the body such as the heart, aorta, and carotids and is carried to the brain), (3) lacunar infarction (due to disease of small penetrating arteries in the brain),[123] and (4) watershed infarcts, also known as border zone infarcts (due to hypoperfusion in the most distal arterial territories; often these occur in situations of prolonged hypotension and perioperatively).[16,123]

Hemorrhagic Stroke

Hemorrhagic stroke is the other form of stroke and is less common than ischemic stroke. It occurs where a blood vessel bursts within the brain (intracerebral hemorrhage) or around the membrane surrounding the brain (subarachnoid hemorrhage).[123] Hemorrhagic stroke is associated with extremely high rates of mortality compared to ischemic stroke. The proportion of this type of stroke is higher in Asian and black populations compared to the white population,[124,125] probably due to environmental differences (eg, lifestyles, diet)[124] and genetic predisposition to hypertension and ischemic stroke risk.[126]

Recently, clinical interest has focused on microbleeding, which is found in a very high percentage of macrobleedings (60%), but has also been reported in about 34% of patients with ischemic stroke and in about 5% of healthy adults.[127]

Vessel disease plays a crucial role in intracerebral hemorrhage, because generally vessel rupture is a consequence of a change in the vessel's structure. Vessel pathology is mainly characterized by the death and the subsequent loss of smooth muscular cells and collagen deposition that can lead to the vessel disruption.[128,129]

In intraparenchymal hemorrhage there are different explanations for the cellular damage. Some experiments have shown that there is a microvascular compression that decreases the regional blood flow in the perihematoma area, with a resultant ischemia in the perihematoma region.[130] Others have shown a perihematoma toxicity mediated by blood and iron in the brain rather than microvasculature compression.[131]

In SAH the main pathophysiologic process is that of early brain injury through a cascade of events cumulating in global cerebral ischemia and subsequent cell death, blood-brain barrier disruption, and brain edema.[132] Another pathophysiologic process that can lead to secondary ischemia in the brain after SAH is the association between early brain injury and cerebral vasospasm.

Ischemic stroke can transform into ICH when microvascular integrity is lost and neurovascular homeostasis is disrupted.[133] Approximately one-third of ischemic strokes will undergo some degree of hemorrhagic transformation (HT).[134] HT expands brain edema and leads to the displacement and disruption of brain structures and an increase in intracranial pressure, and induces apoptotic neuronal and glial cell death.[135]

STROKE PREVENTION

The improved detection and modification of stroke risk factors is a key to reducing both first and recurrent strokes (primary and secondary prevention) (Figure 1–1). About 80% of ischemic strokes are first events, which make primary prevention immensely important, as this could have a huge impact on the total incidence, burden, and cost of stroke. The implementation of effective primary and secondary prevention strategies are likely to have an enormous benefit in reducing the burden of stroke.

The risk factors for stroke are usually categorized as modifiable and nonmodifiable (Table 1–2). Hypertension is the single most important modifiable risk factor

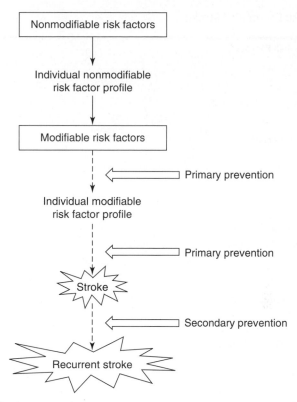

Figure 1–1. Stroke prevention.

for stroke.[136-138] Rothwell and colleagues[137] have shown that the visit-to-visit variability in systolic blood pressure and maximum systolic blood pressure are strong predictors of stroke, independent of the mean systolic blood pressure (on clinic readings) or ambulatory blood pressure monitoring.

Although there is little that can be done to control nonmodifiable risk factors, such as age, sex, ethnicity, and genetic determinants, it is important to focus on managing the modifiable risk factors in this group of individuals to ensure that the risk is not increased still further. The latest guidelines for primary prevention in stroke recommend strict pharmacological control of risk factors such as hypertension, diabetes, dyslipidemia, and atrial fibrillation in association with lifestyle modification.[36]

It has been shown that healthy lifestyle relating to weight, diet, regular exercise, low alcohol consumption, and not smoking is associated with a lower risk of stroke, particularly ischemic stroke.[139] A meta-analysis showed that moderate or high levels of physical activity reduce the risk of both ischemic and hemorrhagic strokes,[140] probably by reducing the cardiovascular risk profile. Promotion of healthy lifestyles should be a theme for public health education programs. A future approach to primary stroke prevention could be through a polypill approach, particularly for cardiovascular risk factors.[141] Polypill is estimated to reduce the incidence of first

Table 1–2. Risk Factors for Stroke

Nonmodifiable Risk Factors
Age
Sex
Race/ethnicity
Heredity/eenetics
Low birth weight
Modifiable Fisk Factors
Hypertension
Prior TIA
Atrial fibrillation
Diabetes
Carotid stenosis
Coronary and peripheral vessel disease
Cardiac diseases (eg, left ventricular hypertrophy)
Hypercholesterolemia
Metabolic syndrome
Obesity
Sleep-disordered breathing
Migraine
Hyperhomocysteinemia
Elevated plasma levels of C-reactive protein, Lp(a)
Hypercoagulability (eg, Leiden V factor)
Antiphospholipid antibodies
Hyperuricemia
Infections (eg, endocarditis)
Cigarette smoking
Alcohol abuse
Hormone replacement therapy
Oral contraceptives
Physical inactivity
Drug abuse (eg, cocaine)
Diet
Low socioeconomic status

TIA, transient ischemic attack.

ischemic stroke by 50%, which would translate into 400,000 fewer strokes in the United States alone every year.[142]

Data from the Framingham study showed a decrease in the incidence of stroke in the last 50 years due to improvements in knowledge of risk factors and in prevention. However, lifetime risk has not declined at the same degree because of the improved life expectancy, so there is a need for ongoing interventions in improving preventive measures and knowledge about stroke prevention.[143] It is likely that the most promising strategies for preventing stroke could be through a comprehensive approach involving setting up prevention clinics, improving diagnostic tools to identify asymptomatic subjects at risk, and improving public knowledge of stroke risk factors as well as the importance of stroke prevention.

URGENCY OF TREATMENT

Secondary Prevention

Patients with acute ischemic stroke are at a high risk of early stroke recurrence in the first week and the risk declines over time.[144,145] The early risk of recurrence has been shown to be approximately 10% at one week, between 2% and 4% at one month, and around 5% annually.[146-148] The very early increased risk of recurrent stroke justifies the need for early secondary prevention, as the risk can be reduced if patients are assessed and treated urgently. It has been shown that at least 95% of recurrent strokes could be prevented through a comprehensive and multifactorial approach involving the use of antiplatelet therapy, reduction of elevated cholesterol, treatment of hypertension, blood sugar control, anticoagulation for atrial fibrillation, carotid endarterectomy (CEA), and/or lifestyle changes.[149]

A transient ischemic attack (TIA) leads to an early high risk of stroke and other vascular events, but with evidence for prevention through urgent management. It has been shown that the risk of stroke after a TIA is about 10.5% with half of the strokes occurring in two days' time after the TIA. The overall risk of cardiovascular events, deaths, or recurrent TIA is about 17% within 90 days, with the greatest risk apparent in the first week.[150,151] A systematic review and meta-analysis of 18 studies of early risk of stroke after TIA, involving 10,126 TIA patients, reported a 3.1% (95% CI, 2.0-4.1) risk at two days and 5.2% (95% CI, 3.9-6.5) at seven days, with risk ranging from 0% to 12.8% at seven days.[152] The highest risks of stroke after TIA were observed in population-based studies without urgent treatment, with intermediate risks in routine clinics and emergency departments, and the lowest risks were observed in studies performed in specialist stroke services offering emergency access and treatment to patients with TIA. Studies have demonstrated the need for urgency of assessment and treatment in reducing the recurrence of stroke after a TIA or a minor stroke. For example, a prospective population-based study (the Early Use of Existing Preventive Strategies of Stroke [EXPRESS] trial) demonstrated how the early initiation of preventive treatments after TIAs or minor stroke was associated with an 80% reduction in the risk of early recurrent stroke.[144] The benefit of urgent and intensive treatment of TIA patients was also confirmed in the observational SOS-TIA study.[153]

Similarly, the FASTER (FAST Assessment of Stroke and Transient Ischemic Attack to Prevent Early Recurrence) study demonstrated a 90-day stroke risk reduction by approximately 30% (from 10.8% to 7.1%) with dual clopidogrel and aspirin compared with aspirin alone in patients who have experienced a TIA or minor stroke within 24 hours of acute ischemic stroke.[154] Large artery disease, particularly carotid stenosis, is another condition with increased risk of preventable stroke after recent TIA or minor stroke. A meta-analysis of ischemic subtype using the TOAST classification, involving 1709 patients with 30 recurrences at seven days, demonstrated remarkable variability for recurrent stroke among the different stroke subtypes.[155] Patients with stroke due to large-artery atherosclerosis had the highest odds of recurrence at seven days (odds ratio [OR] 3.3; 95% CI, 1.5-7.0) compared with other subtypes of stroke. Three large trials, the North American

Symptomatic Carotid Endarterectomy Trial (NASCET),[156] the European Carotid Surgery Trial (ECST),[157] and the Veterans Affairs Cooperative Study (VACS)[158] have shown the benefit of early endarterectomy in reducing recurrent stroke risk in symptomatic patients with high-grade carotid stenosis (>70%). In pooled data from the ECST and NASCET, the benefit is much greater if patients are operated on within the first two weeks after their initial event.[159] The absolute risk reduction (ARR) of ipsilateral stroke at five years and any stroke or death within 30 days after CEA was 9.2 in the group operated on in the first two weeks, decreasing to an ARR of 6.4 in the two- to four-week period, and 2.9 in the period from 4 to 12 weeks. No benefit was noted for CEA when performed more than 12 weeks from the last event. However, there is no demonstrated surgical benefit in terms of reduction of stroke risk for patients with stenosis less than 50% from any of the trials. In borderline cases a complex and multidisciplinary approach is required.

Acute Stroke

The "penumbra" is the term used for the reversibly injured brain tissue around the ischemic core, which is a key target for therapeutic intervention in patients with acute ischemic stroke.[160] The assumption here is that the core area of damage (infarction) will not be salvaged, but if blood flow is swiftly restored the penumbral tissues (the area that surrounds the core) may be saved. Positron emission tomography (PET) studies first provided the evidence supporting the existence of ischemic penumbra in patients with stroke, demonstrating substantial volumes of ischemic penumbra for up to 48 hours after the onset of stroke symptoms.[161] The use of PET and now magnetic resonance imaging (MRI) and computed tomography (CT) in identifying and quantifying the ischemic penumbra is a fast-developing area with broad implications for the future of acute stroke, because there is widespread agreement that this potentially salvageable ischemic tissue is the target of acute stroke therapies.[162] The goal when treating ischemic stroke is to salvage the penumbra as much and as early as possible. Approaches that can be used to salvage the penumbra include restoring blood flow distal to the occlusion (recanalization) and/or the use of strategies that can protect and minimize the harmful effect of ischemia on neurons (neuroprotection).

The phrase "time is brain," as coined by Saver, highlights the urgent need for stroke treatment as it is estimated that about two million neurons die each minute that an ischemic stroke goes untreated.[163] After deprivation of oxygen, some neurons die within minutes and irreversible brain injury occurs immediately, wiping out the function of these cells permanently. However, surrounding the area of necrosis or death of neurons is an area in which the blood supply is marginally sufficient to keep these cells alive (ischemic penumbra), but if no reperfusion occurs further injury is added and time-related death occurs.[164] Therefore, "time is brain" stresses the need for urgent intervention, as brain is lost if time to treatment is delayed. Rapid therapeutic intervention would result in the restoration of cerebral perfusion, salvaging threatened ischemic tissue and yielding improvement in clinical outcome.[165]

Numerous studies have shown that the time interval between symptom onset and induction of therapy is important because as time from stroke onset increases, not only does the risk of ICH increase, but the therapeutic efficacy also decreases, with resultant poor clinical outcome.[166-168]

Apart from the need for the early assessment and initiation of therapy by physicians, there are prehospital issues, such as the need for improved public awareness of the importance of early recognition of stroke symptoms and the benefits of early treatment. The lack of public knowledge regarding stroke symptoms and the need for a rapid response are some of the prime factors that may contribute to delays in seeking treatment for stroke.[169] Stroke needs to be recognized as a potentially fatal but treatable condition, like myocardial infarction, by the patient, relatives, or on-scene bystanders. The patient must be transported to the hospital in the shortest time possible (onset-to-arrival time). Similarly, on arrival to the hospital, assessment of stroke should be as fast as possible, and in cases of ischemic stroke treatment commenced urgently, particularly in suitable patients without contraindications to treatment. Therefore, good awareness of stroke symptoms should facilitate early admission to the hospital and immediate initiation of therapeutic intervention.

REFERENCES

1. Strong K, Mathers C, Bonita R. Preventing strokes: saving lives around the world. *Lancet Neurol.* 2007;6:182-187.
2. Mensah GA. Global burden of cardiovascular disease. Epidemiology of stroke and high blood pressure in Africa. *Heart.* 2008;94:697-705.
3. Feigin VL. Stroke in developing countries: can the epidemic be stopped and outcomes improved? *Lancet Neurol.* 2007;6:94-97.
4. World Health Organization. *The Global Burden of Disease: 2004 Update.* Geneva: World Health Organization; 2008.
5. Murray CJL, Lopez AD. Global mortality, disability and the contribution of risk factors. Global burden of the disease study. *Lancet.* 1997;349:1436-1442.
6. Di Carlo A. Human and economic burden of stroke. *Age Ageing.* 2009;38:4-5.
7. Feigin VL, Lawes CM, Bennett DA, Barker-Collo SL, Parag V. Worldwide stroke incidence and early case fatality reported in 56 population-based studies: a systematic review. *Lancet Neurol.* 2009;8(4):355-369.
8. Rothwell PM, Coull AJ, Giles MF, et al. Changes in stroke incidence, mortality, case-fatality, severity, and risk factors in Oxfordshire, UK, from 1981 to 2004 (Oxford Vascular Study). *Lancet.* 2004;363:1925-1933.
9. Numminen H, Kotila M, Waltimo O, Aho K, Kaste M. Declining incidence and mortality rates of stroke in Finland from 1972 to 1991: results of the three population-based stroke registers. *Stroke.* 1996;27:1487-1491.
10. Brown RD, Whisnant JP, Sicks JD, O'Fallon WM, Wiebers DO. Stroke incidence, prevalence, and survival: secular trends in Rochester, Minnesota, through 1989. *Stroke.* 1996;27:373-380.
11. Anderson CS, Carter KN, Hackett ML, et al. Trends in stroke incidence in Auckland, New Zealand, during 1981 to 2003. *Stroke.* 2005;36(10):2087-2093.
12. Kubo M, Kiyohara Y, Ninomiya T, et al. Decreasing incidence of lacunar vs other types of cerebral infarction in a Japanese population. *Neurology.* 2006;66:1539-1544.
13. Islam MS, Anderson CS, Hankey GJ, et al. Trends in incidence and outcome of stroke in Perth, Western Australia, during 1989 to 2001: the Perth Community Stroke Study. *Stroke.* 2008;39(3):776-782.
14. Bejot Y, Osseby GV, Aboa-éboulé C, et al. Dijon's vanishing lead with regard to low incidence of stroke. *Eur J Neurol.* 2009;16:324-329.
15. Terent A. Trends in stroke incidence and 10-year survival in Soderhamn, Sweden, 1975-2001. *Stroke.* 2003;34(6):1353-1358.

16. Feigin VL, Lawes CM, Bennett DA, Anderson CS. Stroke epidemiology: a review of population-based studies of incidence, prevalence, and case-fatality in the late 20th century. *Lancet Neurol.* 2003;2(1):43-53.

17. Kleindorfer D, Broderick J, Khoury J, et al. The unchanging incidence and case-fatality of stroke in the 1990s: a population-based study. *Stroke.* 2006;37:2473-2478.

18. Medin J, Nordlund A, Ekberg K. Increasing stroke incidence in Sweden between 1989 and 2000 among persons aged 30 to 65 years: evidence from the Swedish Hospital Discharge Register. *Stroke.* 2004;35:1047-1051.

19. Lloyd-Jones D, Adams RJ, Brown TM, et al. Executive summary: heart disease and stroke statistics—2010 update: a report from the American Heart Association. *Circulation.* 2010;121:948.

20. American Heart Association. *2002 Heart and Stroke Facts Statistical Update.* Dallas: American Heart Association; 2001.

21. Rich DQ, Gaziano JM, Kurth T. Geographic patterns in overall and specific cardiovascular disease incidence in apparently healthy men in the United States. *Stroke.* 2007;38:2221.

22. Glymour MM, Kosheleva A, Boden-Albala B. Birth and adult residence in the stroke belt independently predict stroke mortality. *Neurology.* 2009;73:1858.

23. Casper ML, Wing S, Anda RF, et al. The shifting stroke belt. Changes in the geographic pattern of stroke mortality in the United States, 1962 to 1988. *Stroke.* 1995;26:755.

24. Truelsen T, Piechowski-Jozwiak B, Bonita R, Mathers C, Bogousslavsky J, Boysen G. Stroke incidence and prevalence in Europe: a review of available data. *Eur J Neurol.* 2006;13:581-598.

25. The European Registers of Stroke (EROS) Investigators. Incidence of stroke in Europe at the beginning of the 21st century. *Stroke.* 2009;40:1557-1563.

26. Sarti C, Stegmayr B, Tolonen H, et al. Are changes in mortality from stroke caused by changes in stroke event rates or case fatality? Results from the WHO MONICA Project. *Stroke.* 2003;34(8):1833-1840.

27. WHO MONICA Project. Stroke trends in the WHO MONICA Project. *Stroke.* 1997;28:500-506.

28. WHO MONICA Project. Stroke incidence and mortality correlated to stroke risk factors in the WHO MONICA Project. *Stroke.* 1997;28:1367-1374.

29. Mihalka L, Smolanka V, Bulecza B, Mulesa S, Berezki D. A population study of stroke in West Ukraine: incidence, stroke services, and 30-day case fatality. *Stroke.* 2001;32:2227-2231.

30. Feigin VL, Wiebers DO, Whisnant JP, O'Fallan WM. Stroke incidence and 30-day case-fatality rates in Novosibirsk, Russia, 1982 through 1992. *Stroke.* 1995;26:924-929.

31. Giroud M, Beuriat P, Vion P, D'Athis PH, Dusserre L, Dumas R. Stroke in a French prospective population study. *Neuroepidemiology.* 1989;8:97-104.

32. Ryglewicz D, Hier DB, Wiszniewska M, et al. Ischemic strokes are more severe in Poland than in the United States. *Neurology.* 2000;54:513-515.

33. Brainin M, Bornstein N, Boysen G, Demarin V, for the EFNS task Force on Acute Neurologyogical Care. Acute neurological stroke care in Europe: results of the European Stroke Care Inventory. *Eur J Neurol.* 2000;7:5-10.

34. Brainin M, Olsen TS, Chamorro A, et al. Organization of stroke care: education, referral, emergency management and imaging, stroke units and rehabilitation. *Cerebrovasc Dis.* 2004;(Suppl 2):1-14.

35. Department of Health. *National Stroke Strategy.* Crown London. 2007. http://www.dh.gov.uk/en/publicationsandstatistics/Publications (accessed January 12, 2011.)

36. Goldstein LB, Bushnell CD, Adams RJ, et al. Guidelines for the primary prevention of stroke: a guideline for healthcare professionals from the American Heart Association/American Stroke Association. *Stroke.* 2011;42(2):517-584.

37. Rothwell PM, Coull AJ, Silver LE, et al. Population-based study of event-rate, incidence, case fatality, and mortality for all acute vascular events in all arterial territories (Oxford Vascular Study). *Lancet.* 2005;366:1773-1783.

38. Rojas JI, Zurru MC, Romano M, Patrucco L, Cristiano E. Acute ischemic stroke and transient ischemic attack in the very old—risk factor profile and stroke subtype between patients older than 80 years and patients aged less than 80 years. *Eur J Neurol.* 2007;14:895-899.

39. Centers for Disease Control. State-specific mortality from stroke and distribution of place of death—United States, 1999. *MMWR Morb Mortal Wkly Rep.* 2002;51:429-433.

40. Powell JL, Cook IG. Global ageing in comparative perspective: a critical discussion. *Int J Sociol Soc Policy.* 2009;29:388-400.

41. Amlie-Lefond C, Sebire G, Fullerton H. Recent developments in childhood arterial ischaemic stroke. *Lancet Neurol.* 2008;7:425-435.

42. Rojas JL, Zurrú MC, Romano M, Patrucco L, Cristiano E. Acute ischemic stroke and transient ischemic attack in the very old—risk factor profile and stroke subtype between patients older than 80 years and patients aged less than 80 years. *Eur J Neurol.* 2007;14(8):895-899.

43. Arboix A, Garcia-Eroles L, Massons J, Oliveres M, Targa C. Acute stroke in very old people: clinical features and predictors of in-hospital mortality. *J Am Geriatr Soc.* 2000;48:36-41.

44. Sacco RL. Stroke risk factors: an overview. In: Norris JW, Hachinski V, eds. *Stroke Prevention.* New York: Oxford University Press; 2001:17-42.

45. Elkind MSV. Stroke in the elderly. *Mt Sinai J Med.* 2003;70:27-37.

46. Appelros P, Stegmayr B Terént A. Sex differences in stroke epidemiology: a systematic review. *Stroke.* 2009;40:1082-1090.

47. Arboix A, Oliveres M, Garcìa-Eroles L, Maragall C, Massons J, Targa C. Acute cerebrovascular disease in women. *Eur J Neurol.* 2001;45:199-205.

48. Di Carlo A, Lamassa M, Pracucci G, et al. Stroke in every old. *Stroke.* 1999;30:2313-2319.

49. Kammersgaard LP, Jorgensen HS, Reith J, Nakayama H, Pedersen PM, Olsen TS. Short- and long-term prognosis for very old stroke patients: Copenhagen stroke study. *Age Ageing.* 2004;33:149-154.

50. Hajat C, Heuschmann PU, Coshall C, et al. Incidence of aetiological subtype of stroke in a multi-ethnic population based study: the south London Stroke Register. *J Neurol Neurosurg Psychiatry.* 2011;82(5):527-533.

51. Schneider AT, Kissela B, Woo D, et al. Ischemic stroke subtypes: a population-based study of incidence rates among blacks and whites. *Stroke.* 2004;35:1552.

52. Wolfe CD, Rudd AG, Howard R, et al. Incidence and case fatality rates of stroke subtypes in a multiethnic population: the South London Stroke Register. *J Neurol Neurosurg Psychiatry.* 2002;72:211-216.

53. White H, Boden-Albala B, Wand C, et al. Ischemic stroke subtype incidence among whites, blacks and Hispanics: the Northern Manhattan Study. *Circulation.* 2005;111:1327.

54. Morgenstern LB, Smith MA, Lisabeth LD, et al. Excess stroke in Mexican Americans compared with non-Hispanic whites: the Brain Attack Surveillance in Corpus Christi Project. *Am J Epidemiol.* 2004;160:376-383.

55. Zhang Y, Galloway JM, Welty TK, et al. Incidence and risk factors for stroke in American Indians: the Strong Heart Study. *Circulation.* 2008;118:1577.

56. Sarti C, Rastenyte D, Cepaitis Z, Tuomilehto J. International trend in mortality from stroke, 1968 to 1994. *Stroke.* 2000;31:1588-1601.

57. Levi F, Lucchini F, Negri E, La Vecchia C. Trends in mortality from cardiovascular and cerebrovascular diseases in Europe and other areas of the world. *Heart.* 2002;88:119-124.

58. Dai S, Bancej C, Bienek A, Walsh P, Stewart P, Wielgosz A. Chronic Disease Surveillance Division, Centre for Chronic Disease Prevention and Control, Public Health Agency of Canada. Report summary. Tracking heart disease and stroke in Canada 2009. *Chronic Dis Can.* 2009;29(4):192-193. http://www.phac-aspc.gc.ca/publicat/cdic-mcbc/31-1/summary (accessed January 15, 2011.)

59. Lloyd-Jones D, Adams R, Carnethon M, et al. Heart disease and stroke statistics 2009 update: a report from the American Heart Association Statistics Committee and Stroke Statistics Subcommittee. *Circulation.* 2009;119:480-486.

60. Tu JV, Nardi L, Fang J, Liu J, Khalid L, Johansen H, for the Canadian Cardiovascular Outcomes Research Team. National Trends in rates of death and hospital admissions related to acute myocardial infarction, heart failure and stroke, 1994-2004. *CMAJ.* 2009;180(13):E120-E127.

61. Asplund K. What MONICA told us about stroke. *Lancet Neurol.* 2005;4(1):64-68.

62. The National Institute of Neurological Disorders and stroke rt-PA Stroke Study Group. Tissue plasminogen activator for acute ischaemic stroke. *N Engl J Med.* 1995;333:1581-1587.

63. Smith WS, Sung G, Saver J, et al. Mechanical thrombectomy for acute ischemic stroke: final results of the multi MERCI trial. *Stroke.* 2008;39:1205-1212.

64. The Penumbra Stroke Trial Investigators. Safety and effectiveness of a new generation of mechanical devices for clot removal in intracranial large vessel occlusive disease. *Stroke.* 2009;40:2761-2768.

65. Chen ZM, Sandercock P, Pan HC, et al. Indications for early aspirin use in acute stroke: a combined analysis of 40,000 randomised patients from the Chinese Acute Stroke Trial and the International Stroke Trial. On behalf of the CAST and IST collaborative groups. *Stroke.* 2000;31:1240-1249.

66. Stroke Unit Trialists' Collaboration. The Cochrane Library. Organised inpatient (stroke unit) care for stroke (Cochrane Review). Stroke Unit Trialist's Collaboration. *Cochrane Database Syst Rev.* 2007;4:CD000197.

67. Vahedi K, Hofmeijer J, Juttler E, et al. Early decompressive surgery in malignant infarction of the middle cerebral artery: a pooled analysis of three randomised controlled trials. *Lancet Neurol.* 2007;6:215-222.

68. Hofmeijer J, Kappelle LJ, Algra A, Amelink GJ, van Gijn J, van der Worp HB; for HAMLET investigator. Surgical decompression for space-occupying cerebral infarction (the Hemicraniectomy after Middle Cerebral Artery infarction with Life-threatening Edema Trial (HAMLET). *Lancet Neurol.* 2009;8(4):326-333.

69. Hankey GJ, Jamrozik K, Broadhurst RJ, et al. Five-year survival after first-ever stroke and related prognostic factors in the Perth Community Stroke Study. *Stroke.* 2000;31:2080-2086.

70. Wolf CD, Giroud M, Kolominsky-Rabas P, et al. Variations in stroke incidence and survival in 3 areas of Europe. *Stroke.* 2000;31:2074-2079.

71. Saposnik G, Hill MD, O'Donnell M, Fang J, Hachinski V, Kapral MK on behalf of the investigators of the Registry of the Canadian Stroke Network for the Stroke Outcome Research Canada (SORCan) Working Group. Variables associated with 7-day, 30-day, and 1-year fatality after ischemic stroke. *Stroke.* 2008;39:2318-2324.

72. Bae HJ, Yoon DS, Lee J, et al. In-hospital medical complications and long-term mortality after ischemic stroke. *Stroke.* 2005;36(11):2441-2445.

73. Hardie K, Jamrozik K, Hankey GJ, Broadhurst RJ, Anderson C. Trends in five-year survival and risk of recurrent stroke after first-ever stroke in the Perth Community Stroke Study. *Cerebrovasc Dis.* 2005;19:179-185.

74. Lavados PM, Sacks C, Prina L, et al. Incidence, 30-day case-fatality rate, and prognosis of stroke in Iquique, Chile: a 2-year community-based prospective study (PISCIS project). *Lancet.* 2005;365(9478):2206-2215.

75. Bamford J, Sandercock P, Dennis M, Warlow C, Burn J. Classification and natural history of clinically identifiable subtypes of cerebral infarction. *Lancet.* 1991;337:1521-1526.

76. Appelros P, Nydevik I, Viitanen M. Poor outcome after first-ever stroke: predictors for death, dependency, and recurrent stroke within the first year. *Stroke.* 2003;34:122-126.

77. Handschu R, Haslbeck M, Hartmann A, et al. Mortality prediction in critical care for acute stroke: severity of illness—score or coma-scale. *J Neurol.* 2005;252:1249-1254.

78. Eriksson SE, Olsson JE. Survival and recurrent strokes in patients with different subtypes of stroke: a fourteen-year follow-up study. *Cerebrovasc Dis.* 2001;12:171-180.

79. Vernino S, Brown RD Jr, Sejvar JJ, Sicks JD, Petty GW, O'Fallon WM. Cause-specific mortality after first cerebral infarction: a population-based study. *Stroke.* 2003;34:1828-1832.

80. Warlow C, Dennis MS, van Gijn J, et al. *A Practical Approach to the Management and Transient Ischaemic Attack. Stroke Practical Management.* 3rd ed. Oxford: Blackwell Publishing: 2008.

81. Thom T, Haase N, Rosamond W, et al. Heart disease and stroke statistics 2006 update: a report from the American Heart Association Statistics Committee and Stroke Statistics Subcommittee. *Circulation.* 2006;113(14):85-151.

82. Rosamond W, Flegal K, Furie K, et al. Heart disease and stroke statistics—2008 update: a report from the American Heart Association Statistics Committee and Stroke Statistics Subcommittee. *Circulation.* 2008;117(4):e25-e146.

83. Lanska DJ. Geographic distribution of stroke mortality in the United States: 1939-1941 to 1979-1981. *Neurology.* 1993;43:1839.

84. *European Cardiovascular Disease Statistics 2008.* Brussels: European Heart Network; 2008.

85. Asplund K. Stroke in Europe: widening gap between East and West. *Cerebrovasc Dis.* 1996;6:3-6.

86. Kulesh SD, Filina NA, Frantava NM, et al. Incidence and case-fatality of stroke on the east border of the European Union. The Grodno Stroke Study. *Stroke.* 2010;41:2726-2730.

87. Scarborough P, Peto V, Bhatnagar P, et al. Stroke statistics. 2009 edition. British Heart Foundation Statistis Database. www.heartstats.org (accessed January 15, 2011).

88. Lopez AD, Mathers CD, Ezzati M, Jamison DT, Murray CJ. Global and regional burden of disease and risk factors, 2001: systematic analysis of population health data. *Lancet.* 2006;367:1747-1757.

89. Howard G, Anderson R, Sorlie P, Andrews V, Backlund E, Burke GL. Ethnic differences in stroke mortality between non-Hispanic whites, Hispanic whites, and blacks: the National Longitudinal Mortality Study. *Stroke.* 1994;25:2120-2125.

90. Giles WH, Kittner SJ, Hebel JR, Losonczy KG, Sherwin RW. Determinants of black-white differences in the risk of cerebral infarction. *Arch Intern Med.* 1995;155:1319-1324.

91. Spence JD. Physiologic tailoring of treatment in resistant hypertension. *Curr Cardiol Rev.* 2010;6:119-123.

92. Evers SM, Stuijs JN, Ament AJ, Van Genugten ML, Jager JH, Van Den Bos GAM. International comparison of stroke cost studies. *Stroke.* 2004;35:1209-1215.

93. Demaerschalk BM, Hwang HM, Leung G. US cost burden of ischemic stroke: a systematic literature review. *Am J Manag Care.* 2010;16(7):525-533.

94. Saka O, McGuire A, Wolfe CD. Cost of stroke in the United Kingdom. *Age Ageing.* 2009;38:27-32.

95. Di Carlo A, Lamassa M, Pracucci G, et al. Stroke in the very old. *Stroke.* 1999;30:2313-2319.

96. Tanne D, Turgeman D, Alder Y. Management of acute ischaemic stroke in the elderly. *Drugs.* 2001;61(10):1439-1453.

97. Arboix A, Garcia-Eroles L, Massons J, Oliveres M, Targa C. Acute stroke in very old people: clinical features and predictors of in-hospital mortality. *J Am Geriatr Soc.* 2000;48:36-41.

98. Bamford J, Sandercock P, Dennis M, Burn J, Warlow C. A prospective study of acute cerebrovascular disease in the community—the Oxfordshire Community Stroke Project 1981-86. 2. Incidence, case fatality rates and overall outcome at one year of cerebral infarction, primary intracerebral and subarachnoid hemorrhage. *J Neurol Neurosurg Psychiatry.* 1990;53:16-22.

99. Jacobs BS, Boden-Albala B, Lin IF, Sacco RL. Stroke in the young in the Northern Manhattan Stroke Study. *Stroke.* 2002;33:2789-2793.

100. Adams HP Jr, Bendixen BH, Kappelle LJ, et al. Classification of subtype of acute ischemic stroke. Definitions for use in a multicenter clinical trial. TOAST. Trial of Org 10172 in Acute Stroke Treatment. *Stroke.* 1993;24(1):35-41.

101. Bamford J, Sandercock P, Dennis M, Burn J, Warlow C. Classification and natural history of clinically identifiable subtypes of cerebral infarction. *Lancet.* 1991;337:1521-1526.

102. Amarenco P, Bogousslavsky J, Caplan LR, Donnan GA, Hennerici MG. New approach to stroke subtyping: the A-S-C-O (phenotypic) classification of stroke. *Cerebrovasc Dis.* 2009;27:502-508.

103. Simard JM, Kent TA, Chen M, Tarasov KV, Gerzanich V. Brain oedema in focal ischaemia: molecular pathophysiology and theoretical implications. *Lancet Neurol.* 2007;6:258-268.

104. Martin RL, Lloyd HG, Cowan AI. The early events of oxygen and glucose deprivation: setting the scene for neuronal death? *Trends Neurosci.* 1994;17(6):251-257.

105. Hossmann KA. Viability thresholds and the penumbra of focal ischemia. *Ann Neurol.* 1994;36:557-565.

106. Ooboshi H, Sadoshima S, Yao H, Nakahara T, Uchimura H, Fujishima M. Inhibition of ischemia-induced dopamine release by omega-conotoxin, a calcium channel blocker, in the striatum of spontaneously hypertensive rats: in vivo brain dialysis study. *J Neurochem.* 1992;58(1):298-303.

107. Choi DW, Rothman SM. The role of glutamate neurotoxicity in hypoxic-ischemic neuronal death. *Ann Rev Neurosci.* 1990;13:171-182.

108. DeGirolami U, Crowell RM, Marcoux FW. Selective necrosis and total necrosis in focal cerebral ischemia. Neuropathologic observations on experimental middle cerebral artery occlusion in the macaque monkey. *J Neuropathol Exp Neurol.* 1984;43(1):57-71.

109. Choi DW. Calcium-mediated neurotoxicity: relationship to specific channel types and role in ischemic damage. *Trends Neurosci.* 1988;11(10):465-469.

110. Iadecola C, Zhang F, Casey R, Nagayama M, Ross ME. Delayed reduction of ischemic brain injury and neurological deficits in mice lacking the inducible nitric oxide synthase gene. *J Neurosci.* 1997;17(23):9157-9164.

111. Yu W, Niwa T, Miura Y, et al. Calmodulin overexpression causes Ca(2+)-dependent apoptosis of pancreatic beta cells, which can be prevented by inhibition of nitric oxide synthase. *Lab Invest.* 2002;82(9):1229-1239.

112. Pacher P, Beckman JS, Liaudet L. Nitric oxide and peroxynitrite in health and disease. *Physiol Rev.* 2007;87(1):315-424.

113. Leist M, Nicotera P. Apoptosis versus necrosis: the shape of neuronal cell death. *Results Probl Cell Differ.* 1998;24:105-135.

114. Ayata C, Ropper AH. Ischaemic brain oedema. *J Clin Neurosci.* 2002;9:113-124.

115. Kontos HA. Oxygen radicals in cerebral ischemia: the 2001 Willis lecture. *Stroke.* 2001;32(11):2712-2716.

116. Pulsinelli WA, Brierley JB, Plum F. Temporal profile of neuronal damage in a model of transient forebrain ischemia. *Ann Neurol.* 1982;11:491-498.

117. Kirino T. Delayed neuronal death in the gerbil hippocampus following ischemia. *Brain Res.* 1982;239:57-69.

118. Rosenberg GA, Yang Y. Vasogenic edema due to tight junction disruption by matrix metalloproteinases in cerebral ischemia. *Neurosurg Focus.* 2007;22:E4.

119. Astrup J, Siesjo BK, Symon L. Thresholds in cerebral ischemia—the ischemic penumbra. *Stroke.* 1981;12:723-725.

120. Barton JC, von Kummer R, del Zoppo GJ. Treatment of acute ischemic stroke. Challenging the concept of a rigid and universal time window. *Stroke.* 1995;26:2219-2221.

121. Barton JC. Perfusion thresholds in human cerebral ischemia: historical perspective and therapeutic implications. *Cerebrovasc Dis.* 2001;11(S1):2-8.

122. Moustafa RR, Barton JC. Pathophysiology of ischaemic stroke: insights from imaging and implications for therapy and drug discovery. *Br J Pharmacol.* 1998;153(s1):s44-s54.

123. Mohr J. Lacunar stroke. *Hypertension.* 1986;8:349-356.

124. Zhang LF, Yang J, Hong Z, et al. Proportion of different subtypes of stroke in China. *Stroke.* 2003;34:2091-2096.

125. Quresh AL, Mandelow AD, Hanley DF. Intracerebral hemorrhage. *Lancet.* 2009;373:1632-1644.

126. Nakase T, Mizuno T, Harada S, et al. Angiotensinogen gene polymorphism as a risk factor for ischemic stroke. *J Clin Neurosci.* 2007;14:943-947.

127. Cordonnier C, Al-Shahi Salman R, Wardlaw J. Spontaneous brain microbleeds: systematic review, subgroup analyses and standards for study design and reporting. *Brain.* 2007;130:1988-2003.

128. Pantoni L. Cerebral small vessel disease: from pathogenesis and clinical characteristics to therapeutic challenges. *Lancet Neurol.* 2010;9:689-701.

129. Auer RN, Sutherland GR. Primary intracerebral hemorrhage: pathophysiology. *Can J Neurol Sci.* 2005;32(Suppl 2):S3-S12.

130. Shah QA, Ezzeddine MA, Qureshi AI. Acute hypertension in intracerebral hemorrhage: pathophysiology and treatment. *J Neurol Sci.* 2007;261(1-2):74-79.

131. Elijovich L, Patel PV, Hemphill JC III. Intracerebral hemorrhage. *Semin Neurol.* 2008;28(5):657-667.

132. Cahill WJ, Calvert JH, Zhang JH. Mechanism of early brain injury after subarachnoid hemorrhage. *J Cerebr Blood Flow Metab.* 2006;26:1341-1353.

133. Wang X, Lo EH. Triggers and mediators of hemorrhagic transformation in cerebral ischemia. *Mol Neurobiol.* 2003;28:229-244.

134. Lyden PD, Zivin JA. Hemorrhagic transformation after cerebral ischemia: mechanisms and incidence. *Cerebrovasc Brain Metab Rev.* 1993;5:1-16.

135. Felberg RA, Grotta JC, Shirzadi AL, et al. Cell death in experimental intracerebral hemorrhage: the "black hole" model of hemorrhagic damage. *Ann Neurol.* 2002;51:517-524.

136. Wolf PA, D'Agostino RB, O'Neal MA, et al. Secular trends in stroke incidence and mortality. The Framingham Study. *Stroke.* 1992;23(11):1551-1555.

137. Rothwell PM, Howord SC, Dolan E, et al. Prognostic significance of visit-to-visit variability, maximum systolic blood pressure, and episodic hypertension. *Lancet.* 2010;375:895-905.

138. Lawes CM, Vander HS, Rodgers A, for the International Society of Hypertension. Global burden of blood-pressure-related disease, 2001. *Lancet.* 2008;371:1513-1518.

139. Chiuve SE, Rexrode KM, Spiegelman D, Logroscino G, Manson JE, Rimm EB. Primary prevention of stroke by healthy lifestyle. *Circulation.* 2008;118(9):947-954.

140. Lee CD, Folsom AR, Blair SN. Physical activity and stroke risk: a meta-analysis. *Stroke.* 2003;34(10):2475-2481.

141. Wald DS, Wald NJ. The polypill in the primary prevention of cardiovascular disease. *Fundam Clin Pharmacol.* 2010;24(1):29-35.

142. Kernan WN, Launer LJ, Goldstein LB. What is the future of stroke prevention?: debate: polypill versus personalized risk factor modification. *Stroke.* 2010;41:35-38.

143. Carandang R, Seshadri S, Beiser A, et al. Trends in incidence, lifetime risk, severity, and 30-day mortality of stroke over the past 50 years. *JAMA.* 2006;296(24):2939-2946.

144. Rothwell PM, Giles MF, Chandratheva A, et al. Effect of urgent treatment of transient ischaemic attack and minor stroke on early recurrent stroke (EXPRESS study): a prospective population-based sequential comparison. *Lancet.* 2007;370:1432-1442.

145. Lovett JK, Dennis MS, Sandercock PAG, Bamford J, Warlow CP, Rothwell PM. Very early risk of stroke after a first transient ischemic attack. *Stroke.* 2003;34:138-140.

146. Pendlebury ST, Rothwell PM. Risk of recurrent stroke, other vascular events and dementia after transient ischaemic attack and stroke. *Cerebrovasc Dis.* 2009;27(Suppl 3):1-11.
147. Feng W, Hendry RM, Adams RJ. Risk of recurrent stroke, myocardial infarction, or death in hospitalized stroke patients. *Neurology.* 2010;74:588-593.
148. Dhamoon MS, Sciacca RR, Rundek T, Sacco RL, Elkind MSV. Recurrent stroke and cardiac risks after first ischaemic stroke: the Northern Manhattan Study. *Neurology.* 2006;66:641-646.
149. Hackam DG, Spence JD. Combining multiple approaches for the secondary prevention of vascular events after stroke: a quantitative modeling study. *Stroke.* 2007;38:1881-1885.
150. Johnston SC, Gress DR, Browner WS, Sidney S. Short-term prognosis after emergency department diagnosis of TIA. *JAMA.* 2000;284(22):2901-2906.
151. Rothwell PM, Warlow CP. Timing of TIAs preceding stroke time window for prevention is very short. *Neurology.* 2005;64:817-820.
152. Giles MF, Rothwell PM. Risk of stroke early after transient ischaemic attack: a systematic review and meta-analysis. *Lancet Neurol.* 2007;6:1063-1072.
153. Lavallée PC, Meseguer E, Abboud H, et al. A transient ischaemic attack clinic with round-the-clock access (SOS-TIA): feasibility and effects. *Lancet Neurol.* 2007;6:953-960.
154. Kennedy J, Hill MD, Ryckborst KJ, et al. Fast Assessment of Stroke and Transient Ischaemic Attack to Prevent Early Recurrence (FASTER): a randomised controlled pilot trial. *Lancet Neurol.* 2007;6(11):961-969.
155. Lovett JK, Coull AJ, Rothwell PM. Early risk of recurrence by subtype of ischaemic stroke in population-based incidence studies. *Neurology.* 2004;62:569-579.
156. North American Symptomatic Carotid Endarterectomy Trials Collaborators. Beneficial effect of carotid endarterectomy in symptomatic patients with high-grade carotid stenosis. *N Engl J Med.* 1991;325(7):445-453.
157. Randomised trial of endarterectomy for recently symptomatic carotid stenosis: final results of the MRC European Carotid Surgery Trial (ECST). *Lancet.* 1998;351(9113):1379-1387.
158. Mayberg MR, Wilson SE, Yatsu F, et al. Carotid endarterectomy and prevention of cerebral ischemia in symptomatic carotid stenosis. *JAMA.* 1991;266:3289-3294.
159. Rothwell PM, Eliasziw M, Guutnikov SA, et al. Endarterectomy for symptomatic carotid stenosis in relation to clinical subgroups and timing of surgery. *Lancet.* 2004;363:915-924.
160. Astrup J, Sorensen PM, Sorensen HR. Inhibition of cerebral oxygen and glucose consumption in the dog by hypothermia, pentobarbital, and lidocaine. *Anesthesiology.* 1981;55:263-268.
161. Ly JV, Zavala JA, Donnan GA, Neuroprotection and thrombolysis: combination therapy in acute ischaemic strokle. *Exp Opin Pharmacother.* 2006;7:1571-1581.
162. Fisher M. The ischemic penumbra: a new opportunuty for neuroprotection. *Cerebrovasc Dis.* 2006;21(Suppl 2):64-70.
163. Saver JL. Time is brain—quantified. *Stroke.* 2006;37:263.
164. Mergenthaler P, Dirnagl U, Meisel A. Pathophysiology of stroke: lessons from animal models. *Metab Brain Dis.* 2004;19:151-167.
165. Rha JH, Saver JL. The impact of recanalization on iachaemic stroke outcome. A meta-analysis. *Stroke.* 2007;38:967-973.
166. Hacke W, Kaste M, Olsen TS, Orgogozo JM, Bogousslavsky J, for the European Stroke Initiative Writing Committee. European Stroke Initiative (EUSI) recommendations for stroke management. *Eur J Neurol.* 2000;7:607-623.
167. Schellinger PD, Fiebach JB, Mohr A, Ringleb PA, Jansen O, Hacke W. Thrombolytic therapy for ischaemic stroke: a review: part 1: intra-venous thrombolysis. *Crit Care Med.* 2001;29:1812-1818.
168. Schellinger PD, Fiebach JB, Mohr A, Ringleb PA, Jansen O, Hacke W. Thrombolytic therapy for ischaemic stroke: a review: part 11: intra-arterial thrombolysis, vertebrobasilar stroke, phase 1V trails, and stroke imaging. *Crit Care Med.* 2001;29:1819-1825.
169. Jones SP, Jenkinson AJ, Leathley MJ, Watkins CL. Stroke knowledge and awareness: an integrative review of the evidence. *Age Ageing.* 2010;39:11-22.

Potential for Stroke Prevention

Fernando D. Testai
Philip B. Gorelick

INTRODUCTION

During the past 60 years numerous observational epidemiological study and clinical trial results have emerged that have led to major advances in stroke prevention.[1] Knowledge about common or traditional stroke risk factors has evolved from sites around the world.[2-7] Furthermore, international multicenter clinical trials have been carried out on first or recurrent stroke prevention interventions such as blood pressure lowering,[8] extracranial-intracranial artery bypass,[9] carotid endarterectomy,[10,11] angioplasty and stenting,[12,13] antiplatelet therapy,[14-19] anticoagulant therapy to prevent recurrent ischemic stroke,[20,21] and anticoagulant therapy for stroke prevention in atrial fibrillation.[22-25] Risk factors for stroke are now well defined, and it is estimated that approximately 90% of ischemic stroke risk can be explained by 10 traditional factors (Table 2–1).[26] In addition, novel stroke risk markers and factors are being elucidated that include genetic links to stroke.[27,28] Finally, new communication platforms are available to readily link what were once remotely located investigators and local sites into cohesive stroke observational study and clinical trial networks.[29]

In this chapter, we explore the potential for stroke prevention and discuss the following key topics: rationale and traditional approaches to stroke prevention, the concepts of continuum of risk, stroke risk in the absence of traditional factors,

Table 2–1. Odds Ratio (OR) and Population Attributable Risk (PAR) of
10 Factors Estimated to Account for 90% of Ischemic Stroke Risk

Risk Factor	OR (99% confidence interval)	PAR (%) (99% confidence interval)
1. Hypertension	2.64 (2.26-3.08)	34.6 (30.4-39.1)
2. Current smoking	2.09 (1.75-2.51)	18.9 (15.3-23.1)
3. Waist-to-hip ratio	1.65 (1.36-1.99)	26.5 (18.8-36.0)
4. Diet risk score	1.35 (1.11-1.64)	18.8 (11.2-29.7)
5. Regular exercise	0.69 (0.53-0.90)	28.5 (14.5-48.5)
6. Diabetes mellitus	1.36 (1.10-1.68)	5.0 (2.6-9.5)
7. Alcohol: (>30/month or binge)	1.51 (1.18-1.92)	3.8 (0.9-14.4)
8. Psychosocial stress and depression	1.30 (1.06-1.60) 1.35 (1.10-1.66)	4.6 (2.1-9.6) 5.2 (2.7-9.8)
9. Cardiac causes	2.38 (1.77-3.20)	6.7 (4.8-9.1)
10. Ratio of apolipo- protein B to A1	1.89 (1.49-2.40)	24.9 (15.7-37.1)

population attributable risk, an agenda for worldwide stroke prevention, and what
may be in store for future stroke prevention.

RATIONALE FOR STROKE PREVENTION, TRADITIONAL APPROACHES TO PREVENTION, AND ECONOMIC CONSIDERATIONS

Rationale for Stroke Prevention

Interest in health, healthy living, and a healthy environment has been, at least in part,
an outgrowth of rising prosperity that liberates some persons from practical demands of
everyday life.[30] Rose concluded in his monograph, *The Strategy of Preventive Medicine*,
after taking into consideration economic and humanitarian arguments for and
against prevention, that it was better to be healthy than ill or dead, and this was a
sufficient and the only real argument for preventive medicine. Furthermore, in this
treatise Rose concluded that the task of preventive medicine was a matter for societies and their individual members to decide and not a matter of telling people what
they should do. In a review of making choices and how individuals and society do
this, Thaler and Sunstein popularized the term used by the late Milton Friedman,
"libertarian paternalism." This term emphasizes freedom of choice to a path of
healthy behavior influenced by efforts of institutions in the private sector and govern-
ment to steer people to choices that will improve their lives.[31]

Traditional Approaches to Stroke Prevention

The strategies for stroke prevention have been traditionally grouped into two main
categories: the mass approach and the high-risk approach. The mass approach

targets the general population and is usually organized by major governing bodies as it utilizes public education, legislation, and economic measures with the goal of modifying lifestyle behavior and discouraging exposure to discretionary risk factors such as smoking, alcohol consumption, and salt intake. This approach may offer little benefit to those individuals with mild levels of a given risk factor as they are at a relatively low risk for disease. It has the potential to have a substantial impact, however, on the population as it may shift the distribution or prevalence of a particular risk factor in a favorable direction. The mass approach may be more effective when the risk factor is highly prevalent in the population, and there is a strong risk factor–disease association.

The mass approach is complemented by the high-risk approach. The latter approach is usually administered by practicing physicians and concentrates on those individuals with high levels of a risk factor who are identified through screening procedures. Intervention is carried out with the goal of treating the risk factor(s), and there is ongoing monitoring. The cost of screening to identify such high-risk persons in a population may be substantial. Furthermore, persons at lower risk will not benefit from such an approach. Because persons are at high risk, the interventions generally involve administration of medication in addition to lifestyle modification.[32] Because of the limitations noted above for each of the traditional stroke prevention approaches, the mass and high-risk approaches are viewed as complementary strategies.

Stroke Burden, Financial Costs, and Related Issues in Stroke Prevention

Despite major technological advances, stroke remains among the leading causes of death and disability worldwide. Statistics published by the American Heart Association illustrate the public health burden associated with this condition. It is estimated that almost 800,000 Americans suffer a stroke every year and that, on average, a stroke occurs in the United States every 40 seconds.[33] The one-month stroke-fatality rate for individuals 65 years of age or older is estimated to be 12%, and this increases steeply with age (Table 2–2). Among stroke survivors, a substantial proportion may have significant residual deficits (Table 2–3), and 15% to 30% are permanently disabled. These factors along with increasing contemporary medical costs help to explain the alarming total annual cost associated with this condition, which is currently estimated to be $74 billion in the United States. Over the years, a decrease in annual stroke rates has been observed. With an

Table 2–2. Thirty-Day Stroke Mortality Rate by Age

Age (years)	Mortality
65-74	9%
74-84	13.1%
≥85	23%

Table 2-3. Disabilities Observed in Individuals 65 Years of Age or Older at 6 Months After Ischemic Stroke

Type of Disability	Rate
Hemiparesis	50%
Unable to walk without some assistance	30%
Dependent on activities of daily living	26%
Aphasia	19%
Depressive symptoms	35%
Institutionalized in a nursing home	26%

increase in the prevalence of vascular risk factors (eg, hypertension, diabetes, and obesity), however, concern for a possible rebound in the rate of cerebrovascular disease mortality and incidence has been raised.[34]

Given these circumstances, stroke prevention has emerged as a possible opportunity to reduce the economic impact of this disorder. It has been estimated, for example, that the prevention of 25% of strokes would save 10 times more of the stroke-related cost than doubling the use of thrombolytic therapy.[35] In addition, recurrent stroke is a potential target for cost savings. As many as a quarter of strokes are recurrent ones, and the risk of stroke is greatest shortly after the patient experiences a stroke or a transient ischemic attack (TIA). Furthermore, up to 10.5% of patients who suffer a TIA will suffer a stroke within 90 days, with about half of these occurring within the first 48 hours after the initial presentation.[36,37]

Also, stroke and myocardial infarction share similar risk factors, and therefore stroke survivors have an elevated risk of suffering cardiovascular complications and their economic sequela.[38] The Northern Manhattan Study illustrates the former concept. In this study, the age- and sex-adjusted five-year risk of fatal and nonfatal recurrent stroke was 18.3%, and the five-year risk of myocardial infarction or fatal cardiac events was 8.6%.[39]

In another study, Roberts et al illustrate the economic impact of the concurrence of the comorbidities, stroke and cardiac events. Using a database from a large US managed–care health plan, the authors demonstrated that hospitalized ischemic stroke patients have both substantially higher stroke and nonstroke cardiovascular medical costs and hospitalizations than matched hospitalized nonstroke controls (Table 2–4).[40]

The identification of stroke-prone patients, particularly those with TIAs, and the early initiation of treatment have potential financial benefits by reduction of subsequent stroke events, rehospitalization, rehabilitation, and long-term care costs.[41] In the Early use of Existing Preventive Strategies for Stroke (EXPRESS) study, for example, expedited assessment and treatment of patients with TIA or minor stroke, resulted in an 80% reduction in the 90-day risk of subsequent stroke.[42] A similar observation was found in the SOS-TIA study. In this observational study, the rapid evaluation and initiation of treatment of TIA patients

Table 2–4. Mean Cumulative Costs[a] per Patient After 6 and 12 Months of Follow-Up for Stroke-Related and Non-Stroke-Related Cardiovascular Medical Services for Stroke[b] and Control Cohorts[c]

	6 Months[d]		12 Months[d]	
	Stroke	**Control**	**Stroke**	**Control**
All-causes health-related cost	5613	3492	6544	4406
Stroke-related cost	1756	50	2109	68
Non-stroke-related cardiovascular medical services[e]	1433	658	2203	1167

[a]Costs are reported in US dollars and were adjusted for inflation to 2005.
[b]Stroke cohort was composed of individuals hospitalized for ischemic stroke between January 1, 2002, and December 31, 2005.
[c]Control group was composed of patients hospitalized for a noncardiovascular event during the same period.
[d]All the comparisons between the stroke and the control cohorts were statistically significant with a $P < .01$.
[e]Include myocardial infarction, angina, revascularization, and heart failure.

resulted in lower recurrence of stroke, myocardial infarction, and vascular death rates than historical controls.[43]

It must be keep in mind, however, that it may be challenging to maintain long-term stroke prevention medication adherence rates among those with prior TIA or stroke and consequently, stroke rates may increase over time. In the EXPRESS study, for example, mortality and progression from disability at baseline to no disability at six months were not modified by expedited evaluation.[44]

In relation to TIA patients, an important question is, which subgroup of TIA patients are at high risk of stroke and thus may require expedited evaluation and treatment? Risk-stratification tools for this purpose, such as the ABCD2 score, have been developed. This score incorporates the following features: age (A), blood pressure (B), select clinical stroke features (C), and history of diabetes mellitus (D) and duration (D) of the TIA (Table 2–5). The ABCD2 score has been shown to predict 2-, 7-, and 90-day stroke risk after TIA. Furthermore, it has been suggested that individuals with ABCD2 scores above 4 may require hospital admission for rapid diagnosis and treatment, as they have a very high early risk of stroke, whereas those deemed to be at low risk may be evaluated in a timely manner in an ambulatory setting (Table 2–6).[45] The ABCD2 score was recently modified to take into account imaging findings (diffusion-weighted brain magnetic resonance imaging [MRI] for acute infarction and imaging for carotid stenosis), which were shown to be useful additional component predictors to heighten overall prediction with the scoring system. For example, compared to the ABCD2 score, the 90-day prediction of stroke by the new score (called ABCD3-I) improved by almost 40%.[46] Limitations of the ABCD2 scoring system for prediction of stroke after TIA have been published, and further validation studies may be required.[47-49]

Table 2–5. ABCD Score Based on Presentation After TIA

Risk Factor	Points
Age	
≥60	1
Blood pressure	
Systolic BP ≥140 mm Hg or diastolic BP ≥90 mm Hg	1
Clinical features	
Unilateral weakness ± speech impairment, or	2
Speech impairment without unilateral weakness	1
Duration	
≥60 min	2
10-59 min	1
Diabetes	1
Total	0-7

BP, blood pressure; TIA, transient ischemic attack.

Accurate recognition of stroke symptoms in the population at large has been lacking and is a major barrier to timely identification and treatment to prevent stroke or stroke recurrence. Due to the transient and often painless nature of a TIA, individuals with TIA do not always recognize themselves as being at risk of having a potentially irreversible neurological event. The population-based Oxford Vascular Study investigated causes for delay in seeking medical attention of TIA patients. In this study as many as 70% of the individuals did not recognize their symptoms as being consistent with stroke.[50] Also, in a random telephone survey done in noninstitutionalized US residents 18 years of age or older, 2.3% of the 10,112 participants reported being told by a physician that they had a TIA. Of these, only 64% sought medical attention within 24 hours of the event.[51] As proper recognition of cerebral ischemic symptoms is a first necessary step in seeking early medical attention, public education campaigns should continue to raise awareness about TIA symptoms and its risks, emphasizing that TIA constitutes a medical emergency that requires immediate medical attention.

Table 2–6. Risk of Stroke After TIA Predicted by the ABCD Score

ABCD Score	Risk of Stroke	2-Day	7-Day	90-Day
0-3	Low	1	1.2	3.1
4-5	Moderate	4.1	5.7	9.8
6-7	High	8.1	11.7	17.8

TIA, transient ischemic attack.

CONCEPT OF CONTINUUM OF RISK AND GLOBAL OR OVERALL RISK

It has been common practice in guidelines statements to set a categorical target in an individual patient for management of a risk factor. This provides a simple and useful guide for the practitioner who is engaged in risk factor control in office practice or in the inpatient setting. Now, let us apply the principle of a categorical target to an example of risk factor control in hypertension. In the United States, the Seventh Report of the Joint National Committee on Detection, Prevention, Evaluation, and Treatment of High Blood Pressure (JNC 7) recommended a blood pressure target of less than 140/90 mm Hg for uncomplicated hypertensive persons.[52] Upon further inspection of the association between blood pressure and stroke, it turns out that based on observational epidemiological studies there is a positive and direct continuous relationship between blood pressure and stroke down to at least levels of blood pressure of 115/75 mm Hg—an example of continuum of risk.[53] In addition, this relationship may be modified by such factors as age, whereby older persons are at higher risk than younger persons at similar systolic blood pressure levels. The continuum of risk concept suggests, therefore, that it might be beneficial to lower blood pressure to levels much below the categorical cut point of 140/90 mm Hg as recommended in the JNC 7 guideline in an attempt to further reduce stroke risk.[54]

Further study is needed, however, before we change our blood pressure practice management to lower blood pressure targets more than the JNC 7 recommended cut point. In patients with type 2 diabetes mellitus in the Action to Control Cardiovascular Risk in Diabetes (ACCORD), for example, targeting a systolic blood pressure to less than 120 mm Hg when compared to a target of less than 140 mm Hg did not reduce the risk of fatal and nonfatal major cardiovascular events, although any or nonfatal stroke was significantly reduced.[55] Furthermore, in the Cochrane Database of Systematic Reviews, lowering blood pressure below 140/90 mm Hg may not be beneficial in relation to reducing mortality or morbidity.[56] Therefore, a key message is that the benefit of blood pressure lowering has been most obvious in patients with higher blood pressure levels. These concerns reignite controversy over the J-shaped curve and blood pressure, especially among those with coronary artery disease.

Finally, our approach to the treatment of risk factors in an individual patient has evolved over time.[57] Whereas we once screened for and considered individual stroke risk factors for treatment in isolation of one another, we now recommend using risk calculators (eg, Framingham Stroke Risk Profile) to determine overall or global risk for an individual to assist us in the decision-making process for stroke preventives.[58] This approach allows us to place an individual into a specific risk stratum (eg, high, medium, or low risk) and determine annual risk over time. For those in low risk strata, for example, a physician might recommend lifestyle change, at least initially, as the primary means of prevention, whereas those in the highest risk category will likely need a combined approach of lifestyle modification and administration of medication to reduce risk of stroke.[1]

DIFFERENCE IN RISK WHEN TRADITIONAL RISK FACTORS ARE OR ARE NOT PRESENT

By convention a *risk factor* (1) elevates risk of a target disease; (2) is closely associated with the target disease based on an epidemiological measurement of risk such as relative risk (RR) or odds ratio (OR); (3) is a causal factor for the target disease; and (4) when the appropriate intervention is applied to reduce or lower the risk factor, the risk of disease is lessened.[1] The term *risk marker*, on the other hand, has been used to denote a factor that increases risk for a target disease but does not, as of yet, have an intervention that lowers the risk of the target disease.[59]

As noted in Table 2–1, various factors may be potent risks for stroke. Hypertension, for example, may confer a three- to four-fold risk for stroke and has proven to be one of the most consistent modifiable risk factors for stroke.[1] Therefore, it comes as no surprise that control of hypertension is one of the most important means to achieve stroke prevention. The global burden of blood pressure–related diseases, especially stroke and ischemic heart disease, is high in low-, middle-, and high-income countries.[60] Raised blood pressure is a prevalent problem worldwide and is associated with a high relative risk, and thus a high population attributable risk (PAR), which is discussed in more detail below.

Another focus of interest is outcome in the presence of healthy lifestyle factors (or in the absence of traditional stroke risk factors). Not surprisingly, the risk of stroke is low in the presence of healthful lifestyle factors, as noted in Table 2–7 and as evidenced in several major studies in relation to cardiovascular disease risk.[61] It is uncommon, however, to find persons without traditional cardiovascular risk factors or those with completely healthy lifestyles as people age. For example, such persons without risk factors may constitute only 5% to 10% of the population. In contrast, based on the Framingham Study findings, the lifetime risk of developing hypertension is about 90%.[62] Thus it may be difficult to escape hypertension and some of the other traditional cardiovascular risk factors (eg, diabetes mellitus) if a person lives long enough. To add further importance to a person's overall vascular risk factor profile, in the Honolulu Heart Program, the absence of key traditional

Table 2–7. Healthy Lifestyle Factors and Influence on Stroke Risk

Five Lifestyle Factors of Interest
1. Absence of current smoking
2. 30 minutes or more of modest or vigorous physical activity each day
3. Healthy diet (based on diet score in upper 40%)
4. Moderate alcohol consumption
5. Optimal body mass index (BMI) <25 kg/m^2 in midlife
Influence If All 5 Low-Risk Factors
Ischemic stroke risk for women or men:
1. Relative risk ~0.20 (95% CI, ~0.10-0.40)
2. Population attributable risk ~53 (95% CI, ~17-76)

CI, confidence interval.

cardiovascular risks was associated with healthful aging and a general lack of cognitive and physical disability.[63]

RANKING THE IMPORTANCE OF STROKE RISK FACTORS: POPULATION ATTRIBUTABLE RISK

Epidemiological data have shown the impact of risk factor control and lifestyle modification on the occurrence of stroke and have led to the development of effective prevention strategies (Table 2–8).[64] By using a quantitative modeling approach, Hackam and Spence estimated that the combination of dietary modification, exercise, and use of aspirin, statins, and antihypertensive agents in stroke or TIA survivors may reduce the cumulative relative risk of stroke by 80%.[65] PAR (ie, the proportion of a disease that can be attributed to a particular comorbid condition) is an epidemiologic measure that takes into account the prevalence and relative risk of a particular factor of interest and can be used to rank risk factors in order of importance. In the international INTERSTROKE study, 10 modifiable factors were found to account for 90% of the risk of stroke (Table 2–1), and five of these accounted for more than 80% of the global risk of stroke. These latter factors are reviewed in the following.

Hypertension

It is estimated that 1 in 3 adults in the United States has hypertension, and 1 in 4 has prehypertension.[66] Hypertension, the most important modifiable risk factor for cerebrovascular disease, is associated with a two- to three-fold or greater increase in the risk of stroke and accounts for almost a third of total stroke risk.[26] The physiopathology of stroke in hypertension has been linked to lipohyalinosis of the small vessels in lacunar infarction, to Charcot-Bouchard microaneurysm

Table 2–8. Meta-analyses Investigating the Efficacy of Secondary Stroke Prevention Strategies

Strategy	Relative Risk
Dietary modification	0.56 (0.42-0.74)
Exercise	0.72 (0.54-0.95)
Aspirin	0.78 (0.71-0.85)
Statins	0.79 (0.77-0.81)
Antihypertensives	0.79 (0.66-0.95)
Aspirin/dipyridamole	0.82 (0.74-0.91)
Intensified antihypertensives	0.85 (0.76-0.95)
Intensified statins	0.84 (0.80-0.89)
Carotid endarterectomy	0.52 (0.40-0.64)
Oral anticoagulants	0.55 (0.37-0.82)
Smoking cessation	0.64 (0.58-0.71)
Glycemic control	0.81 (0.73-0.91)

formation and small vessel rupture in intracerebral hemorrhage,[67] and to atherosclerotic mechanisms in other stroke subtypes.

Several studies illustrate the importance of blood pressure control in stroke prevention. In the PROGRESS trial, for example, average reduction of 12 mm Hg for systolic blood pressure and 5 mm Hg for diastolic blood pressure using perindopril 4 mg with indapamide 2 to 2.5 mg daily resulted in a 43% reduction in the risk of stroke. This study provided evidence that lowering blood pressure is safe and highly effective for recurrent stroke prevention in both hypertensive and nonhypertensive persons.[68] In addition, evidence for the prevention of a first stroke by blood pressure control has been overwhelming.[1]

Campaigns aimed at the early detection and treatment of hypertension may result in a dramatic reduction in the incidence of stroke. In London, Ontario, Canada, for example, a hypertension identification and follow-up program conducted between 1978 and 1985 led to a high degree of hypertensive control; during this time, the stroke admissions in the same geographic area decreased by 50%.[69]

It has been proposed that some antihypertensive treatments could reduce the rate of stroke and improve stroke outcome by mechanisms other than blood pressure reduction. Angiotensin receptor blockers, in particular, may have neuroprotective properties, and their role in the treatment of patients with acute ischemia has been under investigation.[70] Although appealing, the benefit of potential pleiotropic effects of particular drug classes has not been conclusively proven. Therefore, achievement of blood pressure control continues to be the most important factor to reduce the risk of stroke.

Smoking

Current smoking has been shown to double the risk of stroke and accounts for almost 20% of stroke risk.[26] In addition, environmental exposure to smoke is recognized as a risk factor for stroke. In the Melbourne Stroke Risk Factor Study, spouses of smokers were found to have double the risk of stroke compared with spouses of nonsmokers.[71] Mechanistically, smoking may lead to stroke by increasing platelet aggregability, blood viscosity, and fibrinogen levels, or by causing vascular endothelial damage and vasoconstriction.[72-74] After smoking cessation the risk of stroke decreases and by five years of smoking cessation approaches the level of nonsmokers. Much of the benefit of smoking cessation has been proposed to occur within the first 6 months postcessation.[75,76]

Anthropometrical Factors

Obesity has been established as an independent cardiovascular risk factor. In the INTERSTROKE study waist-to-hip ratio (WTHR), but not body mass index (BMI), was associated with stroke. In this study, elevated WTHR accounted for 26.5% of the strokes, and individuals with ratios in the second and third tertiles had ORs for stroke of 1.42 (99% confidence interval [CI], 1.18-1.71) and 1.65 (99% CI, 1.36-1.99), respectively, compared with those in the first tertile. This observation is in agreement with other studies. In the Northern Manhattan Stroke

Study (NOMASS), for example, waist-to-hip ratio was an independent risk factor for stroke even after adjusting for vascular risk factors and BMI.[77]

The relationship between BMI and stroke, on the other hand, has not been as well established.[78-81] Obesity is defined as a BMI 30 kg/m² or greater. In the United States the rate of obesity increased from 30.5% in the period 1999 to 2000 to 34.3% in the period 2003 to 2004, and it is estimated that if the trend in the growth of obesity continues, as many as 51% of the US adult population will be obese by 2030.[33] Although there is no large study addressing whether weight control reduces the risk of recurrent stroke, losing weight is recommended as it improves the control of vascular risk factors typically associated with obesity such as hypertension, diabetes, insulin resistance, dyslipidemia, and physical inactivity.

Diet

Certain dietary patterns may be predictive of or protective against cardiovascular disease. The Cretan Mediterranean diet, for example, is rich in olive and canola oils, and has low levels of trans fatty acids. In the Lyon Diet Heart Study, 605 persons post–myocardial infarction were randomized to follow a typical cardiac diet or the Cretan Mediterranean diet. In a follow-up period of four years, the rate of cardiac and total death in the Cretan Mediterranean diet group was decreased by 70% compared with controls.[82] Also, in the Nurses' Health Study healthy women (n = 74,886) were followed from 1984 to 2004, and adherence to the Mediterranean diet was associated with a lower rate of coronary heart disease, stroke, and cardiovascular death.[83]

In comparison to the Mediterranean diet, the typical Western diet has an elevated content of fried foods, salty snacks, eggs, and meat. In the INTERSTROKE study, individuals were assigned a diet risk score on the basis of the intake of food that predict (eg, Western diet) or protect (eg, fruits and vegetables) against cardiovascular disease.[26] High diet risk score accounted for 18.8% of the strokes, and individuals with diet risk scores in the second and third tertiles had ORs for stroke of 1.35 (99% CI, 1.12-1.61) and 1.35 (99% CI, 1.31-1.64), respectively, compared with those in the first tertile. According to food grouping, fruit and fish consumption reduced the risk of stroke, whereas the typical components of the Western diet, such as red meat, organ meats, eggs, and fried foods, pizza, and salty snacks, were linked to an increased stroke risk.[26]

Physical Activity

Epidemiological studies have described the beneficial effects of physical activity in the prevention of stroke. In a meta-analysis performed by Lee et al, for example, the stroke risk in active or fit individuals was 25% lower than in their inactive or unfit counterparts. When subdivided by degree of activity, moderately active individuals had a 20% lower risk and highly active individuals had a 27% lower risk of stroke incidence or mortality than low-activity individuals.[84] Exercise may decrease the risk of stroke by lowering blood pressure and weight, increasing vasodilation, and improving tissue oxygenation and glucose tolerance. Furthermore, physical activity optimizes physical performance and functional capacity, and reduces the levels of circulating inflammatory markers.[85,86]

Overall, the above examples illustrate the importance of key stroke risk factors and the potential for stroke risk reduction and a consequent reduction in the public health burden of stroke. A combination of the mass and high-risk approaches is necessary to achieve optimal stroke prevention. Therefore, individuals, health care professionals and providers, governmental agencies, and stroke prevention advocacy organizations are all key elements of the stroke prevention paradigm.

A GLOBAL STROKE PREVENTION AGENDA

In February 2010, an international group of stroke experts and contributors from allied fields gathered in San Antonio, Texas, to establish agendas in a number of key areas related to stroke, including stroke prevention. The meeting was dubbed a "synergium" or opportunity to work together to achieve important and shared goals in stroke prevention, treatment, diagnosis, and recovery.[87] Table 2–9 captures important elements of the global agenda for stroke prevention that emanated from the meeting.[87]

FUTURE STROKE PREVENTION

What might the landscape be like for stroke prevention in the future? We now share with the readers a vision of possible future stroke prevention practices. We anticipate that stroke prevention, like other chronic disease prevention, will move in the direction of self-management when feasible.[88] Patients are an essential component of the prevention equation and may serve in an important capacity to prevent and treat chronic diseases as they accept a stakeholder share in the process. Overall, the preventive field likely will be catalyzed by Internet access to learning tools and messaging about stroke prevention for both physicians and patients alike. The availability of remote monitoring techniques may lead to a layering or hierarchy of care such that patients will be placed in a maintenance phase of prevention that will be managed through self-help techniques, during which time physician assistants or nurse practitioners will apply social learning and behavioral techniques to encourage prevention. However, once the patient profile becomes more complex and challenging to manage, case managers will refer the patient to the primary care physician who will intensify risk factor intervention and prevention methods and consult specialists when they can no longer accountably manage the patient in relation to reaching prespecified benchmarks of prevention or care.

Table 2–9. Key Elements of an Agenda for Stroke Prevention

3 Steps to Influence Stroke Prevention
1. Establish a global chronic disease prevention initiative that includes stroke experts (eg, leadership body, collaborations, cost-effective research)
2. Promote the population approach to stroke prevention (eg, shift to preventive health and education; employ community health workers; stress adherence, incentives for successes, and global vascular screening tools; and establish effective ways to modify behavior)
3. Use traditional and novel public health communication techniques (eg, social media/marketing, centralized web system for chronic disease prevention, central "power grid" for messaging)

Specially trained laypersons from the community may be employed at this stage to intensify preventive care or treatment.

We anticipate that because of similarities in mechanistic pathways for a number of chronic diseases (eg, innate inflammatory pathways), patients may be screened and placed in chronic disease networks of like mechanism.[89] For example, a cardiovascular prevention or health maintenance network may be established in which those prone to stroke, coronary artery disease, and other cardiovascular diseases are placed. Similarly, a cancer chronic disease prevention network may evolve, as well as one for neuropsychiatric disorders. This will offer many advantages including that of proper or focused screening and surveillance for individuals within a network, education of health care providers about the induction and active treatment phases of specific chronic diseases, application of specific prevention and treatment measures for individuals, and the establishment and availability of a cohort of patients who belong to a specific health network that may be utilized to catalyze research and test new and important hypotheses about disease causation and treatment. Such a network approach might be an ideal setting for the study of comparative effectiveness research. Figure 2–1 is a potential model of how a chronic disease or health maintenance network might be organized and linked together.

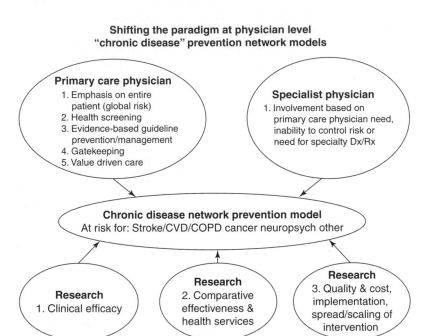

Dx/Rx - Diagnosis/treatment; CVD/COPD = Cardiovascular disease/chronic obstructive pulmonary disease, Neuropsych = Neuropsychological disease

Figure 2–1. Chronic disease prevention or health maintenance network model. CVD/COPD, cardiovascular disease/chronic obstructive pulmonary disease; Dx/Rx, diagnosis/treatment; Neuropsych, neuropsychological disease.

REFERENCES

1. Gorelick PB. The future of stroke prevention by risk factor modification. *Handb Clin Neurol.* 2009;94:1261-1276.
2. Wolf PA, Kannel WB, Verter J. Current status of risk factors for stroke. *Neurol Clin.* 1983;1:317-343.
3. Whisnant JP, Wiebers DO, O'Fallon WM, Sicks JD, Frye RL. A population-based model of risk factors for ischemic stroke. *Neurology.* 1996;47:1420-1428.
4. Northern Manhattan Stroke Study Collaborators, Sacco RL, Boden-Albala B, et al. Stroke incidence among white, black, and hispanic residents of an urban community. The Northern Manhattan Stroke Study. *Am J Epidemiol.* 1998;147:259-268.
5. Rothwell PM, Giles MF, Flossman E, et al. A simple score (ABCD) to identify individuals at high early risk of stroke transient ischemic attack. *Lancet.* 2005;366:29-36.
6. Hankey GJ, Jamrozik K, Broadhurst RJ, et al. Long-term risk of first recurrent stroke in the Pert Community Stroke Study. *Stroke.* 1998;29:2491-2500.
7. Udea K, Omae T, Hirota Y, et al. Decreasing trend in incidence and mortality from stroke in Hisayama residents, Japan. *Stroke.* 1981;12:154-160.
8. Veterans Administration Cooperative Study Group on Antihypertensive Agents. Effects of treatment on morbidity in hypertension. Results in patients with diastolic blood pressure averaging 115 through 129 mm Hg. *JAMA.* 1967;202:1028-1034.
9. The EC/IC bypass study group. Failure of extracranial-intracranial arterial bypass to reduce the risk of ischemic stroke. Results of an international randomized trial. *N Engl J Med.* 1985;313:1191-1200.
10. North American Symptomatic Carotid Endarterectomy Trial Collaborators. Beneficial effect of carotid endarterectomy in symptomatic patients with high-grade carotid stenosis. *N Engl J Med.* 1991;325: 445-453.
11. Warlow CP. MRC European Carotid Surgery Trial: interim results for symptomatic patients with severe (70-99%) or with mild (0-29%) stenosis. *Lancet.* 1991;337:1235-1243.
12. Brott TG, Hobson RI, Howard G, et al, for the CREST Investigators. Stenting versus endarterectomy for treatment of carotid-artery stenosis. *N Engl J Med.* 2010;363:11-23.
13. International Carotid Stenting Study Investigators. Carotid artery stenting compared with endarterectomy in patients with symptomatic carotid stenosis (International Carotid Stenting Study): an interim analysis of a randomized controlled trial. *Lancet.* 2010;375:985-997.
14. Canadian Cooperative Study Group. A randomized trial of aspirin and sulfinpyrazone in threatened stroke. *N Engl J Med.* 1978;299:53-59.
15. Steering Committee of the Physicians' Health Study Research Group. Final report on the aspirin component of the ongoing Physicians' Health Study. *N Engl J Med.* 1989;321:129-135.
16. Gorelick PB, Richardson D, Kelly M, et al. Aspirin and ticlopidine for prevention of stroke in blacks. A randomized trial. *JAMA.* 2003;289:2847-2957.
17. Sacco RL, Diener HC, Yusuf S, et al. Aspirin and extended-release dipyridamole versus clopidogrel for recurrent stroke. *N Engl J Med.* 2008;359:1238-1251.
18. The ESPRIT Study Group. Aspirin plus dipyridamole versus aspirin alone after cerebral ischaemia of arterial origin (ESPRIT): a randomised controlled trial. *Lancet.* 2006;367:1665-1673.
19. Shinohara Y, Katayama Y, Uchiyama S, et al, for the CSPS 2 group. Cilostazol for prevention of secondary stroke (CSPS 2): an aspirin-controlled, double-blind, randomized non-inferiority trial. *Lancet Neurol.* 2010;9:959-968.
20. Mohr JP, Thompson JLP, Lazar RM, et al, for the Warfarin-Aspirin Recurrent Stroke Study Group. A comparison of warfarin and aspirin for the prevention of recurrent ischemic stroke. *N Engl J Med.* 2001;345:1444-1451.
21. Chimowitz MI, Lynn MJ, Howlett-Smith MS, et al, for the Warfarin–Aspirin Symptomatic Intracranial Disease Trial Investigators. Comparison of warfarin and aspirin for symptomatic intracranial artery stenosis. *N Engl J Med.* 2005;352:1305-1316.
22. Stroke Prevention in Atrial Fibrillation Study Group Investigators. Preliminary report of the Stroke Prevention in Atrial Fibrillation Study. *N Engl J Med.* 1990;322:863-868.
23. The Boston Area Anticoagulation Trial for Atrial Fibrillation Investigators. The effect of low-dose warfarin on the risk of stroke in patients with nonrheumatic atrial fibrillation. *N Engl J Med.* 1990;323: 1505-1511.

24. Mant J, Hobbs FDR, Fletcher K, et al. Warfarin versus aspirin for stroke prevention in an elderly community population with atrial fibrillation (the Birmingham Atrial Fibrillation Treatment of the Aged Study [BAFTA]). *Lancet.* 2007;370:493-503.

25. Connolly SJ, Ezekowitz MD, Yusuf S, et al. Dabigatran versus warfarin in patients with atrial fibrillation. *N Engl J Med.* 2009;361:1139-1151.

26. O'Donnell MJ, Xavier D, Liu L, et al. Risk factors for ischemic and intracerebral hemorrhagic stroke in 22 countries (the INTERSTROKE study): a case-control study. *Lancet.* 2010;376:112-123.

27. Gorelick PB. Lipoprotein-associated phospholipase A2 and stroke risk. *Am J Cardiol.* 2008;101(12A): 34F-40F.

28. Meschia J. Stroke genome-wide association studies: the large numbers imperative. *Stroke.* 2010;41: 579-580.

29. The VITATOPS Trial Study Group. B vitamins in patients with recent transient ischemic attack or stroke in the VITAmins TO Prevent Stroke (VITATOPS) trial: a randomized, double-blind, parallel, placebo-controlled trial. *Lancet Neurol.* 2010;9:855-865.

30. Rose G. *The Strategy of Preventive Medicine.* New York: Oxford Medical Publications; 1994:1-135.

31. Thaler RH, Sunstein CR. *Nudge: Improving Decisions About Health, Wealth and Happiness.* New York: Penguin Books; 2009:1-312.

32. Gorelick PB. Stroke prevention. An opportunity for efficient utilization of health care resources during the coming decade. *Stroke.* 1994;25:220-224.

33. Lloyd-Jones D, Adams RJ, Brown TM, et al. Heart disease and stroke statistics—2010 update: a report from the American Heart Association. *Circulation.* 2010;121(7):e46-e215.

34. http://www.americanheart.org/downloadable/heart/1265665152970DS-3241%20HeartStroke Update_2010.pdf (accessed November 5, 2010).

35. http://www.health.gov.on.ca/english/public/pub/ministry_reports/stroke/strokereport.pdf (accessed November 5, 2010).

36. Johnston SC, Gress DR, Browner WS, Sidney S. Short-term prognosis after emergency department diagnosis of TIA. *JAMA.* 2000;284:2901-2906.

37. Chandratheva A, Mehta Z, Geraghty OC, Marquardt L, Rothwell PM; Oxford Vascular Study. Population-based study of risk and predictors of stroke in the first few hours after a TIA. *Neurology.* 2009;72:1941-1947.

38. Adams RJ, Chimowitz MI, Alpert JS, et al. Coronary risk evaluation in patients with transient ischemic attack and ischemic stroke: a scientific statement for healthcare professionals from the Stroke Council and the Council on Clinical Cardiology of the American Heart Association/American Stroke Association. *Circulation.* 2003;108:1278-1290.

39. Dhamoon MS, Sciacca RR, Rundek T, Sacco RL, Elkind MS. Recurrent stroke and cardiac risks after first ischemic stroke: the Northern Manhattan Study. *Neurology.* 2006;66:641-646.

40. Roberts CS, Gorelick PB, Ye X, Harley C, Goldberg GA. Additional stroke-related and non-stroke-related cardiovascular costs and hospitalizations in managed-care patients after ischemic stroke. *Stroke.* 2009;40:1425-1432.

41. Cadilhac DA, Carter RC, Thrift AG, Dewey HM. Why invest in a national public health program for stroke? An example using Australian data to estimate the potential benefits and cost implications. *Health Policy.* 2007;83:287-294.

42. Rothwell PM, Giles MF, Chandratheva A, et al. Effect of urgent treatment of transient ischaemic attack and minor stroke on early recurrent stroke (EXPRESS study): a prospective population-based sequential comparison. *Lancet.* 2007;370:1432-1442.

43. Lavallée PC, Meseguer E, Abboud H, et al. A transient ischaemic attack clinic with round-the-clock access (SOS-TIA): feasibility and effects. *Lancet Neurol.* 2007;6:953-960.

44. Luengo-Fernandez R, Gray AM, Rothwell PM. Effect of urgent treatment for transient ischaemic attack and minor stroke on disability and hospital costs (EXPRESS study): a prospective population-based sequential comparison. *Lancet Neurol.* 2009;8:235-243.

45. Johnston SC, Rothwell PM, Nguyen-Huynh MN, et al. Validation and refinement of scores to predict very early stroke risk after transient ischaemic attack. *Lancet.* 2007;369:283-292.

46. Merwick A, Albers GW, Amarenco P, et al. Addition of brain and carotid imaging to the ABCD2 score to identify patients at early risk of stroke after transient ischaemic attack: a multicentre observational study. *Lancet Neurol.* 2010;9:1060-1069.

47. Sheehan OC, Kyne L, Kelly LA, et al. Population-based study of ABCD2 score, carotid stenosis, and atrial fibrillation for early stroke prediction after transient ischemic attack: the North Dublin TIA study. *Stroke*. 2010;41:844-850.

48. Lou M, Safdar A, Edlow JA, et al. Can ABCD score predict the need for in-hospital intervention in patients with transient ischemic attacks? *Int J Emerg Med*. 2010;3:75-80.

49. Stead LG, Suravaram S, Bellolio MF, et al. An assessment of the incremental value of the ABCD2 score in the emergency department evaluation of transient ischemic attack. *Ann Emerg Med*. 2011;57(1):46-51.

50. Chandratheva A, Lasserson DS, Geraghty OC, Rothwell PM; Oxford Vascular Study. Population-based study of behavior immediately after transient ischemic attack and minor stroke in 1000 consecutive patients: lessons for public education. *Stroke*. 2010;41:1108-1114.

51. Johnston SC, Fayad PB, Gorelick PB, et al. Prevalence and knowledge of transient ischemic attack among US adults. *Neurology*. 2003;60:1429-1434.

52. Chobanian A, Bakris G, Black H, et al. The National High Blood Pressure Education Coordinating Committee. Seventh Report of the Joint National Committee on Detection, Prevention, Evaluation and Treatment of High Blood Pressure. The JNC 7 Report. *JAMA*. 2003;289:2560-2572.

53. Lawes CMM, Bennett DA, Feigin VL, Rodgers A. Blood pressure and stroke. An overview of published reviews. *Stroke*. 2004;35:1024-1033.

54. Chrysant SG, Chrysant GS. Effectiveness of lowering blood pressure to prevent stroke versus coronary events. *Am J Cardiol*. 2010;106:825-829.

55. The ACCORD Study Group. Effects of intensive blood-pressure control in type 2 diabetes mellitus. *N Engl J Med*. 2010;362:1575-1585.

56. Arguedas JA, Perez MI, Wright JM. Treatment blood pressure targets for hypertension. *Cochrane Database Syst Rev*. 2009;3:CD004349.

57. Gorelick PB. Stroke prevention therapy beyond antithrombotics: unifying mechanisms in ischemic stroke pathogenesis and implications for therapy. An invited review. *Stroke*. 2002;33:862-875.

58. Elkind MSV. Implications of stroke prevention trials. Treatment of global risk. *Neurology*. 2005;65:17-21.

59. Borer JS. Heart rate: from risk marker to risk factor. *Eur Heart J Suppl*. 2008;10(Suppl F):F2-F6.

60. Lawes CMM, Hoorn SV, Rodgers A; for the International Society of Hypertension. Global burden of blood-pressure-related disease, 2001. *Lancet*. 2008;371:1513-1518.

61. Greenland P, Knoll MD, Stamler J, et al. Major risk factors as antecedents of fatal and nonfatal coronary heart disease events. *JAMA*. 2003;290:891-897.

62. Vasan RS, Beiser A, Seshadri S, et al. Residual lifetime risk for developing hypertension in middle aged women and men: The Framingham Heart Study. *JAMA*. 2002;287:1003-1010.

63. Reed DM, Foley DJ, White LR, Heimovitz H, Burchfiel CM, Masaki K. Predictors of healthy aging in men with high life expectancies. *Am J Public Health*. 1998;88:1463-1468.

64. Furie KL, Kasner SE, Adams RJ, et al. Guidelines for the prevention of stroke in patients with stroke or transient ischemic attack. A guideline for healthcare professionals from the American Heart Association/American Stroke Association. *Stroke*. 2011;42(1):227-276.

65. Hackam DG, Spence JD. Combining multiple approaches for the secondary prevention of vascular events after stroke: a quantitative modeling study. *Stroke*. 2007;38:1881-1885.

66. Fields LE, Burt VL, Cutler JA, Hughes J, Roccella EJ, Sorlie P. The burden of adult hypertension in the United States 1999 to 2000: a rising tide. *Hypertension*. 2004;44:398-404.

67. Fisher CM. Hypertensive cerebral hemorrhage. Demonstration of the source of bleeding. *J Neuropathol Exp Neurol*. 2003;62:104-107.

68. PROGRESS Collaborative Group. Randomised trial of a perindopril-based blood-pressure-lowering regimen among 6,105 individuals with previous stroke or transient ischaemic attack. *Lancet*. 2001;358:1033-1041.

69. Spence JD. Antihypertensive drugs and prevention of atherosclerotic stroke. *Stroke*. 1986;17:808-810.

70. Sandset EC, Murray G, Boysen G, et al. Angiotensin receptor blockade in acute stroke. The Scandinavian Candesartan Acute Stroke Trial: rationale, methods and design of a multicentre, randomised- and placebo-controlled clinical trial (NCT00120003). *Int J Stroke*. 2010;5:423-427.

71. You RX, Thrift AG, McNeil JJ, Davis SM, Donnan GA. Ischemic stroke risk and passive exposure to spouses' cigarette smoking. Melbourne Stroke Risk Factor Study (MERFS) Group. *Am J Public Health*. 1999;89:572-575.

72. O'Donnell CJ, Larson MG, Feng D, et al. Genetic and environmental contributions to platelet aggregation: the Framingham heart study. *Circulation.* 2001;103:3051-3056.

73. Wilhelmsen L, Svärdsudd K, Korsan-Bengtsen K, Larsson B, Welin L, Tibblin G. Fibrinogen as a risk factor for stroke and myocardial infarction. *N Engl J Med.* 1984;311:501-505.

74. Kool MJ, Hoeks AP, Struijker Boudier HA, Reneman RS, Van Bortel LM. Short- and long-term effects of smoking on arterial wall properties in habitual smokers. *J Am Coll Cardiol.* 1993;22:1881-1886.

75. Kawachi I, Colditz GA, Stampfer MJ, et al. Smoking cessation and decreased risk of stroke in women. *JAMA.* 1993;269:232-236.

76. Wannamethee SG, Shaper AG, Whincup PH, Walker M. Smoking cessation and the risk of stroke in middle-aged men. *JAMA.* 1995;274:155-160.

77. Suk SH, Sacco RL, Boden-Albala B, et al. Abdominal obesity and risk of ischemic stroke: the Northern Manhattan Stroke Study. *Stroke.* 2003;34:1586-1592.

78. Abbott RD, Behrens GR, Sharp DS, et al. Body mass index and thromboembolic stroke in nonsmoking men in older middle age. The Honolulu Heart Program. *Stroke.* 1994;25:2370-2376.

79. DiPietro L, Ostfeld AM, Rosner GL. Adiposity and stroke among older adults of low socioeconomic status: the Chicago Stroke Study. *Am J Public Health.* 1994;84:14-19.

80. Kurth T, Gaziano JM, Berger K, et al. Body mass index and the risk of stroke in men. *Arch Intern Med.* 2002;162:2557-2562.

81. Selmer R, Tverdal A. Body mass index and cardiovascular mortality at different levels of blood pressure: a prospective study of Norwegian men and women. *J Epidemiol Community Health.* 1995;49:265-270.

82. de Lorgeril M, Salen P, Martin JL, Monjaud I, Delaye J, Mamelle N. Mediterranean diet, traditional risk factors, and the rate of cardiovascular complications after myocardial infarction: final report of the Lyon Diet Heart Study. *Circulation.* 1999;99:779-785.

83. Fung TT, Rexrode KM, Mantzoros CS, Manson JE, Willett WC, Hu FB. Mediterranean diet and incidence of and mortality from coronary heart disease and stroke in women. *Circulation.* 2009;119: 1093-1100.

84. Lee CD, Folsom AR, Blair SN. Physical activity and stroke risk: a meta-analysis. *Stroke.* 2003;34: 2475-2481.

85. Ranković G, Milicić B, Savić T, Dindić B, Mancev Z, Pesić G. Effects of physical exercise on inflammatory parameters and risk for repeated acute coronary syndrome in patients with ischemic heart disease. *Vojnosanit Pregl.* 2009;66:44-48.

86. Schumacher A, Peersen K, Sommervoll L, Seljeflot I, Arnesen H, Otterstad JE. Physical performance is associated with markers of vascular inflammation in patients with coronary heart disease. *Eur J Cardiovasc Prev Rehabil.* 2006;13:356-362.

87. Hachinski V, Donnan GA, Gorelick PB, et al. Stroke: working toward a prioritized world agenda. *Stroke.* 2010;41:1084-1099.

88. Wennberg D, Marr A, Lang L, O'Malley S, Bennett G. A randomized trial of telephone care-management strategy. *N Engl J Med.* 2010;363:1245-1255.

89. del Zoppo G, Gorelick PB, Eisert W. Innate inflammation as the common pathway of risk factors leading to TIAs and stroke. *Ann NY Acad Sci.* 2010;1207:8-10.

Section 2

Preventing Stroke

Nutrition, Diabetes, and Stroke Prevention

3

J. David Spence

TOPICS

INTRODUCTION

Lifestyle is much more important than many physicians recognize. This is illustrated well in a 2008 analysis[1] of data from the Health Professionals Follow-Up Study and the Nurses' Health Study. There were data on 43,685 men from the Health Professionals Follow-Up Study, and 71,243 women from the Nurses' Health Study. A low-risk lifestyle was defined as not smoking, a body mass index (BMI) below 25 kg/m^2, 30 minutes or more of moderate activity per day, modest alcohol consumption (men, 5-30 g/d; women, 5-15 g/d), and scoring within the top 40% of a healthy diet score. Compared with participants who had none of these beneficial factors, women with all five low-risk factors had a relative risk of 21% for any stroke and 19% for ischemic stroke; men with all five low-risk factors had a 31% risk of any stroke and 20% risk of ischemic stroke. In women, not adhering to a low-risk lifestyle accounted for 47% of total stroke and 54% of ischemic stroke. In men, 35% of total and 52% of ischemic stroke were attributed to unhealthy lifestyle. In 2004, the US Centers for Disease Control estimated that half of all deaths could be attributed to preventable behaviors.[2]

Other chapters discuss smoking cessation and exercise. In this chapter the focus is on weight loss, the composition of the diet, and effects of vitamins and antioxidants.

IMPORTANCE OF DIET

In the era of powerful statin drugs to lower cholesterol, many patients and even many physicians seem to think that there is not much point in paying attention to diet, which only lowers fasting serum cholesterol by around 10%, whereas statins reduce fasting LDL cholesterol by around 50%. However, nothing could be further from the truth. Diet is not about fasting blood levels, it is about the 16 to 18 hours of the day that we spend in a nonfasting state.[3]

Obesity, Weight Loss, and Maintenance of Weight Loss

Obesity is a significant predictor of mortality, and of stroke. Even childhood obesity carries a significant risk of mortality, both from endogenous causes (from disease or self-inflicted injury such as acute alcohol intoxication or drug use) and exogenous causes (accidents or homicide). In a cohort of 4857 American Indian children without diabetes who were followed for almost 24 years,[4] the relative risk of the highest quartile of BMI to the lowest was 2.3 for exogenous causes of death and 1.73 for endogenous causes. Obesity, glucose intolerance, and hypertension in childhood were strongly associated with increased rates of premature death in this cohort.

Obesity also strongly predicted mortality in a 2010 analysis[5] of pooled data from 19 prospective studies with data on 1.46 million white adults with a median follow-up of 10 years. As shown in Figure 3–1, a BMI above the reference range strongly increases risk in a graded fashion.

The effect of obesity on incident stroke was studied in a meta-analysis of 25 studies,[6] with 2,274,961 participants and 30,757 events. Factors controlled for in subgroup analyses and meta-regression analyses were sex, population average age, body

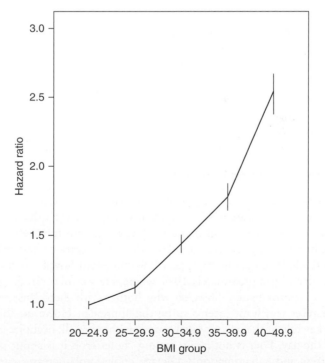

Figure 3–1. Mortality by body mass index (BMI). Mortality increases in an exponential fashion as BMI increases from normal levels to morbid obesity.

mass index and blood pressure, year of recruitment, year of study publication, and duration of follow-up. After adjusting for all these factors, obesity remained a significant independent predictor of ischemic stroke, with a relative risk (RR) of 1.22 (95% confidence interval [CI], 1.05-1.41) for overweight and 1.64 (95% CI, 1.36-1.99).

The prevalence of obesity, insulin resistance, and diabetes are increasing, particularly in economically advantaged societies, to the extent that obesity has been called "the new tobacco." In 2004, the Centers for Disease Control predicted[2] that by approximately 2005, obesity would overtake tobacco as the leading preventable cause of death.

Many patients have the mistaken belief that they have been gaining weight because of an injury such as a sprained ankle; the tendency to underestimate the importance of caloric intake in obesity is surprisingly widespread. However, the arithmetic of obesity is straightforward and is based on the first law of thermodynamics: energy can neither be created nor destroyed. One pound of fat contains 3500 calories. On average, sedentary people only burn approximately 10 calories per pound, so a person who weighs 250 pounds has been consuming, on average, about 2500 calories per day. We only burn about 100 calories walking a mile. So to lose a pound, we can either walk 35 miles or cut out 500 calories per day for a week (7 × 500 = 3500 calories). Someone who needs to lose 20 pounds needs to permanently reduce caloric intake by approximately 200 calories per day, or walk two miles per day. To lose 50 pounds would require walking 1750 miles, or cutting out 500 calories a day for a year.

Assuming that most sedentary city dwellers are not realistically going to increase their exercise to that extent, the reality is that to maintain significant weight loss requires a *permanent* reduction of caloric intake, to approximately 10 calories per day per pound of target weight. This is best done by increasing the intake of low-calorie foods and reducing the intake of high-calorie foods.

Much is made in the lay press about the benefits of a low-carbohydrate diet; however, the common interpretation of this diet is dangerous, as it is high in animal fat and cholesterol. Controlled trials have shown that, on average, weight loss depends more on calorie intake than on the composition of the diet.[7]

Dietary Cholesterol and Egg Yolk

There is a widespread tendency to assume that dietary cholesterol, including egg yolk, is harmless. This dangerous error may be in part or largely due to propaganda from egg marketers.[8] The notion that dietary cholesterol is relatively unimportant seems to be based on the relatively modest effects of dietary cholesterol on fasting levels of LDL cholesterol. On average, a low-cholesterol/low-fat diet only lowers fasting cholesterol by approximately 10%, whereas powerful statin drugs can lower cholesterol by approximately 50%, so why bother with diet? "Just take a statin and eat whatever you want" seems to be the approach. However, this approach ignores the key role of the postprandial state, which, after all, occupies about three-quarters of the day. Diet is not about fasting cholesterol, it is about postprandial oxidative stress and inflammation.[9] Dietary cholesterol increases cardiovascular mortality,[10,11] and elevated serum cholesterol increases both cardiovascular mortality[12] and overall mortality.[13] Dietary cholesterol, fat, and refined sugars increase postprandial oxidative stress and inflammation,[8] and a high-fat/high-cholesterol meal impairs endothelial function for about four hours.[14] There are good reasons for long-standing recommendations to keep daily cholesterol intake below 200 mg/d.[8] A single large egg yolk contains 237 mg of cholesterol—more than a day's worth of cholesterol; indeed more than a Hardee's Monster Thickburger,[15] which contains more than four days' worth of meat, according to the Mediterranean diet described below. In patients at risk of vascular disease, dietary cholesterol should be kept below 200 mg/d; this means that egg yolks should be avoided by such people. Patients at risk of vascular disease should learn to make a tasty omelette or frittata using egg whites or egg white–based substitutes such as Egg Beaters, Egg Creations, or Better Than Eggs.[16]

The Cretan Mediterranean Diet

The diet that has been shown in a randomized trial to be most effective at preventing heart attacks and strokes is the Mediterranean diet—not just any Mediterranean diet, but the diet from Crete. In the Lyon Diet Heart Study,[17] patients who survived a myocardial infarction were randomized to a Cretan Mediterranean diet or to a "prudent Western diet" that was consistent with the NCEP Step 1 diet and is the diet recommended by the American Heart Association (AHA) for healthy people. Despite no difference in fasting cholesterol levels or alcohol intake between the two diets, patients randomized to the Mediterranean diet had 70% fewer cardiovascular events during a mean follow-up of 27 months.[17] As Willett and Stampfer point out,[18] the low-fat diet that is generally recommended for vascular risk reduction was "drawn from thin air" by committees trying to design a diet that would lower fasting serum cholesterol. In the Seven Countries Study, it was observed that cardiovascular mortality was much lower on Crete than elsewhere, despite a high fat intake—40% of calories from fat—but the fat consisted mainly of beneficial olive oil.[18] The Cretan Mediterranean diet is good for the arteries because it is both high in beneficial foods and low in harmful foods. It is high in whole grains; high in beneficial oils such as olive and canola; high in fruits, vegetables, lentils, and nuts; and low in cholesterol and animal fat. Ancel Keys, who led the Seven Countries Study, pointed out in a retrospective paper[19] that "the heart of this diet is mainly vegetarian, and differs from American and northern European diets in that it is much lower in meat and dairy products and uses fruit for dessert." The diet recommended for patients at risk of cardiovascular events is described in Table 3–1: a high intake of beneficial oils such as olive and canola, a high intake of fruits, vegetables, lentils, beans and nuts, and a low intake of cholesterol and animal flesh.[3,8,16]

Diabetes and Stroke Prevention

Diabetes mellitus affects a growing proportion of the adult US population, and 15%-33% of patients with ischemic stroke.[20] Among 11,092 participants without diabetes in the Atherosclerosis Risk in Communities (ARIC) study,[21] the level of glycosylated hemoglobin strongly predicted risk (Figure 3–2); participants with levels 6.5% or greater had a hazard ratio (HR) of 3.68 (95% CI, 2.56-5.30) after

Table 3–1. The Diet Recommended for Patients at Risk of Cardiovascular Events

High intake of olive oil, canola oil
High intake of whole grains, vegetables, fruit, legumes
NO egg yolks → egg whites, Egg Beaters, etc
Meat of any animal: 4 oz every OTHER day[a]
Avoid deep-fried foods, hydrogenated oils (trans fats)

[a] For most North Americans, it is easier to save up the meat and have a decent piece of meat every other day than to keep to 2 oz per day. Meat is anything with eyes, a face, or a mother, so it includes chicken and fish. To accomplish this, patients need to think of their meatless day not as a punishment day, but as a gourmet cooking class day: "Having fun learning how to make healthy eating tasty."

adjustment for age, sex, and race. Diabetes independently increases risk of stroke by 1.8- to nearly 6-fold.[22] Although randomized trials of glycemic control alone have not shown a reduction of stroke risk, or even an increase of cardiovascular mortality, intensive management of multiple risk factors does reduce the risk of stroke in diabetics.[22]

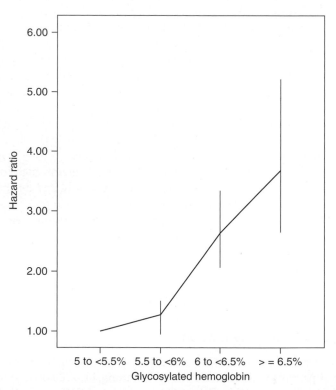

Figure 3–2. Risk of ischemic stroke by glycosylated hemoglobin level. In people who are not yet diabetic, the level of glycosylated hemoglobin strongly predicts risk of ischemic stroke, more steeply than the risk of coronary disease or all-cause mortality.

The metabolic syndrome (at least three of centrally distributed obesity, elevated triglycerides, low high-density lipoprotein cholesterol [HDL-C] concentrations, hypertension, and hyperglycemia) and insulin resistance increase the risk of cardiovascular events, including stroke. Weight loss and exercise are most important in treating insulin resistance, but are difficult to implement. Drugs that are agonists at peroxisome proliferator–activated receptors (PPARs) are promising for the management of insulin resistance,[23,24] and indeed pioglitazone, a PPAR γ agonist, reduced stroke in the PROspective pioglitazone Clinical Trial In macroVascular Events (PROACTIVE) trial.[25] Among 5238 patients with type 2 diabetes and macrovascular disease, pioglitazone was associated with a 47% reduction of recurrent stroke (HR 0.53; 95% CI, 0.34-0.85) and a 28% relative reduction of stroke, vascular death, or myocardial infarction (HR 0.72; 95% CI, 053-1.00). The Insulin Resistance after Stroke (IRIS) trial (Clinicaltrials.gov, number NCT00091949) is under way to test the effect of pioglitazone in secondary stroke patients in the setting of insulin resistance before the occurrence of diabetes.

A sadly neglected issue is the dietary management of diabetes. In my experience most diabetics are prescribed too many calories (and consume even more), and the instructions they receive regarding intake of protein (often three 100-gram servings per day) are too often interpreted by patients as meaning three pieces of meat (each of which is much larger than 100 grams). The Dietary Intervention Randomized Controlled Trial (DIRECT)[26] compared a low-fat, low-carbohydrate diet and the Cretan Mediterranean diet in 322 moderately obese residents of a nuclear facility in Israel. Participants were randomized to one of the three diets, and meals, provided in the cafeteria, were color-coded; this approach achieved remarkable adherence, unmatched in dietary studies: 95% adherence at one year and 87% at two years. Blood levels of glucose and insulin, and insulin resistance were significantly better among diabetics on the Mediterranean diet.[26] Weight loss was better on the Mediterranean and low-carbohydrate diet, and the change in carotid artery volume was similar on the three diets. Regression of three-dimensional vessel wall volume[27] was proportional to weight loss and blood pressure reduction.

The role of diabetes management in stroke prevention was well reviewed in both of the recent AHA guidelines on stroke prevention.[20,22]

VITAMINS AND ANTIOXIDANTS

An unhealthy diet cannot be remedied by administration of vitamin and antioxidant supplements. It seems likely that the failure of single supplements such as vitamin C or vitamin E[28,29] may be related to interactions between antioxidants. A diet high in whole grains, fruits, and vegetables provides a much broader range of beneficial substances than would be provided in a pill. In general, fruits and vegetables get their color and flavor from antioxidants and bioflavonoids. For example, if you buy naringin from Sigma Chemicals you will find that it is a greenish powder that has the taste of grapefruit—likewise hesperidin in oranges; resveratrol in red grapes; lycopene in tomatoes, strawberries, and watermelon; anthocyanin in blueberries; and so on. A useful slogan, therefore, is "we should eat fruits and vegetables of all colors." An important exception is vitamin B$_{12}$.

Vitamin Therapy for Homocysteine

Although "folate therapy" has not proven to be effective for reducing the risk of cardiovascular events, a special case can be made for vitamin B_{12}.

There is an important problem with underestimation of the prevalence of B_{12} deficiency in the elderly. Much of this results from failure to understand that a "normal" serum B_{12} does not define adequacy of B_{12}. Serum B_{12} is total B_{12} (active and inactive, with 20% or less being active) so it is not sensitive for B_{12} deficiency. In Europe, measurement of active B_{12} is assessed by measurement of holotranscobalamin, to assess metabolic B_{12} deficiency.[30]

Metabolic B_{12} deficiency is specifically defined by elevation of methylmalonic acid levels (or in folate-replete subjects by elevation of plasma homocysteine).[31] It is present in approximately 20% of the elderly,[32] so the "normal" range (the 95% of the population within two standard deviations of the mean) includes, in the elderly, quite a few people with B_{12} deficiency (about 17.5% of those in the "normal" range).

Helga Refsum at Oxford, and colleagues, recently showed[33] that to be 95% confident that metabolic B_{12} deficiency can be excluded, serum B_{12} needs to be above 400 pmol/L. In my vascular patients, metabolic B_{12} deficiency is present in 12% of those below age 50, in 13% of those aged 50 to 71, and in 30% of those over age 70.[34] Figure 3–3 shows the "normal" distribution of serum B_{12} among my patients; it can be seen that it is clearly not adequate!

B_{12} deficiency raises levels of total homocysteine (tHcy),[31] which is a clotting factor that increases the risk of deep vein thrombosis, retinal vein thrombosis, and cerebral vein thrombosis, and quadruples the risk of stroke in patients with atrial fibrillation. Stroke attributable to atrial fibrillation increases steeply with age— from 1.5% of stroke at age 50 to approximately 25% by age 85, and both vitamin B_{12} deficiency and plasma levels of tHcy increase steeply with age. This is probably why reduction of homocysteine is important in stroke prevention, even though it has not reduced myocardial infarction.[35]

Just as with folate deficiency, B_{12} deficiency can cause atrophy of intestinal villi,[36] preventing absorption of oral B_{12}. This can be restored in many (or maybe most) patients with a couple of injections of B_{12}, so that thereafter B_{12} can be absorbed from tablets.

If the serum B_{12} is not above 400 pmol/L with oral B_{12}, it may be necessary to give several B_{12} injections (eg, 1000 µg subcutaneously on four occasions at weekly intervals) to restore the intestinal villi. After that is done, if the serum B_{12} remains above 400 pmol/L, then B_{12} shots won't be needed in most cases.

Monthly injections are usually not adequate to maintain serum B_{12} levels above 400 (because it is water soluble and excreted in the urine); injections may need to be more frequent, so for most patients daily B_{12}, 1200 µg extended release, or 1000 µg sublingually, once or twice a day, is better.

Harmful Effects of B Vitamins

We recently found that in patients with diabetic nephropathy, high doses of folic acid, pyridoxine, and cyanocobalamin were harmful[37]—they accelerated impairment

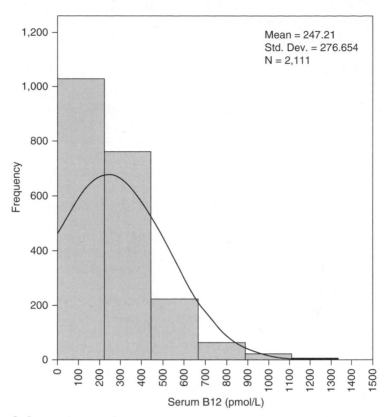

Figure 3–3. Distribution of serum B$_{12}$ in patients attending my vascular prevention clinics. Serum B$_{12}$ levels in patients attending my stroke prevention clinic are surprisingly low. To be confident that a patient does not have metabolic B$_{12}$ deficiency (defined by elevation of methylmalonic acid), the serum B$_{12}$ needs to be above 400 pmol/L. Metabolic B$_{12}$ deficiency is present in 12% of my patients aged younger then 50, 13% of those aged 50 to 71, and 30% of those aged older than 71.

of renal function and doubled cardiovascular events, among patients with a glomerular filtration rate (GFR) less then 50.

Possible mechanisms by which high-dose vitamins could be harmful in patients with renal failure include accumulation of folic acid unmetabolized to tetrahydrofolate, leading to excess production of asymmetric dimethylarginine (ADMA), a nitric oxide antagonist, and accumulation of cyanide from cyanocobalamin, leading to consumption of hydrogen sulphide (an endothelium-derived relaxing factor similar to nitric oxide, in the formation of thiocyanate. Koyama et al.[38] showed in dialysis patients that administration of methylcobalamin lowered levels of both tHcy and ADMA.

In patients with renal failure it may therefore be prudent to use methylcobalamin and tetrahydrofolate,[39] and to consider thiols such as mesna[40] to lower levels of homocysteine, rather than using high doses of traditional B vitamins. In dialysis patients, overnight daily dialysis is effective in reducing levels of tHcy.

CONCLUSION

Diet is far more important than most physicians seem to think it is; statin therapy is not a substitute for a healthy diet, because diet is mainly about the postprandial state. A Cretan Mediterranean diet, low in cholesterol, trans fats and meat, and high in beneficial oils, fruits, vegetables, and legumes is the most effective diet for reducing cardiovascular disease, delaying the onset of diabetes and for the treatment of diabetes. Vitamin B_{12} deficiency is much commoner in the elderly than most physicians realize, and in the wake of folic acid fortification, the response to B vitamins for lowering of homocysteine is dependent on vitamin B_{12} and on renal function.

REFERENCES

1. Chiuve SE, Rexrode KM, Spiegelman D, Logroscino G, Manson JE, Rimm EB. Primary prevention of stroke by healthy lifestyle. *Circulation.* 2008;118:947-954.
2. Mokdad AH, Marks JS, Stroup DF, Gerberding JL. Actual causes of death in the United States, 2000. *JAMA.* 2004;291:1238-1245.
3. Spence JD. Fasting lipids: the carrot in the snowman. *Can J Cardiol.* 2003;19:890-892.
4. Franks PW, Hanson RL, Knowler WC, Sievers ML, Bennett PH, Looker HC. Childhood obesity, other cardiovascular risk factors, and premature death. *N Engl J Med.* 2010;362:485-493.
5. Berrington de GA, Hartge P, Cerhan JR, et al. Body-mass index and mortality among 1.46 million white adults. *N Engl J Med.* 2010;363:2211-2219.
6. Strazzullo P, D'Elia L, Cairella G, Garbagnati F, Cappuccio FP, Scalfi L. Excess body weight and incidence of stroke: meta-analysis of prospective studies with 2 million participants. *Stroke.* 2010;41:e418-e426.
7. Sacks FM, Bray GA, Carey VJ, et al. Comparison of weight-loss diets with different compositions of fat, protein, and carbohydrates. *N Engl J Med.* 2009;360:859-873.
8. Spence JD, Jenkins DJ, Davignon J. Dietary cholesterol and egg yolks: not for patients at risk of vascular disease. *Can J Cardiol.* 2010;26:e336-e339.
9. Spence JD. Fasting lipids: the carrot in the snowman. *Can J Cardiol.* 2003;19:890-892.
10. Kushi LH, Lew RA, Stare FJ, et al. Diet and 20-year mortality from coronary heart disease. The Ireland-Boston Diet-Heart Study. *N Engl J Med.* 1985;312:811-818.
11. Shekelle RB, Shryock AM, Paul O, et al. Diet, serum cholesterol, and death from coronary heart disease. The Western Electric study. *N Engl J Med.* 1981;304:65-70.
12. Menotti A, Lanti M, Kromhout D, et al. Homogeneity in the relationship of serum cholesterol to coronary deaths across different cultures: 40-year follow-up of the Seven Countries Study. *Eur J Cardiovasc Prev Rehabil.* 2008;15:719-725.
13. Strandberg TE, Strandberg A, Rantanen K, Salomaa VV, Pitkälä K, Miettinen TA. Low cholesterol, mortality, and quality of life in old age during a 39-year follow-up. *J Am Coll Cardiol.* 2004;44:1002-1008.
14. Vogel RA, Corretti MC, Plotnick GD. Effect of a single high-fat meal on endothelial function in healthy subjects. *Am J Cardiol.* 1997;79:350-354.
15. Hardee's Monster Thickburger. http://www.hardees.com/menu/lunch-and-dinner/23-lb-monster-thickburger/ (accessed September 23, 2009).
16. Spence JD. *How to Prevent Your Stroke.* Nashville: Vanderbilt University Press; 2006.
17. Renaud S, de Lorgeril M, Delaye J, et al. Cretan Mediterranean diet for prevention of coronary heart disease. *Am J Clin Nutr.* 1995;61:1360S-1367S.

18. Willett WC, Stampfer MJ. Rebuild the food pyramid. *Scientific American.* 2003;64-71.
19. Keys A. Mediterranean diet and public health: personal reflections. *Am J Clin Nutr.* 1995;61: 1321S-1323S.
20. Furie KL, Kasner SE, Adams RJ, et al. Guidelines for the prevention of stroke in patients with stroke or transient ischemic attack: a guideline for healthcare professionals from the American Heart Association/ American Stroke Association. *Stroke.* 2011;42:227-276.
21. Selvin E, Steffes MW, Zhu H, et al. Glycated hemoglobin, diabetes, and cardiovascular risk in nondiabetic adults. *N Engl J Med.* 2010;362:800-811.
22. Goldstein LB, Bushnell CD, Adams RJ, et al. Guidelines for the primary prevention of stroke: a guideline for healthcare professionals from the American Heart Association/American Stroke Association. *Stroke.* 2011;42:517-584.
23. Blaschke F, Takata Y, Caglayan E, Law RE, Hsueh WA. Obesity, peroxisome proliferator-activated receptor, and atherosclerosis in type 2 diabetes. *Arterioscler Thromb Vasc Biol.* 2006;26:28-40.
24. Robinson E, Grieve DJ. Significance of peroxisome proliferator-activated receptors in the cardiovascular system in health and disease. *Pharmacol Ther.* 2009;122:246-263.
25. Wilcox R, Bousser MG, Betteridge DJ, et al. Effects of pioglitazone in patients with type 2 diabetes with or without previous stroke: results from PROactive (PROspective pioglitAzone Clinical Trial In macroVascular Events 04). *Stroke.* 2007;38:865-873.
26. Shai I, Schwarzfuchs D, Henkin Y, et al. Weight loss with a low-carbohydrate, Mediterranean, or low-fat diet. *N Engl J Med.* 2008;359:229-241.
27. Shai I, Spence JD, Schwarzfuchs D, et al. Dietary intervention to reverse carotid atherosclerosis. *Circulation.* 2010;121:1200-1208.
28. Lee IM, Cook NR, Gaziano JM, et al. Vitamin E in the primary prevention of cardiovascular disease and cancer: the Women's Health Study: a randomized controlled trial. *JAMA.* 2005;294:56-65.
29. Lonn E, Yusuf S, Dzavik V, et al. Effects of ramipril and vitamin E on atherosclerosis: the study to evaluate carotid ultrasound changes in patients treated with ramipril and vitamin E (SECURE). *Circulation.* 2001;103:919-925.
30. Clarke R, Sherliker P, Hin H, et al. Detection of vitamin B_{12} deficiency in older people by measuring vitamin B_{12} or the active fraction of vitamin B_{12}, holotranscobalamin. *Clin Chem.* 2007;53:963-970.
31. Robertson J, Iemolo F, Stabler SP, Allen RH, Spence JD. Increased importance of Vitamin B_{12} for total homocysteine and carotid plaque in the era of folate fortification of the grain supply. *CMAJ.* 2005;172:1569-1573.
32. Andres E, Loukili NH, Noel E, et al. Vitamin B_{12} (cobalamin) deficiency in elderly patients. *CMAJ.* 2004;171:251-259.
33. Vogiatzoglou A, Oulhaj A, Smith AD, et al. Determinants of plasma methylmalonic acid in a large population: implications for assessment of vitamin B_{12} status. *Clin Chem.* 2009;55:2198-2206.
34. Spence JD. Nutrition and stroke prevention. *Stroke.* 2006;37:2430-2435.
35. Spence JD. Homocysteine-lowering therapy: a role in stroke prevention? *Lancet Neurol.* 2007;7:830-838.
36. Arvanitakis C. Functional and morphological abnormalities of the small intestinal mucosa in pernicious anemia—a prospective study. *Acta Hepatogastroenterol (Stuttg).* 1978;25:313-318.
37. House AA, Eliasziw M, Cattran DC, et al. Effect of B-vitamin therapy on progression of diabetic nephropathy: a randomized controlled trial. *JAMA.* 2010;303:1603-1609.
38. Koyama K, Ito A, Yamamoto J et al. Randomized controlled trial of the effect of short-term coadministration of methylcobalamin and folate on serum ADMA concentration in patients receiving long-term hemodialysis. *Am J Kidney Dis.* 2010;55:1069-1078.
39. Spence JD, Eliasziw M, House AA. B-vitamin therapy for diabetic nephropathy: reply. *JAMA.* 2010;304:636-637.
40. Urquhart BL, Freeman DJ, Spence JD, House AA. The effect of mesna on plasma total homocysteine concentration in hemodialysis patients. *Am J Kidney Dis.* 2007;49:109-117.

Smoking Cessation

Andrew Pipe

SMOKING—DOGMAS, MISCONCEPTIONS, AND EMERGING CLINICAL REALITIES

The importance of smoking cessation in the prevention and management of cardiovascular disease is constantly acknowledged.[1] One-half of all smokers will die prematurely as a result of their addiction to nicotine, and one billion unnecessary deaths are predicted to occur in the 21st century as a result of the pandemic of tobacco diseases.[2] Until recently, approaches to assisting our smoker-patients with the management of their tenacious addiction have been hampered by the persistence of dogmas and misconceptions.[3,4] Far from being a "habit" or a "lifestyle choice" smoking is an addiction, and the onset and perpetuation of regular smoking is reflective of a profound transformation in the neurophysiology of a smoker.[5]

Nicotine has been identified as the most addictive of the substances with addiction potential that are accessible in the community. The inhalation of tobacco smoke results in the delivery of nicotine to the arterial system (via the pulmonary circulation) where it is rapidly transported to addiction centers in the brain. There, the stimulation of an array of nicotine receptors (particularly the $\alpha_4\beta_2$ receptor) initiates a cascade of neurotransmitter activity culminating in the release of dopamine in the mid- and forebrain. Within days of "learning" to inhale tobacco smoke an upregulation of nicotine receptors begins; thereafter the maintenance of a state of "neurophysiologic equanimity" requires the regular readministration of nicotine.[6,7] The delivery of that nicotine is facilitated by a perversely designed drug-delivery device—the cigarette—that is precisely engineered to deliver an aliquot of nicotine as rapidly as possible. Falling levels of nicotine produce characteristic symptoms of withdrawal accentuating the desire for a cigarette—a desire that is abetted by the conditioning that occurs as a result of the association of smoking with a variety of settings, circumstances, and situations. The likelihood of becoming a smoker may be a function of a variety of metabolic and genomic factors: those who metabolize nicotine rapidly (an inherited trait) are much more likely to become smokers and experience more difficulty in attempting cessation (Figure 4–1).[8,9]

Withdrawal, craving, stress, and environmental cues prompt smoking, which leads to the sequential activation, desensitization, and ultimate inactivation of nicotine receptors, ultimately resulting in withdrawal and a repetition of the smoking cycle (Figure 4–2).

Sadly, most clinicians have, until recently, been blissfully unaware of the many common pharmacodynamic and neurophysiologic factors that surround smoking behavior.[10] The outdated view of smoking as a "habit" that anyone should be able to address ("provided they are self-disciplined, responsible, insightful and intelligent enough!") has precluded any broader consideration of the array of common medical, pharmacodynamic, and physiological factors that are integral to smoking behavior.[11] Many do not recognize the association between depression and smoking—cigarette smoke contains small amounts of monoamine oxidase inhibitors (MAOIs) that are self-administered hundreds of times a day and afford a degree of relief to those experiencing depression. Not surprisingly, smoking cessation may result in the appearance of depressive symptoms in some patients.[12,13] Schizophrenics, who are typically very heavy smokers, derive relief from their symptoms when smoking as a result of the stimulation of certain nicotine receptors (the α_7 receptors) producing a reduction in the multiplicity of visual, auditory, and other stimuli that constantly assail them.[14-16] The relationship between pregnancy and nicotine metabolism is largely unappreciated—pregnancy increases the rate of nicotine metabolism—suggesting that cessation may be more difficult for the pregnant woman.[17] A commonly encountered phenomenon is the interaction between smoking and caffeine consumption: the polycyclic aromatic hydrocarbons (PCAHs) found in cigarette smoke stimulate a variety of the CYP450 enzymes including those responsible for the metabolism of numerous medications, as well as caffeine.[18] Caffeine levels rise significantly in the absence of any increase in caffeine intake in the days following smoking cessation, with obvious implications for the comfort—and likelihood of cessation success—of the would-be nonsmoker. An appreciation of such realities permits recognition of the need to be more insightful in assisting with cessation, and to provide more than admonishment regarding a regrettable "habit."

Tobacco addiction is the leading cause of preventable disease, disability, and death in the developed world; it is therefore important that we develop and apply

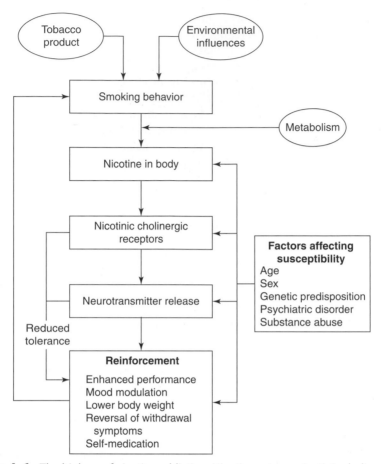

Figure 4–1. The biology of nicotine addiction. Nicotine acts on nicotinic cholinergic receptors, triggering the release of neurotransmitters that produce psychoactive effects that are rewarding. With repeated exposure, tolerance develops to many of the effects of nicotine, thereby reducing its primary reinforcing effects and inducing physical dependence (ie, withdrawal symptoms in the absence of nicotine). Smoking behavior is influenced by pharmacologic feedback and by environmental factors such as smoking cues, friends who smoke, stress, and product advertising. Levels of nicotine in the body in relation to a particular level of nicotine intake from smoking are modulated by the rate of nicotine metabolism, which occurs in the liver largely by means of the enzyme CYP2A6. Other factors that influence smoking behavior include age, sex, genetics, mental illness, and substance abuse. (Reproduced with permission from Benowitz NL. Nicotine addiction. *N Engl J Med.* 2010;362(24):2295-2303.)

systematic approaches to the identification and treatment of smokers in all clinical settings.[4,19,20] Increasingly, there is recognition that assistance with smoking cessation is a fundamental responsibility of all clinicians who treat smokers and their smoking-related diseases.[4,21] Given the burden of cerebrovascular disease engendered by tobacco addiction, this has particular relevance for the neurologist.[3]

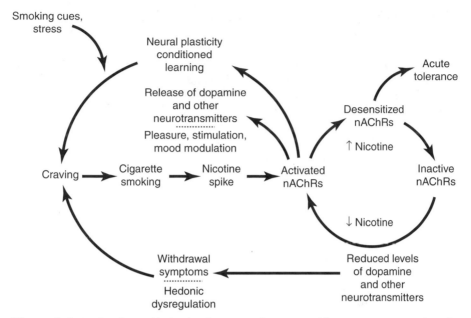

Figure 4–2. Molecular and behavioral aspects of nicotine addiction. Craving—induced by smoking cues, stressors, or a desire to relieve withdrawal symptoms—triggers the act of smoking a cigarette, which delivers a spike of nicotine to the brain. Nicotinic cholinergic receptors (nAChRs) are activated, resulting in the release of dopamine and other neurotransmitters, which in turn cause pleasure, stimulation, and mood modulation. Receptor activation also results in the development of new neural circuits (neural plasticity) and, in association with environmental cues, behavioral conditioning. After being activated by nicotine, nAChRs ultimately become desensitized to it, which results in short-term tolerance of nicotine and reduced satisfaction from smoking. In the time between smoking cigarettes, or after quitting tobacco use, brain nicotine levels decline, which leads to reduced levels of dopamine and other neurotransmitters and to withdrawal symptoms, including craving. In the absence of nicotine, nAChRs regain their sensitivity to nicotine and become reactivated in response to a new dose. (Reproduced with permission from Benowitz NL. Nicotine addiction. *N Engl J Med*. 2010;362(24):2295-2303.)

SMOKING AND THE EPIDEMIOLOGY OF CEREBROVASCULAR DISEASE

Smoking has been described as a "crucial independent determinant of stroke."[22] The significant, substantial, and causal relationships between smoking, exposure to tobacco smoke, and cerebrovascular disease have been recognized for many years and in many settings.[22-48] Up to one-quarter of all strokes have been attributed to cigarette smoking.[49] A prospective examination of a large cohort of Swedish women revealed that the risk of stroke was elevated four-fold in smokers.[50]

Smoking does not discriminate in the genesis of stroke morbidity or mortality: ischemic and hemorrhagic strokes are both directly related to tobacco addiction.[51-53] There is a clear relationship between smoking and the incidence of subarachnoid hemorrhage.[33,54,55] Silent cerebral infarctions are noted to be more frequent among smokers.[56] The risk of stroke is increased in young women smokers and a clear dose-response relationship is evident.[57] The often tragic consequences of a combination of estrogen-containing oral contraceptives, smoking, and stroke in young women are well known but have been attenuated with a reduction in the estrogen content of contemporary oral contraceptives; postmenopausal hormonal replacement also carries risk of stroke.[58-60]

Some investigators have noted a 40% increase in the relative risk of stroke among those who use smokeless tobacco products.[41,61] Others have noted the need for further research to clarify the relationship between smokeless tobacco and stroke.[62]

Smoking is highly predictive of stroke mortality; daily smoking has been observed to more than triple the risk of a fatal stroke.[51,52,63,64] Conversely, the benefits of smoking cessation in reducing the risk of primary or repeat stroke are substantial and accrue rapidly—within five years of cessation the risk of a stroke is that of a nonsmoker.[25,65-67]

It has been noted that it is difficult to identify any other condition that is as prevalent, lethal, and yet so prone to neglect as tobacco addiction.[20] Unfortunately, the significantly increased risk of stroke associated with smoking, although acknowledged, is not generally addressed with the same vigor that is associated with the management of hypertension or hyperlipidemia. Many clinicians may be unaware of the degree to which those who continue to smoke do not derive the benefits of hypertension control or the management of dyslipidemias.[68-72] Smoking is an undertreated risk factor for cerebrovascular disease.[3] The tragic reality is that "the more you smoke, the more you stroke."[73]

SMOKING AND THE PATHOPHYSIOLOGY OF CEREBROVASCULAR DISEASE

The mechanisms by which smoking contributes to the vascular pathology that under-lies, and foreshadows, the development of a stroke have long been appreciated.[74]

It is recognized that up to 60% to 70% of patients experiencing a subarach-noid hemorrhage (SAH) are smokers.[75,76] The risk of SAH is almost tripled in smokers.[27] There is a causal relationship between smoking and the development of aneurysms and their subsequent rupture that is independent of other risk factors.[75]

Tobacco smoke is a chemical "cocktail" made up of thousands of "ingredients" that, on entering the arterial circulation, exert an array of toxic, damaging effects leading to the initiation and progression of atherosclerosis.[77] Atheromatous lesions develop within blood vessels as the consequence of a combination of pathophysi-ologic processes that disrupt vasomotor function, damage the vessel wall, accentu-ate the effects of elevated lipoproteins, and stimulate platelet aggregation and thrombosis. Cigarette smoking plays a distinct role in each. The consequences of cigarette smoke reduce the availability of nitric oxide disrupting the normal vasomotor responses of the blood vessel wall; accelerate vascular inflammation contributing to an accumulation of leukocytes on endothelial surfaces; stimulate the deposition of inflammatory and proinflammatory materials within the vessel wall; elevate levels of total cholesterol and low-density lipoprotein cholesterol (LDL) while reducing levels of high-density lipoprotein cholesterol (HDL); increase the oxidation of LDL; accentuate platelet aggregation and adhesion; increase intima-media thickness; increase blood viscosity; reduce the breakdown of thrombi; and stimulate plaque rupture.[78-83] Oxidant gases and their constituents play a major role in the initiation and progression of atheroma.[84] Smoking results in elevated levels of carbon monoxide (CO), resulting in increased levels of carboxyhemoglobin reducing the blood's capacity to carry and release oxygen and consuming nitric oxide (Figure 4–3).

Products of tobacco smoke, in association with transient loss of cerebral blood flow, can significantly affect the integrity of the blood-brain barrier, predisposing to the development of postischemic brain edema—a process that is of major significance given this structure's important role in maintaining brain homeostasis.[85-87]

The benefits of smoking cessation in reducing the risk of cerebrovascular disease are substantial and sustained. The importance of cessation should assume a priority in the primary and secondary prevention of such disease and in the management strategies of all clinicians involved in its treatment.

SECONDHAND SMOKE AND CEREBROVASCULAR DISEASE

Exposure to the tobacco smoke of others confers added risk to the nonsmoker or never-smoker as a consequence of the passive inhalation of the toxic compounds present in such smoke, albeit at lower levels of concentration. It is not surprising that the risk of stroke is elevated in those repeatedly exposed to the smoke of others. Evidence of this causal relationship continues to accumulate. In fact, the failure to exclude nonsmokers or never-smokers who have been exposed to environmental tobacco smoke (ETS) in studies assessing the contribution of smoking to the development of stroke may have led to an underestimation of the adverse effects of smoking.[32] The relationship between passive smoking and ischemic stroke has been clearly described.[32,34,88] Such evidence has accumulated in a variety of societies and settings: in China, women nonsmokers who lived with smoking husbands had an increased prevalence of stroke in direct proportion to the intensity of spousal smoking; their risk is elevated by more than 50%.[35,41] Similar findings have been reported in Germany.[36,39] Meta-analyses of the relationship between passive smoking and stroke continue to demonstrate a "strong, consistent and dose-dependent association . . . suggesting no safe limit of exposure."[42] Although the relative risk of passive smoking may be small, the impact on population health may be substantial.[39] A woman smoker living with a smoker has a risk of stroke that is increased almost six-fold.[36] The benefits of smoking cessation always extend to both the smoker and their spouse.[40]

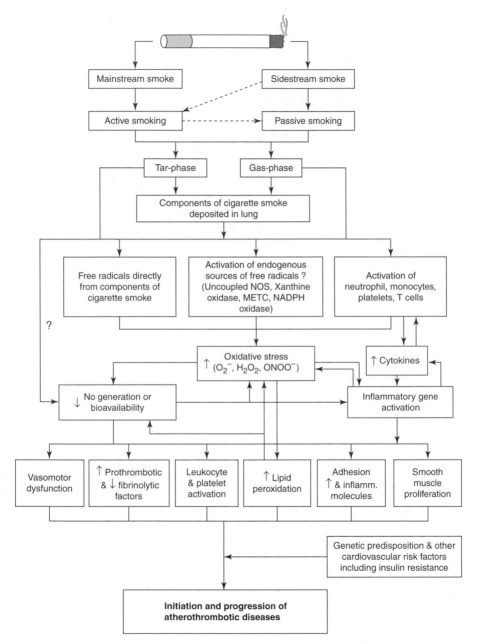

Figure 4–3. Potential pathways and mechanisms for cigarette smoking–mediated cardiovascular dysfunction. (Reproduced with permission from Ambrose JA, Barua RS. The pathophysiology of cigarette smoking and cardiovascular disease. *J Am Coll Cardiol.* 2004;43:1731-1737.)

CEREBROVASCULAR EVENTS—THEIR IMPACT ON THE SMOKER

Smoking contributes to a worsening of the morbidity associated with any cerebrovascular event; much poorer functional outcomes are associated with current or recent smoking.[89-91] It is often assumed that a major health event—a myocardial infarction or a stroke—precipitates smoking cessation. Would that it were so. Despite evidence that these events may result in higher rates of spontaneous cessation, the tenacious realities of tobacco addiction mean that many such patients continue to smoke despite their recognition of the need, and the desire, to stop.[92,93] Sadly, it has been noted that many stroke survivors are unaware of the increased risks associated with ongoing smoking.[94] It has been reported that only 28% of those experiencing a completed stroke are successful in achieving cessation within six months of their event.[92] Others have observed that 43% of smokers quit within three months of a stroke, but only 21% remain abstinent six months after their event.[92] In one stroke-prevention clinic it was observed that only 11% of smokers were able to remain smoke-free one year after initial presentation.[95] Others have described virtually no change in smoking rates in similar settings.[96] The degree of addiction and the presence of other smokers in the home are important predictors of continued smoking in those who have experienced an ischemic stroke.[97] Typically, a majority of smokers make attempts to quit after a stroke but only a minority is able to sustain cessation over the long term.[98,99]

SMOKING CESSATION AND THE PREVENTION OF STROKE

The importance of stroke prevention—both primary and secondary—is universally acknowledged, and the role of smoking cessation is recognized as being of central importance.[23,100-102] The benefits of smoking cessation in reducing the risk of a first stroke accrue rapidly, with the risk returning to that of a nonsmoker in five years.[103] Policy statements and practice guidelines consistently identify smoking cessation as a critical priority for those at cardiovascular risk.[104-107] The adverse impact of continued smoking after a stroke may have been underestimated given the misclassification of smoking histories in previous research.[91,108]

Smoking cessation may be second only to anticoagulation in its potential impact in preventing stroke.[109] Yet it is likely that there is no other risk factor that has been so inadequately addressed. This, in part, reflects a combination of outdated attitudes and minimal understanding of the basis of smoking behaviors; a lack of effective interventions, until recently, to assist smokers struggling to escape their addiction; and limited insight into the ways in which contemporary approaches to smoking cessation can be incorporated into patterns of care in both acute-care and stroke-prevention settings. Systematic approaches to the identification and documentation of the smoking status of all patients, coupled with a similarly systematic approach to ensuring an offer of assistance with cessation at the time of clinical presentation may enable us, in a variety of clinical settings, to be far more effective in addressing this fundamental, formidable risk factor.[4,21,110-115]

THE COST-EFFECTIVENESS OF SMOKING CESSATION

Smoking cessation, it should be appreciated, is the most cost-effective of all the preventive interventions—dramatically so in comparison with many other commonly applied disease prevention strategies.[116-120] Described as the "gold standard" of health care cost-effectiveness, smoking cessation is the only preventive intervention shown to be cost efficient, in a variety of national settings, over a 30-year period.[121-124] The cost per life-year saved through smoking cessation (US$2000-$6000) is a fraction of that expended to achieve the same result through the control of hypertension (US$9000-$26,000 per life-year saved), or dyslipidemia (US$50,000-$196,000 per life-year saved) as a primary prevention strategy.[125-128]

SMOKING CESSATION AND THE STROKE PATIENT

Although we are typically systematic in identifying and documenting hypertension and dyslipidemia among those presenting with transient ischemic attack (TIA) or established stroke, we have been less methodical in establishing a history of current or former tobacco use in most clinical settings. Even asking, "Are you a smoker?" may result in misclassification of the patient who replies, "No," having decided 48 minutes earlier on a gurney in the Emergency Department that today was the day he or she was going to quit. The answer is reflective of misguided optimism rather than an attempt to deceive clinicians. Asking, "Have you used any form of tobacco in the past six months? In the past seven days?" will ensure the accurate identification of smoking status. Clinical protocols, care maps, or other practice templates should incorporate such questions and, most importantly, mandate that positive answers to the questions produce an offer of assistance with cessation if current or recent tobacco use is identified. That assistance should reflect more than simple advice regarding the importance of cessation: most smokers admitted to hospitals will frequently manifest symptoms of nicotine withdrawal within hours of their admission. Those symptoms classically manifest as frustration, uncooperative behavior, and a growing sense of unease and discomfort as the physical symptoms of withdrawal emerge. The use of nicotine replacement therapy (NRT) at the time of admission can significantly reduce such symptoms, enhance patient comfort, facilitate compliance with treatment, and initiate a cessation attempt.

A systematic approach to the treatment of all admitted smokers was developed at the University of Ottawa Heart Institute ("The Ottawa Model") and has proven effective in significantly increasing smoking cessation rates among admitted smoker-patients in that setting (Table 4–1).[114,129] There is increasing recognition of the need for the introduction of such protocols, and evidence continues to emerge of their effectiveness in facilitating cessation while decreasing rates of readmission following an initial hospitalization.[111-113,130-132]

Familiarity with the use of smoking cessation pharmacotherapies, including their titration and combination, is a *sine qua non* for any clinician involved in the care of those who are smokers. The presence of patients smoking outside hospital doors can be seen as an indicator of substandard care of the smoker-patient. Their need for nicotine, and assistance with cessation, can be addressed by the provision of

Table 4–1. The "Ottawa Model" of Smoking Cessation

A systematic approach, embedded in institutional clinical protocols, to
IDENTIFY *Identification of Smoking Status of All Patients*
• "Have you used any form of tobacco in the past 6 months? In the past 7 days?"
DOCUMENT *Documentation of Smoking Status of All Patients*
• Smoking history (pack-years); previous quit attempts; time to first cigarette
ADVISE *Provision of Advice and Cessation Assistance*
• "There is nothing more important than cessation. We can help you with that."
PHARMACOTHERAPY *Provision or Prescription of Appropriate Pharmacotherapy*
• Readily available; prescribed to treat withdrawal; titrated appropriately
FOLLOW-UP *Follow-Up After Hospital Discharge*
• Family physician; public health; automated telephone calls; community resources

From Reid RD, Mullen KA, Slovinec D'Angelo ME, et al. Smoking cessation for hospitalized smokers: an evaluation of the "Ottawa Model." *Nicotine Tob Res.* 2010;12(1):11-18; and Reid RD, Pipe AL, Quinlan B. Promoting smoking cessation during hospitalization for coronary artery disease. *Can J Cardiol.* 2006;22(9):775-780.

NRT or other smoking cessation pharmacotherapies during hospital admission. Such therapy can be continued postdischarge and ongoing follow-up provided by the family practitioner in exactly the same way as ongoing management of hypertension or dyslipidemia. Alternatively, follow-up arrangements may be secured through access to a hospital's smoking cessation service, community smoking-cessation resources, or public-health agencies, and facilitated by the use of voice-recognition telephone technologies or quit-line programs.

The need to improve rates of smoking cessation in those who have experienced stroke is frequently expressed.[94] Systematic approaches to the identification of smokers who have recently experienced a stroke and the provision of cessation assistance at the time of their hospitalization have been identified as providing particular opportunities to contribute to cessation success.[110,133]

ENHANCING SMOKING CESSATION SUCCESS

Guidelines for the development and delivery of successful smoking cessation interventions have consistently emphasized the importance of pharmacotherapy in association with minimal counseling.[120,134,135] Smoking is a tenacious addiction that is accentuated by the degree to which it frequently occurs in association with certain settings, situations, or circumstances. It follows that the provision of strategic, tactical advice regarding the circumstances associated with smoking—and their avoidance—in association with the use of pharmacotherapy proven to reduce or eliminate the craving and withdrawal associated with abstinence from nicotine affords the greatest opportunity for cessation success.

It is useful to consider that smoking cessation be approached in ways similar to the identification and management of other common cardiovascular risk factors.

The identification of a smoker should prompt advice regarding cessation, the prescription of appropriate medications, and arrangements for follow-up and the titration of medication. The provision of clear, unambiguous, nonjudgmental, and personally relevant advice regarding the importance of smoking cessation can be delivered by any clinician efficiently and effectively. When allied with a system that ensures the provision of "best-practice" pharmacotherapy, strategic cessation advice, and an organized approach to follow-up, the chances of cessation success are greatly enhanced.

Most smokers understand why they should not smoke; the majority do not wish to smoke; and many will make a personal quit attempt each year.[136] Clinicians should remember that the mechanisms that impel and maintain smoking behavior reside in the brainstem—not the cerebral cortex. Thus the provision of additional information regarding the health or other dire consequences of continued smoking is likely to have minimal impact. Smokers welcome clear offers of assistance. They value their clinicians' assistance, not their lectures. The consistent identification of the importance of cessation, an acknowledgment to the patient that cessation can be very difficult, and a recognition that relapse to smoking is not indicative of a clinician's failure but rather the manifestation of the power of nicotine addiction will greatly assist all practitioners to become more adept, more confident, and more effective in treating their smoker-patients.

Despite our best efforts some, perhaps many, of our patients will continue to smoke. Many of our patients will also be noncompliant with medications for the treatment of hypertension or dyslipidemia, but we continue to measure blood pressure and lipid levels, and prescribe appropriate medications while encouraging compliance. Similarly, the application of a consistent approach to offering cessation assistance will substantially improve overall smoking cessation performance in most clinical settings. The magnitude of the impact of stopping smoking mandates such an approach.

PHARMACOTHERAPY FOR SMOKING CESSATION

Until recently, conventional approaches to the provision of pharmacotherapy for smoking cessation typically used fixed, declining doses of a medication prescribed for a finite period of time. Such approaches are outdated. In contrast, consider the management of hypertension or dyslipidemia: we would typically introduce, titrate, and often combine medications. They would be used indefinitely, often for life, or until they were no longer necessary. Increasingly, smoking cessation practitioners recognize the need to titrate and combine therapies to optimize the likelihood of success, or minimize the likelihood of side effects, and to continue treatment until no longer needed. Given the magnitude of the risk represented by continued smoking it is appropriate to ensure comparable and optimal use of the available, effective cessation pharmacotherapies.[21] Pharmacotherapy is intended to reduce or eliminate the discomfort of nicotine withdrawal and the irritation of craving over a period of time sufficient to allow a would-be nonsmoker to acquire a repertoire of new, nonsmoking behaviors. For some smokers, it must be recognized that the dose and duration of therapy may need to be modified.

Table 4–2. A Comparison of the Effectiveness of, and Abstinence Rates From Medications and Combinations of Medications Compared to Placebo at 6 Months Post–Quit Date

Medication	Number of Arms	Estimated Odds Ratio (95% CI)	Estimated Abstinence Rate (95% CI)
Varenicline (2 mg/d)	5	3.1 (2.5-3.8)	33.2 (28.9-37.8)
Nicotine nasal spray	4	2.3 (1.7-3.0)	26.7 (21.5-32.7)
Nicotine inhaler	6	2.1 (1.5-2.9)	24.8 (19.1-31.6)
Bupropion SR	26	2.0 (1.8-2.2)	24.2 (22.2-26.4)
Nicotine patch (6-14 wk)	32	1.9 (1.7-2.2)	23.4 (21.3-25.8)
Patch (long term; >14 wk) + ad lib NRT (gum or spray)	3	3.6 (2.5-5.2)	36.5 (28.6-45.3)
Patch + bupropion SR	3	2.5 (1.9-3.4)	28.9 (23.5-35.1)
Patch + inhaler	2	2.2 (1.3-3.6)	25.8 (17.4-36.5)

Adapted from Fiore MC, et al., *Treating Tobacco Use and Dependence: 2008 Update. Clinical Practice Guideline*. Rockville, MD: US Department of Health and Human Services. Public Health Service; 2008.

Many of the effects of nicotine withdrawal may be confused as being side effects of cessation pharmacotherapy. Sleep disturbances, headache, irritability, anxiety, and feelings of depression have all been identified in those who stop smoking; they are frequently experienced, reported, and also misinterpreted by those using pharmacotherapy to aid a cessation attempt.

Three drugs have consistently demonstrated their efficacy in enhancing cessation success: NRT, bupropion SR, and varenicline. Used appropriately they substantially increase the likelihood of sustained cessation (Table 4–2).

Nicotine Replacement Therapy

Commonly available since the early 1980s, NRT was the first pharmacotherapy to establish effectiveness in facilitating smoking cessation.[137] In many communities NRT is available as an over-the-counter medication (OTC) and can be purchased in a variety of retail settings without prescription. It is cheaper than the prescription cessation therapies and its availability was felt to provide optimal access to an important cessation aide. Its unsupervised use may mean, however, that the product is used suboptimally by those who would benefit from modified dosing or who are unaware of the opportunity to combine more than one form of NRT delivery system.

Originally available as a transdermal patch, NRT is now produced as a nasal spray, an "inhaler" (actually a vaporizer), gum, and a lozenge. In each case nicotine is delivered to the venous system via the skin or mucous membranes in a slowly rising manner until a steady state is achieved. There are no extreme elevations of arterial nicotine such as occurs with the inhalation of tobacco smoke; no carbon monoxide, oxidant substances, or any of the several thousand other chemicals are introduced into the circulation. Standard doses of NRT may be insufficient to meet the nicotine "needs" of certain patients, especially those who are heavy smokers.[138] Smoking cessation specialists have learned that the titration of NRT can be particularly helpful in these cases.[139-144] At our institution, for instance, a patient smoking two packs of cigarettes a day will commonly receive two 21-mg NRT patches and be provided with an "inhaler" in order to facilitate titration of nicotine levels to a personalized level of comfort. Provision is made in our standard orders for the dose of NRT to be individualized in every case. This is of particular assistance in ensuring the comfort of very heavy smokers and facilitating the elimination of nicotine withdrawal and its associated behavioral and patient-management challenges. Those who continue to smoke while using conventional doses of NRT are most likely demonstrating that their nicotine "needs" have not been adequately met.

Optimal smoking cessation treatment has been impeded by the persistence of erroneous assumptions and outdated misconceptions. Despite burgeoning evidence to the contrary, many practitioners believe that NRT cannot be used in patients with a history of cardiac disease, which is understandable given that the original trials of these products excluded cardiovascular disease (CVD) patients and thus package inserts and manufacturer's notes preclude the use of NRT in such patient populations. Clinical experience and evidence derived from a variety of settings demonstrate the contrary.[141,145-155] An understanding of the pharmaco-dynamics of nicotine delivery, the differing nicotine doses delivered by a cigarette in comparison to those absorbed with the use of NRT, and the reality that NRT is delivered slowly via the venous system permit the realization that NRT can be used safely in those with cardiac disease.[5,156,157] Most clinicians fail to appreciate that smoking produces dramatic surges of nicotine in the arterial circulation that may be 10-fold higher than venous concentrations; NRT produces no such surges and is free of carbon monoxide, and prothrombotic and proinflammatory substances, all of which are problematic for the smoker with CVD.[151,158]

Smokers titrate their nicotine intake to maintain a certain idiosyncratic "comfort level" of nicotine.[6] The provision of nicotine via patch, gum, or spray to someone who is continuing to smoke will almost always result in an adjustment of smoking levels. This is the basis of the "Reduce to Quit" paradigm in which a smoker is asked to begin to use NRT without any specific adjustment in smoking behavior; the corresponding reduction in cigarette consumption is encouraging to the smoker and enhances the likelihood of a successful smoking cessation attempt, often in association with an increased dose of NRT.[120,159-164]

Ultimately, it is important for all clinicians to recognize that any patient who is intending or continuing to smoke is at much lower at risk while receiving NRT; this has obvious implications for the treatment of hospitalized smokers in general and for stroke patients in particular.

A meta-analysis of pharmacotherapies for smoking cessation has demonstrated that a combination of NRT products (patch plus ad lib gum or spray) was more effective than any other pharmacotherapy or combination pharmacotherapy when compared to placebo—more than tripling the likelihood of sustained cessation (Table 4–2).[120]

In summary, the chances of successful smoking cessation are increased by combining the use of an NRT patch with gum or inhaler; using NRT prior to a formalized quit attempt may also enhance the likelihood of cessation success and, most importantly, there is no evidence that NRT increases the risk of heart attacks.[165]

Bupropion SR

The antidepressant medication bupropion was found, serendipitously, to induce and sustain smoking cessation. It is now recognized that this product blocks the reuptake of dopamine and norepinephrine while also demonstrating some nicotine-receptor blocking activity.[166] It thus serves to simulate the effects of nicotine. This medication, marketed as bupropion SR for smoking cessation, has been demonstrated to be effective in broad populations of smokers.[167-170] It can be used in combination with NRT with enhanced effectiveness.[171] Evidence is now emerging of the effectiveness of a combination of bupropion SR and varenicline.[172]

The use of bupropion SR is contraindicated in those with a history of or propensity for seizures and in those taking monoamine oxidase inhibitors or other medications containing bupropion. The risk of seizure is dose related and is higher when given at doses of 450 mg per day.[173] Bupropion is also marketed as an antidepressant medication and it is important, given the dose-related nature of its side effects, to ensure that patients are not already receiving bupropion before considering this medication for the treatment of nicotine dependency. More commonly encountered side effects include sleep disturbances, dry mouth, headache, and anxiety.[174] Many of these side effects are dose related and can be addressed by a reduction in dose or a change of dose scheduling.

An association between the use of bupropion SR for smoking cessation and neuropsychiatric symptoms including suicidal behavior was noted by the Food and Drug Administration (FDA) in 2009. Large postmarketing studies in the United Kingdom failed to identify evidence of an association between bupropion SR and suicidality.[175,176] Similarly, no evidence of such a relationship was identified in a meta-analysis of bupropion SR's effectiveness in smoking cessation.[177] Nevertheless, it is important for clinicians to be aware of the possibility of these relationships. Other authors have identified a relation between nicotine dependence and rates of suicide attempts; they note that rates of suicide fall when smoking cessation occurs.[178,179]

The use of bupropion SR has been shown to double the likelihood of long-term abstinence when compared to placebo.[120,177]

Varenicline

When delivered to the brainstem, nicotine attaches itself to a variety of nicotine receptors, prominent among which are the $\alpha_4\beta_2$ subtype—the receptor felt to be central to the initiation and maintenance of nicotine addiction. The binding of nicotine to these transmembrane ligand-gated ion channels causes the opening of the channel, an influx of cations resulting in the depolarization of the cell, the initiation of a cascade of neural stimulation across the mesolimbic pathway, and the subsequent release of dopamine and other neurotransmitters in the mid- and forebrain. Repeated exposure to nicotine induces tolerance and initiates the upregulation of nicotine receptors. Varenicline, a structural modification of the naturally occurring plant alkaloid cytisine, binds to the $\alpha_4\beta_2$ receptors even more tenaciously than does nicotine, but causes only a partial opening of the channel, which results in less overall neuronal discharge and reduced levels of dopamine and other neurotransmitter release. The smoker perceives a degree of nicotine stimulation and the release of some dopamine and thus withdrawal symptoms do not appear, or are markedly attenuated, and the urge to smoke disappears. At the same time varenicline occupies the receptor site, preventing the attachment of nicotine and dramatically altering the perceptions that would otherwise occur during smoking. This compound binds only to the $\alpha_4\beta_2$ receptors, does not interact with other medications or the CYP450 pathways, and is excreted virtually unchanged in the urine. In clinical trials varenicline has been shown to triple the likelihood of long-term abstinence when compared to placebo.[120]

Because varenicline stimulates nicotine receptors at many sites, including those in the gut, mild to moderate nausea is its most common side effect and can be managed by taking the medication with a full glass of water in association with a meal. Should nausea persist, a reduction in the dosage from the usual 1.0 mg twice a day to 0.5 mg twice daily commonly addresses the problem with minimal effect on varenicline's ability to induce and maintain cessation.[180]

Following varenicline's introduction, postmarketing reports emerged suggesting that the use of the drug was associated with incidents of mood change and suicidal ideation. These findings have led to additional package warnings indicating a need for clinicians to be aware of these findings, to use caution in prescribing, and to ensure that appropriate advice and follow-up is provided to patients. Ongoing examinations of these phenomena have failed to demonstrate any clear association between the use of varenicline and their appearance, and no causal relationship has been identified. A meta-analysis of the impact of varenicline has concluded that "post marketing safety data raised questions about the association between varenicline, depressed mood, agitation and suicidal behavior or ideation. . . . Thus far, surveillance reports and secondary analyses of trial data lend little support to a causal relationship."[181] A careful reanalysis of all clinical trials involving varenicline also failed to identify any relationship between the use of this drug and psychiatric disturbances, including suicidal ideation and behaviors, and concluded, "There was no significant increase in overall psychiatric disorders, other than sleep disorders and disturbances, in varenicline-treated subjects in this sample of smokers without current psychiatric disorders."[182] The finding of a relationship between smoking and suicidality, and the recognition of a reduction in risk with smoking cessation have been noted previously.[178,179]

A clinical trial of varenicline use in a population of patients with stable CVD demonstrated both effectiveness and safety, and resulted in more than a doubling

Study or subgroup	Treatment Events	Total	Control Events	Total	Weight	Risk ratio M-H, Fixed, 95% CI	Risk ratio M-H, Fixed, 95% CI
Gonzales 2006	77	352	29	344	12.6%	2.59 [1.74, 3.87]	
Jorenby 2006	79	344	35	341	15.1%	2.24 [1.55, 3.24]	
Nakamura 2007	56	155	35	154	15.1%	1.59 [1.11, 2.28]	
Niaura 2008	35	160	12	160	5.2%	2.92 [1.57, 5.41]	
Nides 2006	18	127	6	127	2.6%	3.00 [1.23, 7.31]	
Oncken 2006	58	259	5	129	2.9%	5.78 [2.38, 14.05]	
Rigotti 2010	68	353	26	354	11.1%	2.62 [1.71, 4.02]	
Tashkin 2010	46	248	14	253	6.0%	3.35 [1.89, 5.94]	
Tsai 2007	59	126	27	124	11.7%	2.15 [1.47, 3.15]	
Wang 2009	63	165	42	168	17.9%	1.53 [1.10, 2.12]	
Total (95% CI)		**2289**		**2154**	**100.0%**	**2.31 [2.01, 2.66]**	
Total events	**559**		**231**				

Heterogeneity: Chi^2 = 17.81, df = 9 (P = .04): I* = 49%
Test for overall effect: Z = 11.69 (P < .00001)

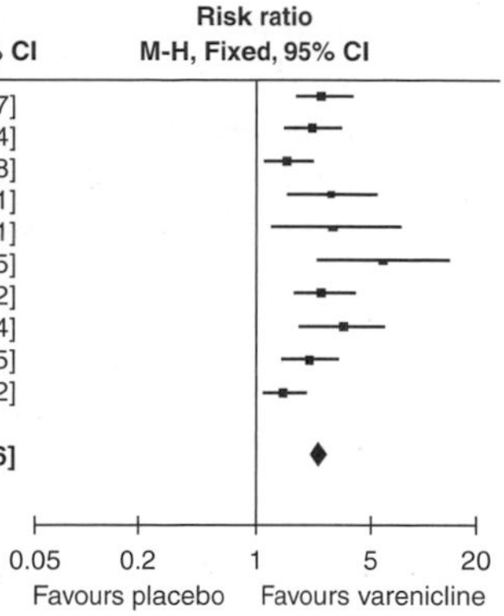

0.05   0.2   1   5   20
Favours placebo   Favours varenicline

Figure 4–4. Forest plot of comparison 1: Varenicline (1.0 mg 2/d) vs placebo, outcome: 1.1 Continuous abstinence at longest follow-up (24+ weeks). (Reproduced with permission from Cahill K, Stead LF, Lancaster T. Nicotine receptor partial agonists for smoking cessation. *Cochrane Database Sys Rev.* 2011;(2):CD006103. DOI: 10.1002/14651858. CD006103.pub5.)

of cessation success when compared to placebo.[183] Recent research suggests that there may be opportunities to combine varenicline with NRT in certain clinical settings; it is speculated that the addition of NRT may permit more complete saturation of all nicotine receptors.[184]

A recent Cochrane report on the overall efficacy of varenicline noted that at standard doses it more than doubled the chances of quitting, while the use of low-dose varenicline roughly doubled the chances of quitting while reducing the severity and number of side effects (Figure 4–4).[181]

Other Approaches and Future Developments

Several other medications have been shown to be effective in smoking cessation.[185] They include nortriptyline and clonidine. Both are effective in approximately doubling the rate of cessation but are accompanied by an array of side effects that limit their general use.[186,187] Other forms of NRT are being developed including a true inhaler and a metered-dose skin-spray technology.[185] Nicotinic receptor agonists (including dianacline, sazetidine-A, and cytisine) continue to be evaluated.[188] Cannabinoid receptor antagonists (rimonabant, surinabant, taranabant) were thought to hold promise for smoking cessation, but have poor safety profiles and have demonstrated limited success in assisting with cessation.[189] Dopamine antagonists and monoamine oxidase inhibitors are also being considered for smoking cessation.[185]

Nicotine vaccines continue to be the focus of research; nicotine is conjugated to larger carrier proteins, but at present the immunological response varies, the vaccine may require multiple injections, and there is a time delay before an immune response is achieved.[185,190] No vaccine is currently available for clinical use.

There is little evidence to support the use of hypnotherapy, acupuncture, or laser therapy for smoking cessation.[191,192]

In many jurisdictions the provision of cost-free pharmacotherapy is being actively considered or has become a reality. It appears that cessation rates are enhanced in settings where the cost of such therapy is borne by the health system or insurers. There is also clear evidence of the cost benefit to system or insurance funders.[193] As these policies become more widespread they will undoubtedly find immediate application within hospital-based cessation programs.

CONCLUSION

The relationship between smoking and the development, complications, and recurrence of stroke is clear and unequivocal. Smoking cessation affords a dramatic opportunity to significantly reduce morbidity and mortality, and increase quality of life following a cerebrovascular event. Until recently, smoking cessation was not seen as the province of the neurologist. The recognition that systematic approaches to the identification and treatment of smokers can significantly enhance the likelihood of cessation affords an opportunity to improve the quality of care provided to all smokers who experience a TIA or stroke. Clinicians involved in the care of smokers should be as familiar with the initiation of a smoking cessation attempt and the management of smoking cessation pharmacotherapy as they are with the prescription and titration of antihypertensive or lipid-lowering medications. The introduction of systematic approaches to the identification, treatment, and follow-up of smokers in stroke-care settings in association with the training of house staff and nurses in smoking cessation practice will greatly enhance our ability to help smokers.

Not all of our patients will stop smoking. But all clinicians can become as adept with the consistent, systematic treatment of nicotine addiction as they are with the management of other classic cerebrovascular risk factors, and many more patients will stop smoking as a result.[21,194]

REFERENCES

1. A clinical practice guideline for treating tobacco use and dependence: a US Public Health Service report. The Tobacco Use and Dependence Clinical Practice Guidelines Panel, Staff and Consortium Represenetatives. *JAMA*. 2000;283(24):3244-3254.
2. Peto R, Lopez AD. The future worldwide health effects of current smoking patterns. In: Koop CE, Pearson CE, Schwarz MR, eds. *Critical Issues in Global Health*. San Francisco: Jossey-Bass; 2001.
3. Erhardt L. Cigarette smoking: an undertreated risk factor for cardiovascular disease. *Atherosclerosis*. 2009;205(1):23-32.
4. Pipe AL, Eisenberg MJ, Gupta A, Reid RD, Suskin NG, Stone JA. Smoking cessation and the cardiovascular specialist: Canadian Cardiovascular Society position paper. *Can J Cardiol*. 2011;27(2):132-137.
5. Benowitz N. Nicotine addiction. *N Engl J Med*. 2010;362:2295-2303.
6. Benowitz NL. Neurobiology of nicotine addiction: implications for smoking cessation treatment. *Am J Med*. 2008;121(4A):S3-S10.
7. De Biasi M, Dani JA. Reward, addiction, withdrawal to nicotine. *Annu Rev Neurosci*. 2011;34:105-130.
8. Bierut LJ. Convergence of genetic findings for nicotine dependence and smoking related diseases with chromosome 15q24-25. *Trends Pharmacol Sci*. 2010;31(1):46-51.
9. Liu JZ, Tozzi F, Waterworth DM, et al. Meta-analysis and imputation refines the association of 15q25 with smoking quantity. *Nat Genet*. 2010;42(5):436-440.

10. Benowitz N. Pharmacology of nicotine addiction, smoking-induced disease, and therapeutics. *Annu Rev Pharmacol Toxicol.* 2009;49:57-71.

11. Pipe AL, Papadakis S, Reid RD. The role of smoking cessation in the prevention of coronary artery disease. *Curr Atheroscler Rep.* 2010;12(2):145-150.

12. Covey LS, Glassman AH, Stetner F. Major depression following smoking cessation. *Am J Psychiatry.* 1997;154(2):263-265.

13. Tsoh JY, Humfleet GL, Munoz RF, Reus VI, Hartz DT, Hall SM. Development of major depression after treatment for smoking cessation. *Am J Psychiatry.* 2000;157(3):368-374.

14. Degenhardt L, Hall W. The relationship between tobacco use, substance-use disorders and mental health: results from the National Survey of Mental Health and Well-being. *Nicotine Tob Res.* 2001;3:225-234.

15. Kang E, Lee J. A longitudinal study on the causal association between smoking and depression. *J Prev Med Public Health.* 2010;43(3):193-204.

16. Lasser K, Boyd JW, Woolhandler S, Himmelstein DU, McCormick D, Bor DH. Smoking and mental illness. A population-based prevalence study. *JAMA.* 2000;284:2602-2610.

17. Dempsey D, Jacob III P, Benowitz NL. Accelerated metabolism of nicotine and cotinine in pregnant smokers. *J Pharmacol Exp Ther.* 2002;301:594-598.

18. Arnaud MJ. Pharmacokinetics and metabolism of natural methylxanthines in animal and man. *Handb Exp Pharmacol.* 2011;200:33-91.

19. Fujiwara H. Smoking is a disease and smokers are patients. *Circ J.* 2010;74(4):628-629.

20. Orleans CT. Increasing the demand for and use of effective smoking-cessation treatments reaping the full health benefits of tobacco-control science and policy gains in our lifetime. *Am J Prev Med.* 2007;33(6):S340-S348.

21. Hurt RD, Ebbert JO, Hays JT, McFadden DD. Treating tobacco dependence in a medical setting. *CA Cancer J Clin.* 2009;59(5):314-326.

22. Paul SL, Thrift AG, Donnan GA. Smoking as a crucial independent determinant of stroke. *Tob Induc Dis.* 2004;2(2):67-80.

23. Ockene IS, Miller NH. Cigarette smoking, cardiovascular disease, and stroke: a statement for health-care professionals from the American Heart Association. American Heart Association task Force on Risk Reduction. *Circulation.* 1997;96:3243-3247.

24. Abbott RD, Yin Y, Reed DM, Yano K. Risk of stroke in male cigarette smokers. *N Engl J Med.* 1986;315(12):717-720.

25. Wolf PA, D'Agostino RB, Kannel WB, Bonita R, Belanger AJ. Cigarette smoking as a risk factor for stroke. The Framingham Study. *JAMA.* 1988;259(7):1025-1029.

26. Gill JS, Shipley MJ, Tsementzis SA, et al. Cigarette smoking. A risk factor for hemorrhagic and non-hemorrhagic stroke. *Arch Intern Med.* 1989;149(9):2053-2057.

27. Shinton R, Beevers G. Meta-analysis of relation between cigarette smoking and stroke. *BMJ.* 1989;298(6676):789-794.

28. Donnan GA, McNeil JJ, Adena MA, Doyle AE, O'Malley HM, Neill GC. Smoking as a risk factor for cerebral ischaemia. *Lancet.* 1989;2(8664):643-647.

29. Robbins AS, Manson JE, Lee IM, Satterfield S, Hennekens CH. Cigarette smoking and stroke in a cohort of U.S. male physicians. *Ann Intern Med.* 1994;120(6):458-462.

30. Hankey GJ, Warlow CP. Treatment and secondary prevention of stroke: evidence, costs, and effects on individuals and populations. *Lancet.* 1999;354(9188):1457-1463.

31. Burns DM. Epidemiology of smoking-induced cardiovascular disease. *Prog Cardiovasc Dis.* 2003;46(1):11-29.

32. Bonita R, Duncan J, Truelsen T, Jackson RT, Beaglehole R. Passive smoking as well as active smoking increases the risk of acute stroke. *Tob Control.* 1999;8(2):156-160.

33. Anderson CS, Feigin V, Bennett D, Lin RB, Hankey G, Jamrozik K. Active and passive smoking and the risk of subarachnoid hemorrhage: an international population-based case-control study. *Stroke.* 2004;35(3):633-637.

34. Iribarren C, Darbinian J, Klatsky AL, Friedman GD. Cohort study of exposure to environmental tobacco smoke and risk of first ischemic stroke and transient ischemic attack. *Neuroepidemiology.* 2004;23(1-2):38-44.

35. Zhang X, Shu XO, Yang G, et al. Association of passive smoking by husbands with prevalence of stroke among Chinese women nonsmokers. *Am J Epidemiol.* 2005;161(3):213-218.

36. Qureshi AI, Suri MF, Kirmani JF, Divani AA. Cigarette smoking among spouses: another risk factor for stroke in women. *Stroke.* 2005;36(9):e74-e76.

37. Lee PN, Forey BA. Environmental tobacco smoke exposure and risk of stroke in nonsmokers: a review with meta-analysis. *J Stroke Cerebrovasc Dis.* 2006;15(5):190-201.

38. Raupach T, Schafer K, Konstantinides S, Andreas S. Secondhand smoke as an acute threat for the cardiovascular system: a change in paradigm. *Eur Heart J.* 2006;27(4):386-392.

39. Heuschmann PU, Heidrich J, Wellmann J, Kraywinkel K, Keil U. Stroke mortality and morbidity attributable to passive smoking in Germany. *Eur J Cardiovasc Prev Rehabil.* 2007;14(6):793-795.

40. Glymour MM, Defries TB, Kawachi I, Avendano M. Spousal smoking and incidence of first stroke: the Health and Retirement Study. *Am J Prev Med.* 2008;35(3):245-248.

41. He Y, Lam TH, Jiang B, et al. Passive smoking and risk of peripheral arterial disease and ischemic stroke in Chinese women who never smoked. *Circulation.* 2008;118(15):1535-1540.

42. Oono IP, Mackay DF, Pell JP. Meta-analysis of the association between secondhand smoke exposure and stroke. *J Public Health (Oxf).* 2011 [Epub ahead of print].

43. Whincup PH, Gilg JA, Emberson JR, et al. Passive smoking and risk of coronary heart disease and stroke: prospective study with cotinine measurement. *BMJ.* 2004;329(7459):200-205.

44. Ueshima H, Choudhury SR, Okayama A, et al. Cigarette smoking as a risk factor for stroke death in Japan: NIPPON DATA80. *Stroke.* 2004;35(8):1836-1841.

45. Martiniuk AL, Lee CM, Lam TH, et al. The fraction of ischaemic heart disease and stroke attributable to smoking in the WHO Western Pacific and South-East Asian regions. *Tob Control.* 2006;15(3):181-188.

46. Haheim LL, Holme I, Hjermann I, Tonstad S. Risk-factor profile for the incidence of subarachnoid and intracerebral haemorrhage, cerebral infarction, and unspecified stroke during 21 years' follow-up in men. *Scand J Public Health.* 2006;34(6):589-597.

47. Kelly TN, Gu D, Chen J, et al. Cigarette smoking and risk of stroke in the chinese adult population. *Stroke.* 2008;39(6):1688-1693.

48. Girot M. Smoking and stroke. *Presse Med.* 2009;38(7-8):1120-1125.

49. Hankey GJ. Smoking and risk of stroke. *J Cardiovasc Risk.* 1999;6(4):207-211.

50. Lu M, Ye W, Adami HO, Weiderpass E. Stroke incidence in women under 60 years of age related to alcohol intake and smoking habit. *Cerebrovasc Dis.* 2008;25(6):517-525.

51. Kurth T, Kase CS, Berger K, Gaziano JM, Cook NR, Buring JE. Smoking and risk of hemorrhagic stroke in women. *Stroke.* 2003;34(12):2792-2795.

52. Kurth T, Kase CS, Berger K, Schaeffner ES, Buring JE, Gaziano JM. Smoking and the risk of hemorrhagic stroke in men. *Stroke.* 2003;34(5):1151-1155.

53. Yamagishi K, Iso H, Kitamura A, et al. Smoking raises the risk of total and ischemic strokes in hypertensive men. *Hypertens Res.* 2003;26(3):209-217.

54. Longstreth WT Jr, Nelson LM, Koepsell TD, van Belle G. Cigarette smoking, alcohol use, and subarachnoid hemorrhage. *Stroke.* 1992;23(9):1242-1249.

55. Feigin VL, Rinkel GJ, Lawes CM, et al. Risk factors for subarachnoid hemorrhage: an updated systematic review of epidemiological studies. *Stroke.* 2005;36(12):2773-2780.

56. Howard G, Wagenknecht LE, Cai J, Cooper L, Kraut MA, Toole JF. Cigarette smoking and other risk factors for silent cerebral infarction in the general population. *Stroke.* 1998;29(5):913-917.

57. Bhat VM, Cole JW, Sorkin JD, et al. Dose-response relationship between cigarette smoking and risk of ischemic stroke in young women. *Stroke.* 2008;39(9):2439-2443.

58. Mishell DR Jr. Cardiovascular risks: perception versus reality. *Contraception.* 1999;59(1 Suppl):21S-24S.

59. Bushnell CD. Oestrogen and stroke in women: assessment of risk. *Lancet Neurol.* 2005;4(11):743-751.

60. Davis PH. Use of oral contraceptives and postmenopausal hormone replacement: evidence on risk of stroke. *Curr Treat Options Neurol.* 2008;10(6):468-474.

61. Boffetta P, Straif K. Use of smokeless tobacco and risk of myocardial infarction and stroke: systematic review with meta-analysis. *BMJ.* 2009;339:b3060.

62. Piano MR, Benowitz NL, Fitzgerald GA, et al. Impact of smokeless tobacco products on cardiovascular disease: implications for policy, prevention, and treatment: a policy statement from the American Heart Association. *Circulation.* 2010;122(15):1520-1544.

63. Myint PK, Welch AA, Bingham SA, et al. Smoking predicts long-term mortality in stroke: the European Prospective Investigation into Cancer (EPIC)-Norfolk Prospective Population Study. *Prev Med.* 2006;42(2):128-131.

64. Haheim LL, Holme I, Hjermann I, Leren P. Smoking habits and risk of fatal stroke: 18 years follow up of the Oslo Study. *J Epidemiol Community Health.* 1996;50(6):621-624.

65. Wannamethee SG, Shaper AG, Whincup PH, Walker M. Smoking cessation and the risk of stroke in middle-aged men. *JAMA.* 1995;274(2):155-160.

66. Kawachi I, Colditz GA, Stampfer MJ, et al. Smoking cessation and decreased risk of stroke in women. *JAMA.* 1993;269(2):232-236.

67. Song YM, Cho HJ. Risk of stroke and myocardial infarction after reduction or cessation of cigarette smoking: a cohort study in korean men. *Stroke.* 2008;39(9):2432-2438.

68. Milionis HJ, Rizos E, Mikhailidis DP. Smoking diminishes the beneficial effect of statins: observations from the landmark trials. *Angiology.* 2001;52(9):575-587.

69. Journath G, Nilsson PM, Petersson U, Paradis BA, Theobald H, Erhardt L. Hypertensive smokers have a worse cardiovascular risk profile than non-smokers in spite of treatment—a national study in Sweden. *Blood Pressure.* 2005;14(3):144-150.

70. Etminan N, Beseoglu K, Steiger HJ, Hanggi D. The impact of hypertension and nicotine on the size of ruptured intracranial aneurysms. *J Neurol Neurosurg Psychiatry.* 2011;82(1):4-7.

71. Hering D, Kucharska W, Kara T, Somers VK, Narkiewicz K. Smoking is associated with chronic sympathetic activation in hypertension. *Blood Pressure.* 2010;19(3):152-155.

72. Frey P, Waters DD, DeMicco DA, et al. Impact of smoking on cardiovascular events in patients with coronary disease receiving contemporary medical therapy (from the Treating to New Targets [TNT] and the Incremental Decrease in End Points Through Aggressive Lipid Lowering [IDEAL] trials). *Am J Cardiol.* 2011;107(2):145-150.

73. Shah RS, Cole JW. Smoking and stroke: the more you smoke the more you stroke. *Expert Rev Cardiovasc Ther.* 2010;8(7):917-932.

74. Rahman MM, Laher I. Structural and functional alteration of blood vessels caused by cigarette smoking: an overview of molecular mechanisms. *Curr Vasc Pharmacol.* 2007;5(4):276-292.

75. Weir BK, Kongable GL, Kassell NF, Schultz JR, Truskowski LL, Sigrest A. Cigarette smoking as a cause of aneurysmal subarachnoid hemorrhage and risk for vasospasm: a report of the Cooperative Aneurysm Study. *J Neurosurg.* 1998;89(3):405-411.

76. Juvela S. Risk factors for multiple intracranial aneurysms. *Stroke.* 2000;31(2):392-397.

77. Howard G, Wagenknecht LE, Burke GL, et al. Cigarette smoking and progression of atherosclerosis: the Atherosclerosis Risk in Communities (ARIC) Study. *JAMA.* 1998;279(2):119-124.

78. Hioki H, Aoki N, Kawano K, et al. Acute effects of cigarette smoking on platelet-dependent thrombin generation. *Eur Heart J.* 2001;22(1):56-61.

79. Ambrose J, Barua R. The pathophysiology of cigarette smoking and cardiovascular disease: an update. *J Am Coll Cardiol.* 2004;43(10):1731-1737.

80. *The Health Consequences of Smoking: A Report of the Surgeon General.* Atlanta: U.S. Department of Health and Human Services, Centers for Disease Control and Prevention, National Center for Chronic Disease Pevention and Health Promotion, Office on Smoking and Health; 2004.

81. Benowitz N. Cigarette smoking and cardiovascular disease: pathophysiology and implications for treatment. *Prog Cardiovasc Dis.* 2003;46(1):91-111.

82. Poredos P, Orehek M, Tratnik E. Smoking is associated with dose-related increase of intima-media thickness and endothelial dysfunction. *Angiology.* 1999;50(3):201-208.

83. Shimada S, Hasegawa K, Wada H, et al. High blood viscosity is closely associated with cigarette smoking and markedly reduced by smoking cessation. *Circ J.* 2010;75(1):185-189.

84. Tonstad S, Johnston JA. Cardiovascular risks associated with smoking: a review for clinicians. *Eur J Cardiovasc Prev Rehabil.* 2006;13:507-514.

85. Hawkins BT, Brown RC, Davis TP. Smoking and ischemic stroke: a role for nicotine? *Trends Pharmacol Sci.* 2002;23(2):78-82.

86. Hossain M, Sathe T, Fazio V, et al. Tobacco smoke: a critical etiological factor for vascular impairment at the blood-brain barrier. *Brain Res.* 2009;1287:192-205.

87. Mazzone P, Tierney W, Hossain M, Puvenna V, Janigro D, Cucullo L. Pathophysiological impact of cigarette smoke exposure on the cerebrovascular system with a focus on the blood-brain barrier: expanding the awareness of smoking toxicity in an underappreciated area. *Int J Environ Res Public Health.* 2010;7(12):4111-4126.

88. You RX, Thrift AG, McNeil JJ, Davis SM, Donnan GA. Ischemic stroke risk and passive exposure to spouses' cigarette smoking. Melbourne Stroke Risk Factor Study (MERFS) Group. *Am J Public Health.* 1999;89(4):572-575.

89. Dagenais GR, Yi Q, Lonn E, Sleight P, Ostergren J, Yusuf S. Impact of cigarette smoking in high-risk patients participating in a clinical trial. A substudy from the Heart Outcomes Prevention Evaluation (HOPE) trial. *Eur J Cardiovasc Prev Rehabil.* 2005;12(1):75-81.

90. Ovbiagele B, Weir CJ, Saver JL, Muir KW, Lees KR. Effect of smoking status on outcome after acute ischemic stroke. *Cerebrovasc Dis.* 2006;21(4):260-265.

91. Xu G, Liu X, Wu W, Zhang R, Yin Q. Recurrence after ischemic stroke in chinese patients: impact of uncontrolled modifiable risk factors. *Cerebrovasc Dis.* 2007;23(2-3):117-120.

92. Bak S, Sindrup SH, Alslev T, Kristensen O, Christensen K, Gaist D. Cessation of smoking after first-ever stroke: a follow-up study. *Stroke.* 2002;33(9):2263-2269.

93. Zillich AJ, Hudmon KS, Damush T. Tobacco use and cessation among veterans recovering from stroke or TIA: a qualitative assessment and implications for rehabilitation. *Top Stroke Rehabil.* 2010;17(2):140-150.

94. Kothari R, Sauerbeck L, Jauch E, et al. Patients' awareness of stroke signs, symptoms, and risk factors. *Stroke.* 1997;28(10):1871-1875.

95. Mouradian MS, Majumdar SR, Senthilselvan A, Khan K, Shuaib A. How well are hypertension, hyperlipidemia, diabetes, and smoking managed after a stroke or transient ischemic attack? *Stroke.* 2002;33(6):1656-1659.

96. Hornnes N, Larsen K, Boysen G. Little change of modifiable risk factors 1 year after stroke: a pilot study. *Int J Stroke.* 2010;5(3):157-162.

97. Sienkiewicz-Jarosz H, Zatorski P, Baranowska A, Ryglewicz D, Bienkowski P. Predictors of smoking abstinence after first-ever ischemic stroke: a 3-month follow-up. *Stroke.* 2009;40(7):2592-2593.

98. Ives SP, Heuschmann PU, Wolfe CD, Redfern J. Patterns of smoking cessation in the first 3 years after stroke: the South London Stroke Register. *Eur J Cardiovasc Prev Rehabil.* 2008;15(3):329-335.

99. Gall SL, Dewey HM, Thrift AG. Smoking cessation at 5 years after stroke in the North East Melbourne stroke incidence study. *Neuroepidemiology.* 2009;32(3):196-200.

100. Sanossian N, Ovbiagele B. Multimodality stroke prevention. *Neurologist.* 2006;12(1):14-31.

101. Spence JD. Stroke prevention in the high-risk patient. *Expert Opin Pharmacother.* 2007;8(12):1851-1859.

102. Spence JD. Secondary stroke prevention. *Nat Rev Neurol.* 2010;6(9):477-486.

103. Lightwood J, Glantz S. Short-term economic and health benefits of smoking cessation: myocardial infarction and stroke. *Circulation.* 1997;96(4):1089-1096.

104. Goldstein LB, Adams R, Alberts MJ, et al. Primary prevention of ischemic stroke: a guideline from the American Heart Association/American Stroke Association Stroke Council: cosponsored by the Atherosclerotic Peripheral Vascular Disease Interdisciplinary Working Group; Cardiovascular Nursing Council; Clinical Cardiology Council; Nutrition, Physical Activity, and Metabolism Council; and the Quality of Care and Outcomes Research Interdisciplinary Working Group. *Circulation.* 2006;113(24):e873-e923.

105. Sacco RL, Adams R, Albers G, et al. Guidelines for prevention of stroke in patients with ischemic stroke or transient ischemic attack: a statement for healthcare professionals from the American Heart Association/American Stroke Association Council on Stroke: co-sponsored by the Council on Cardiovascular Radiology and Intervention: the American Academy of Neurology affirms the value of this guideline. *Stroke.* 2006;37(2):577-617.

106. MacDougall NJ, Amarasinghe S, Muir KW. Secondary prevention of stroke. *Expert Rev Cardiovasc Ther.* 2009;7(9):1103-1115.

107. Ratchford EV, Black JH 3rd. Approach to smoking cessation in the patient with vascular disease. *Curr Treat Options Cardiovasc Med.* 2011;13(2):91-102.

108. Leira EC, Chang KC, Davis PH, et al. Can we predict early recurrence in acute stroke? *Cerebrovasc Dis.* 2004;18(2):139-144.
109. Romero JR, Morris J, Pikula A. Stroke prevention: modifying risk factors. *Ther Adv Cardiovasc Dis.* 2008;2(4):287-303.
110. Ovbiagele B, Saver JL, Fredieu A, et al. In-hospital initiation of secondary stroke prevention therapies yields high rates of adherence at follow-up. *Stroke.* 2004;35(12):2879-2883.
111. Mohiuddin SM, Mooss AN, Hunter CB, Grollmes TL, Cloutier DA, Hilleman DE. Intensive smoking cessation intervention reduces mortality in high-risk smokers with cardiovascular disease. *Chest.* 2007;131(2):446-452.
112. Rigotti NA, Munafo MR, Stead LF. Interventions for smoking cessation in hospitalised patients. *Cochrane Database Syst Rev.* 2007(3):CD001837.
113. Rigotti NA, Munafo MR, Stead LF. Smoking cessation interventions for hospitalized smokers: a systematic review. *Arch Intern Med.* 2008;168(18):1950-1960.
114. Reid RD, Mullen KA, Slovinec D'Angelo ME, et al. Smoking cessation for hospitalized smokers: an evaluation of the "Ottawa Model". *Nicotine Tob Res.* 2010;12(1):11-18.
115. Park ER, Japuntich S, Temel J, et al. A smoking cessation intervention for thoracic surgery and oncology clinics: a pilot trial. 2011;6(6):1059-1065.
116. Godfrey C, Parrott S, Coleman T, Pound E. The cost-effectiveness of the English smoking treatment services: evidence from practice. *Addiction.* 2005;100(Suppl 2):70-83.
117. Solberg LI, Maciosek MV, Edwards NM, Khanchandani HS, Goodman MJ. Repeated tobacco-use screening and intervention in clinical practice: health impact and cost effectiveness. *Am J Prev Med.* 2006;31(1):62-71.
118. Shearer J, Shanahan M. Cost effectiveness analysis of smoking cessation interventions. *Aust N Z J Public Health.* 2006;30(5):428-434.
119. Maciosek MV, Coffield AB, Edwards NM, Flottemesch TJ, Goodman MJ, Solberg LI. Priorities among effective clinical preventive services: results of a systematic review and analysis. *Am J Prev Med.* 2006;31(1):52-61.
120. Fiore MC, Jaen CR, Baker TB, et al. *Treating Tobacco Use and Dependence: 2008 Update. Clinical Practice Guideline.* Rockville, MD: US Dept of Health and Human Services. Public Health Service; 2008.
121. Rasmussen SR, Prescott E, Sorensen TI, Sogaard J. The total lifetime health cost savings of smoking cessation to society. *Eur J Public Health.* 2005;15(6):601-606.
122. Kahn R, Robertson RM, Smith R, Eddy D. The impact of prevention on reducing the burden of cardiovascular disease. *Circulation.* 2008;118(5):576-585.
123. Eddy DM, Peskin B, Shcheprov A, Pawlson G, Shih S, Schaaf D. Effect of smoking cessation advice on cardiovascular disease. *Am J Med Qual.* 2009;24(3):241-249.
124. Cornuz J, Gilbert A, Pinget C, et al. Cost-effectiveness of pharmacotherapies for nicotine dependence in primary care settings: a multinational comparison. *Tob Control.* 2006;15(3):152-159.
125. Brown AI, Garber AM. A concise review of the cost-effectiveness of coronary heart disease prevention. *Med Clin North Am.* 2000;84(1):279-297, xi.
126. Lightwood J. The economics of smoking and cardiovascular disease. *Prog Cardiovasc Dis.* 2003;46(1):39-78.
127. Parrott S, Godfrey C. Economics of smoking cessation. *BMJ.* 2004;328(7445):947-949.
128. Franco OH, der Kinderen AJ, De Laet C, Peeters A, Bonneux L. Primary prevention of cardiovascular disease: cost-effectiveness comparison. *Int J Technol Assess Health Care.* 2007;23(1):71-79.
129. Reid RD, Lipe AL, Quinlan B. Promoting smoking cessation during hospitalization for coronary artery disease. *Can J Cardiol.* 2006;22(9):775-780.
130. Molyneux A, Lewis S, Leivers U, et al. Clinical trial comparing nicotine replacement therapy (NRT) plus brief counselling, brief counselling alone, and minimal intervention on smoking cessation in hospital inpatients. *Thorax.* 2003;58(6):484-488.
131. Bastian LA. Smoking cessation for hospital patients: an opportunity to increase the reach of effective smoking cessation programs. *J Gen Intern Med.* 2008;23(8):1286-1287.
132. Gadomski AM, Gavett J, Krupa N, Tallman N, Jenkins P. Effectiveness of an inpatient smoking cessation program. *J Hosp Med.* 2011;6(1):E1-E8.

133. Ovbiagele B, Kidwell CS, Selco S, Razinia T, Saver JL. Treatment adherence rates one year after initiation of a systematic hospital-based stroke prevention program. *Cerebrovasc Dis.* 2005;20(4):280-282.

134. West R, McNeill A, Raw M. Smoking cessation guidelines for health professionals: an update. Health Education Authority. *Thorax.* 2000;55(12):987-999.

135. McRobbie H, Bullen C, Glover M, Whittaker R, Wallace-Bell M, Fraser T. New Zealand smoking cessation guidelines. *N Z Med J.* 2008;121(1276):57-70.

136. Cinciripini PM, McClure JB. Smoking cessation: recent developments in behavioral and pharmacologic interventions. *Oncology (Williston Park).* 1998;12(2):249-256, 59; discussion 60, 65, 2.

137. Schneider NG, Popek P, Jarvik ME, Gritz ER. The use of nicotine gum during cessation of smoking. *Am J Psychiatry.* 1977;134(4):439-440.

138. Dale L, Hurt R, Offord K, Lawson G, Croghan I, Schroeder D. High-dose nicotine patch therapy. Percentage of replacement and smoking cessation. *JAMA.* 1995;274(17):1353-1358.

139. Hurt RD, Dale LC, Offord KP, et al. Serum nicotine and cotinine levels during nicotine-patch therapy. *Clin Pharmacol Ther.* 1993;54(1):98-106.

140. Fredrickson PA, Hurt RD, Lee GM, et al. High dose transdermal nicotine therapy for heavy smokers: safety, tolerability and measurement of nicotine and cotinine levels. *Psychopharmacology (Berl).* 1995;122(3):215-222.

141. Joseph AM, Norman SM, Ferry LH, et al. The safety of transdermal nicotine as an aid to smoking cessation in patients with cardiac disease. *N Engl J Med.* 1996;335(24):1792-1798.

142. Fiore M, Bailey W, Cohen S, et al. *Treating Tobacco Use and Dependence. Clinical Practice Guideline.* Rockville, MD: U.S. Department of Health and Human Services. Public Health Service; 2000.

143. Silagy C, Lancaster T, Stead L, Mant D, Fowler G. Nicotine replacement therapy for smoking cessation. *Cochrane Database Syst Rev.* 2004(3):CD000146.

144. Ontario Medical Association. Rethinking stop-smoking medications: treatment myths and medical realities. [update 2008]. *Ont Med Rev.* 2008;1:22-34.

145. Nicotine replacement therapy for patients with coronary artery disease. Working Group for the Study of Transdermal Nicotine in Patients with Coronary artery disease. *Arch Intern Med.* 1994;154(9):989-995.

146. Mahmarian JJ, Moye LA, Nasser GA, et al. Nicotine patch therapy in smoking cessation reduces the extent of exercise-induced myocardial ischemia. *J Am Coll Cardiol.* 1997;30(1):125-130.

147. Tzivoni D, Keren A, Meyler S, Khoury Z, Lerer T, Brunel P. Cardiovascular safety of transdermal nicotine patches in patients with coronary artery disease who try to quit smoking. *Cardiovasc Drugs Ther.* 1998;12(3):239-244.

148. Zevin S, Jacob P III, Benowitz NL. Dose-related cardiovascular and endocrine effects of transdermal nicotine. *Clin Pharmacol Ther.* 1998;64(1):87-95.

149. Kimmel SE, Berlin JA, Miles C, Jaskowiak J, Carson JL, Strom BL. Risk of acute first myocardial infarction and use of nicotine patches in a general population. *J Am Coll Cardiol.* 2001;37(5):1297-1302.

150. McRobbie H, Hajek P. Nicotine replacement therapy in patients with cardiovascular disease: guidelines for health professionals. *Addiction.* 2001;96(11):1547-1551.

151. Joseph AM, Fu SS. Safety issues in pharmacotherapy for smoking in patients with cardiovascular disease. *Prog Cardiovasc Dis.* 2003;45(6):429-441.

152. Joseph AM, Fu SS. Smoking cessation for patients with cardiovascular disease: what is the best approach? *Am J Cardiovasc Drugs.* 2003;3(5):339-349.

153. Ford C, Zlabek J. Nicotine replacement therapy and cardiovascular disease. *Mayo Clin Proc.* 2005;80(5):652-656.

154. Meine T, Patel M, Washam J, Pappas P, Jollis J. Safety and effectiveness of transdermal nicotine patch in smokers admitted with acute coronary syndromes. *Am J Cardiol.* 2005;95(8):976-978.

155. Hubbard R, Lewis S, Smith C, et al. Use of nicotine replacement therapy and the risk of acute myocardial infarction, stroke, and death. *Tob Control.* 2005;14(6):416-421.

156. Benowitz N, Gourlay S. Cardiovascular toxicity of nicotine: implications for nicotine replacement therapy. *J Am Coll Cardiol.* 1997;29(7):1422-1431.

157. Benowitz NL. Pharmacology of nicotine: addiction, smoking-induced disease, and therapeutics. *Ann Rev Pharmacol Toxicol.* 2009;49:57-71.

158. Henningfield JE, Stapleton JM, Benowitz NL, Grayson RF, London ED. Higher levels of nicotine in arterial than in venous blood after cigarette smoking. *Drug Alcohol Depend.* 1993;33:23-29.

159. Schuurmans MM, Diacon AH, van Biljon X, Bolliger CT. Effect of pre-treatment with nicotine patch on withdrawal symptoms and abstinence rates in smokers subsequently quitting with the nicotine patch: a randomized controlled trial. *Addiction.* 2004;99(5):634-640.

160. Rose JE, Behm FM, Westman EC, Kukovich P. Precessation treatment with nicotine skin patch facilitates smoking cessation. *Nicotine Tob Res.* 2006;8(1):89-101.

161. Wang D, Connock M, Barton P, Fry-Smith A, Aveyard P, Moore D. 'Cut down to quit' with nicotine replacement therapies in smoking cessation: a systematic review of effectiveness and economic analysis. *Health Technol Assess.* 2008;12(2):iii-iv, ix-xi, 1-135.

162. Moore D, Aveyard P, Connock M, Wang D, Fry-Smith A, Barton P. Effectiveness and safety of nicotine replacement therapy assisted reduction to stop smoking: systematic review and meta-analysis. *BMJ.* 2009;338:b1024.

163. Asfar T, Ebbert JO, Klesges RC, Relyea GE. Do smoking reduction interventions promote cessation in smokers not ready to quit? *Addict Behav.* 2011;36(7):764-768.

164. Chan SS, Leung DY, Abdullah AS, Wong VT, Hedley AJ, Lam TH. A randomized controlled trial of a smoking reduction plus nicotine replacement therapy intervention for smokers not willing to quit smoking. *Addiction.* 2011;106(6):1155-1163.

165. Stead LF, Perera R, Bullen C, Mant D, Lancaster T. Nicotine replacement therapy for smoking cessation. *Cochrane Database Syst Rev.* 2008;(1):CD000146.

166. Benowitz NL. Clinical pharmacology of nicotine: implications for understanding, preventing, and treating tobacco addiction. *Clin Pharmacol Ther.* 2008;83(4):531-541.

167. Hurt RD, Sachs DP, Glover ED, et al. A comparison of sustained-release bupropion and placebo for smoking cessation. *N Engl J Med.* 1997;337(17):1195-1202.

168. Jorenby D. Clinical efficacy of bupropion in the management of smoking cessation. *Drugs.* 2002; 62(Suppl 2):25-35.

169. Tonnesen P, Tonstad S, Hjalmarson A, et al. A multicentre, randomized, double-blind, placebo-controlled, 1-year study of bupropion SR for smoking cessation. *J Intern Med.* 2003;254(2):184-192.

170. Swan GE, McAfee T, Curry SJ, et al. Effectiveness of bupropion sustained release for smoking cessation in a health care setting: a randomized trial. *Arch Intern Med.* 2003;163(19):2337-2344.

171. Jorenby DE, Leischow SJ, Nides MA, et al. A controlled trial of sustained-release bupropion, a nicotine patch, or both for smoking cessation. *N Engl J Med.* 1999;340(9):685-691.

172. Ebbert JO, Croghan IT, Sood A, Schroeder DR, Hays JT, Hurt RD. Varenicline and bupropion sustained-release combination therapy for smoking cessation. *Nicotine Tob Res.* 2009;11(3):234-239.

173. Davidson J. Seizures and bupropion: a review. *J Clin Psychiatry.* 1989;50(7):256-261.

174. Hays JT, Ebbert JO. Adverse effects and tolerability of medications for the treatment of tobacco use and dependence. *Drugs.* 2010;70(18):2357-2372.

175. Boshier A, Wilton LV, Shakir SA. Evaluation of the safety of bupropion (Zyban) for smoking cessation from experience gained in general practice use in England in 2000. *Eur J Clin Pharmacol.* 2003;59(10):767-773.

176. Hubbard R, Lewis S, West J, et al. Bupropion and the risk of sudden death: a self-controlled case-series analysis using The Health Improvement Network. *Thorax.* 2005;60(10):848-850.

177. Hughes JR, Stead LF, Lancaster T. Antidepressants for smoking cessation. *Cochrane Database Syst Rev.* 2007;(1):CD000031.

178. Clarke DE, Eaton WW, Petronis KR, Ko JY, Chatterjee A, Anthony JC. Increased risk of suicidal ideation in smokers and former smokers compared to never smokers: evidence from the Baltimore ECA follow-up study. *Suicide Life Threat Behav.* 2010;40(4):307-318.

179. Yaworski D, Robinson J, Sareen J, Bolton JM. The relation between nicotine dependence and suicide attempts in the general population. *Can J Psychiatry.* 2011;56(3):161-170.

180. Oncken C, Gonzales D, Nides M, et al. Efficacy and safety of the novel selective nicotinic acetylcholine receptor partial agonist, varenicline, for smoking cessation. *Arch Intern Med.* 2006;166(15): 1571-1577.

181. Cahill K, Stead LF, Lancaster T. Nicotine receptor partial agonists for smoking cessation. *Cochrane Database Syst Rev.* 2011;(2):CD006103.

182. Tonstad S, Davies S, Flammer M, Russ C, Hughes J. Psychiatric adverse events in randomized, double-blind, placebo-controlled clinical trials of varenicline: a pooled analysis. *Drug Saf.* 2010;33(4): 289-301.

183. Rigotti NA, Pipe AL, Benowitz NL, Arteaga C, Garza D, Tonstad S. Efficacy and safety of vareni-cline for smoking cessation in patients with cardiovascular disease: a randomized trial. *Circulation.* 2010;121(2):221-229.

184. Ebbert JO, Burke MV, Hays JT, Hurt RD. Combination treatment with varenicline and nicotine replacement therapy. *Nicotine Tob Res.* 2009;11(5):572-576.

185. Polosa R, Benowitz NL. Treatment of nicotine addiction: present therapeutic options and pipeline developments. *Trends Pharmacol Sci.* 2011;32(5):281-289.

186. Hughes JR, Stead LF, Lancaster T. Nortriptyline for smoking cessation: a review. *Nicotine Tob Res.* 2005;7(4):491-499.

187. Gourlay SG, Stead LF, Benowitz NL. Clonidine for smoking cessation. *Cochrane Database Syst Rev.* 2004;(3):CD000058.

188. Rollema H, Shrikhande A, Ward KM, et al. Pre-clinical properties of the alpha4beta2 nicotinic acetylcholine receptor partial agonists varenicline, cytisine and dianicline translate to clinical efficacy for nicotine dependence. *Br J Pharmacol.* 2010;160(2):334-345.

189. Cohen C, Kodas E, Griebel G. CB1 receptor antagonists for the treatment of nicotine addiction. *Pharmacol Biochem Behav.* 2005;81(2):387-395.

190. Maurer P, Bachmann MF. Vaccination against nicotine: an emerging therapy for tobacco dependence. *Exp Opin Investig Drugs.* 2007;16(11):1775-1783.

191. Barnes J, Dong CY, McRobbie H, Walker N, Mehta M, Stead LF. Hypnotherapy for smoking cessation. *Cochrane Database Syst Rev.* 2010;(10):CD001008.

192. White AR, Rampes H, Liu JP, Stead LF, Campbell J. Acupuncture and related interventions for smok-ing cessation. *Cochrane Database Syst Rev.* 2011;(1):CD000009.

193. Tran K, Asakawa K, Cimon K, et al. *Pharmacologic-Based Strategies for Smoking Cessation: Clinical and Cost-Effectiveness Analyses.* Ottawa: Canadian Agency for Drugs and Technologies in Health; 2010.

194. Hatsukami DK, Stead LF, Gupta PC. Tobacco addiction. *Lancet.* 2008;371(9629):2027-2038.

Exercise

5

Neville Suskin
Marilyn MacKay-Lyons

TOPICS

This chapter focuses on the rationale and recommendations for the provision of aerobic and resistance exercise training. Physical therapy for individuals with disabling stroke is described in Chapter 18.

RATIONALE

Despite the link between exercise training and improved cardiovascular fitness and health being well established in the general and cardiac populations,[1-3] sedentary behaviors continue to be prevalent.[4]

Beneficial Effects of Exercise to Decrease Stroke Risk

There are a number of biological reasons why exercise might be beneficial in preventing both primary and recurrent stroke. Individuals at risk of stroke or who have experienced a stroke typically have atherosclerotic lesions throughout their vascular system and often manifest coronary artery disease (CAD). Common risk factors for both stroke and CAD include hypertension, dyslipidemia, diabetes, physical inactivity, obesity, excessive alcohol consumption, and tobacco use.[5] Physical activity exerts a beneficial effect on many of these risk factors.[6-11] An aerobic conditioning program can enhance glucose regulation and promote decreases in body weight and fat stores; blood pressure (BP), particularly in hypertensive patients; C-reactive protein; and levels of total blood cholesterol, serum triglycerides, and low-density lipoprotein cholesterol (LDL-C).[12,13] As well, exercise increases high-density lipoprotein cholesterol (HDL-C) and improves blood rheology and coronary artery endothelial function.[12] Physical activity tends to lower blood pressure and weight,[11] enhance vasodilation,[14] improve glucose tolerance[15] and insulin resistance,[16] and promote cardiovascular health.[6]

In a review of existing studies on physical activity and stroke, moderately or highly active persons had a lower risk of stroke incidence or mortality than did persons with a low level of activity.[8] Moderately active men and women had a 20% lower risk, and those who were highly active had a 27% lower risk. Stroke risk can be reduced with regular leisure-time physical activity in individuals of all ages and both sexes.[17] A 10-year cohort study in over 16,000 healthy men demonstrated an inverse association between increasing baseline cardiorespiratory fitness and stroke mortality, with those in the high-fitness groups experiencing a 68% lower risk of stroke and death than those in the lowest-fitness group.[18] Moreover, the inverse association between aerobic fitness and stroke mortality remained after adjustments for cigarette smoking, alcohol consumption, body mass index, hypertension, diabetes mellitus, and family history of CAD.[18] Recently, the beneficial effect of habitual exercise on the relationship of acute moderate- to vigorous-intensity exercise to the onset of acute stroke was also reported.[19] The risk of acute stroke following moderate to vigorous acute exercise was significantly lower in subjects who were previously physically active compared with those who were not (adverse rate ratio 2 vs 6.8).[19]

The above-mentioned benefits of exercise are consistent with the growing body of evidence that interventions (such as exercise training) that promote plaque stability and favorable changes in vascular wall function have important implications for the medical management of patients after a stroke.[14,20]

Multifactorial risk factor intervention[21] and exercise-based cardiac rehabilitation[1] have been shown in randomized trials to improve risk factors and to reduce morbidity and mortality among cardiovascular patients by 20% to 30%. The Ontario Cardiac Rehabilitation Pilot Project demonstrated the real-world clinical effectiveness of cardiac rehabilitation in which cardiac rehabilitation resulted in 65% more patients categorized at low (<1%) annual risk of death or major cardiac event (including hospital readmission) by cardiac rehabilitation program exit compared to entry. The report also noted that the direct costs for outcomes demonstrated in the Cardiac Rehabilitation Pilot were low compared to other cardiac interventions and to costs for a cardiac-related admission.[22,23]

Interestingly, our own work in patients with CAD has demonstrated that significant improvements in exercise capacity were not associated with improved glucometabolic profile as measured by insulin sensitivity in the absence of weight loss.[24] This finding would suggest that some insulin-sensitizing benefits of physical activity may be mediated via weight loss.

Although there is a paucity of literature pertaining to the effects of exercise training in patients post–transient ischemic attack (TIA), there is emerging evidence of the beneficial effect of exercise training in patients following established stroke resulting in functional capacity that may be comparable to that of age-matched, healthy controls.[25] In a randomized controlled trial (RCT) of 42 hemiparetic stroke survivors, vigorous aerobic exercise training three times per week for 10 weeks resulted in significant improvements in peak oxygen consumption and sensorimotor function; moreover, the latter was significantly related to improvement in aerobic capacity.[26] An RCT of a six-month home exercise training program in 88 men with CAD and disability (two-thirds were stroke survivors) demonstrated significant increases in HDL-C and decreases in total cholesterol (TC) with exercise training.[27]

Neurological deficits following stroke have, not surprisingly, been linked to physical deconditioning.[25] Aerobic exercise and strength training have been recommended by several authors to improve cardiovascular fitness after stroke.[25,28,29] Potential benefits of structured programs of therapeutic exercise following stroke include improved mobility, balance, and endurance.[28] However, although studies have shown that structured exercise programs are not harmful after stroke, there is a lack of appropriately controlled study evidence to support the causality of therapeutic exercise on the reduction of incidence of subsequent stroke.[30] Nevertheless, following stroke, health care provider advice to increase physical activity appears to be effective as a larger percentage of stroke survivors who had received advice to exercise reported actually doing so (76% vs 39%) than stroke survivors who did not receive such advice, and stroke survivors who reported engaging in more exercise had fewer limited activity days than those who did not report exercising after stroke.[31] As well, patients who had sustained a completed stroke 1 to 12 years earlier showed improved risk factors and psychological status after a 10-week exercise program.[32] Moreover, these authors have proposed a randomized trial of 10-week cardiac rehabilitation with stable subjects poststroke, or at least three months post-TIA.[33]

Preliminary support for a multifaceted approach to secondary stroke prevention comes from a modeling study in which the authors concluded that up to 80% of recurrent vascular events in patients with cerebrovascular disease might be prevented by multifactorial risk reduction interventions.[34] A nonrandomized study of a three-month exercise program for patients within six months of a TIA demonstrated improvements in walking endurance and exercise capacity.[35]

Thus, although acknowledging that additional validation by RCTs is required, the American Heart Association has recommended that stroke survivors participate in regular physical activity or exercise training programs (Table 5–1).[25] Supporting this recommendation are the results from a small RCT in patients one year or greater post completed stroke where a limited Cardiac Rehabilitation (CR) program consisting of 10 weeks (16 sessions) of cycle ergometer intervention resulted in a 20% improvement of exercise capacity versus controls.[32]

Consequently, we provide general recommendations concerning structured exercise programming to prevent stroke recurrence based on the recommendations for aerobic training following stroke or TIA. These recommendations are based on recent national consensus processes,[30] and the intervention strategies from two in-progress RCTs specifically evaluating the impact of structured exercise programming on important risk factors related to stroke recurrence following TIA or minor nondisabling led by Mackay-Lyons[29] and Suskin (Cardiac Rehabilitation for TIA Patients, www.ClinTrials.gov, accessed January 5, 2011).

Table 5–1. Physical Activity Counseling and Exercise Training—CR TIA Exercise Programming Strategy

Mode of Exercise	Major Goals	Intensity/Frequency/Duration[a]
Aerobic • Large-muscle activities (eg, walking, treadmill, stationary cycle, combined arm-leg ergometry, arm ergometry, seated stepper)	• Increase independence in ADLs • Increase walking speed/ efficiency • Improve tolerance for prolonged physical activity • Reduce risk of cardiovascular disease	• 60%-70% heart rate reserve or, 50%-80% maximal heart rate or, RPE 11-14 (6-20 scale) • 3-7 d/wk • 20-60 min/session (or multiple 10-min sessions)
Strength • Circuit training • Weight machines • Free weights • Isometric exercise	• Increase independence in ADLs	• 1-3 sets of 10-15 repetitions of 8-10 exercises involving the major muscle groups • 2-3 d/wk
Flexibility • Stretching	• Increase ROM of involved extremities	• 2-3 d/wk (before or after aerobic or strength training) • Hold each stretch for 10-30 s
Neuromuscular • Coordination and balance activities	• Improve level of safety during ADLs	• 2-3 d/wk (consider performing on same day as strength activities)

ADLs, activities of daily living; ROM, range of motion; RPE, rating of perceived exertion.

[a]Recommended intensity, frequency, and duration of exercise depend on each individual patient's level of fitness. Intermittent training sessions may be indicated during the initial weeks of rehabilitation. *From Potempa K, Lopez M, Braun LT, Szidon JP, Fogg L, Tincknell T. Physiological outcomes of aerobic exercise training in hemiparetic stroke patients. Stroke. 1995;26:101-105.*

THE PRE-EXERCISE EVALUATION

All stable patients without contraindications for exercise training should be screened for participation in exercise training following stroke or TIA.

Exercise can be undertaken safely by stroke survivors as long as the exercise prescription has been formulated to minimize the potential adverse effects of exercise via appropriate screening, program design, and patient education.[25] The major potential health hazards of exercise for stroke survivors are musculoskeletal injury and sudden cardiac death. It has therefore been recommended that all stroke survivors undergo a complete medical assessment to identify medical conditions that require special consideration or constitute a contraindication to exercise.[25]

In general, the following are considered absolute contraindications to exercise testing and training[25,36]:

- Acute myocardial infarction (within two days) or unstable angina
- Uncontrolled cardiac arrhythmias causing symptoms or hemodynamic compromise
- Symptomatic severe aortic stenosis
- Uncontrolled symptomatic heart failure
- Acute pulmonary embolus or pulmonary infarction
- Acute myocarditis or pericarditis
- Acute aortic dissection

Although the likelihood of experiencing a fatal cardiac event during exercise training is extremely small,[37] it is usually associated with the presence of CAD. Because up to 75% of stroke victims have coexisting cardiac disease,[38] it is recommended that stroke patients undergo electrocardiogram (ECG)-monitored graded exercise testing as part of a medical evaluation before beginning an exercise program.[39] Generally, graded exercise testing in stroke patients should be conducted in accordance with contemporary guidelines, as detailed elsewhere.[36,40] Briefly, the exercise test protocol for the stroke survivor should assess functional capacity and the cardiovascular response to exercise. The graded exercise test should include continuous 12-lead ECG monitoring and recordings at rest prior to exercise, every minute during exercise, at peak exercise, and at 1-minute intervals for 6 minutes during recovery. Symptoms of chest pain, leg fatigue, and dyspnea should be quantified using an appropriate scale, such as the 6-20 Borg Scale.[36,41] The stress test should be terminated according to usual indications,[36] with modified blood pressure indications[25] given stroke history, as follows: when the subject cannot continue due to symptoms (such as fatigue, dyspnea, or chest pain) or if it is deemed medically necessary due to any of the following clinical findings:

- Greater than 2 mm of horizontal or downsloping ST segment depression
- Persistent 10 mm Hg or greater decline in systolic blood pressure
- A hypertensive (SBP >250 mm Hg, DBP >115 mm Hg) blood pressure response
- The development of significant arrhythmias

The testing mode should be selected or adapted to the needs of the stroke survivor. Often, a standard treadmill walking protocol can be used (with the aid of handrails) such as the Bruce protocol (or a modified version). If required, special protocols are available for stroke survivors, especially those with hemiplegia or paresis.[27] Many testing protocols use arm cycle ergometry with the subject seated to optimize the load.[27] Thus, if flexibility and adaptability are used in the selection of testing protocols, most stroke survivors who are deemed stable for physical activity can undergo exercise testing.[25]

Exercise testing is safe, with less than one potentially life-threatening complication such as myocardial infarction or arrhythmia occurring per 1000 to 10,000 tests.[42,43]

Although studies have reported that patients can be screened for and have exercise training implemented safely within 24 to 48 hours following acute stroke,[44,45] it has been recommended that usual cardiac stress testing strategies can be deployed as soon as 3 weeks after the stroke or TIA.[25]

If an exercise ECG is not performed, lighter-intensity exercise should be prescribed. The reduced exercise intensity may be compensated for by increasing the training frequency, duration, or both.[25]

EXERCISE PROGRAMMING

In general, the latest[30] guidelines from the American Stroke Association for the prevention of recurrent stroke following stroke or TIA are endorsed:

- For patients with ischemic stroke or TIA who are capable of engaging in physical activity, at least 30 minutes of moderate-intensity physical exercise, typically defined as vigorous activity sufficient to break a sweat or noticeably raise heart rate, one to three times a week (eg, walking briskly, using an exercise bicycle) may be considered to reduce the risk factors and comorbid conditions that increase the likelihood of recurrent stroke.
- For those individuals with a disability after ischemic stroke, supervision by a health care professional, such as a physical therapist or cardiac rehabilitation professional, at least on initiation of an exercise regimen, may be considered.

For more specific exercise programming guidance we recommend following a modified version of the 2004[25] American Heart Association Scientific Statement for physical activity and exercise recommendations for stroke survivors:

- Twice-per-week supervised exercise training and twice-per-week supplementary home-based training at an individualized but progressive prescription (Table 5–1).
- In general, exercise training should be aerobic at an intensity of 60% to 70% heart rate reserve, or rate of perceived exertion of 11 to 14 (Borg), five to seven d/wk, at 20 to 60 min/session (or multiple 10-minute sessions).[25,41]

REFERENCES

1. Taylor RS, Brown A, Ebrahim S, et al. Exercise-based rehabilitation for patients with coronary heart disease: systematic review and meta-analysis of randomized controlled trials. *Am J Med.* 2004;116(10):682-692. Available from: http://www.sciencedirect.com/science/article/B6TDC-4CB08F3-6/2/b95aae08edb7-f5e7f2ad50ff6b25198d.

2. Stone JA, Arthur HM; Canadian Association of Cardiac Rehabilitation Guidelines Writing Group. Canadian guidelines for cardiac rehabilitation and cardiovascular disease prevention, second edition, 2004: executive summary. *Can J Cardiol.* 2005;21 Suppl D(0828-282):3D-19D.

3. Leon AS, Franklin BA, Costa F, et al. Cardiac rehabilitation and secondary prevention of coronary heart disease: an American Heart Association scientific statement from the Council on Clinical Cardiology (Subcommittee on Exercise, Cardiac Rehabilitation, and Prevention) and the Council on Nutrition, Physical Activity, and Metabolism (Subcommittee on Physical Activity), in collaboration with the American Association of Cardiovascular and Pulmonary Rehabilitation. *Circulation.* 2005;111(3): 369-376. Available from: http://circ.ahajournals.org/cgi/content/abstract/111/3/369.

4. Katzmarzyk PT, Gledhill N, Shephard RJ. The economic burden of physical inactivity in Canada. *CMAJ.* 2000;163(11):1435-1440. Available from: http://www.cmaj.ca/cgi/content/abstract/163/11/1435.

5. Wolf PA, Clagett GP, Easton JD, et al. Preventing ischemic stroke in patients with prior stroke and transient ischemic attack: a statement for healthcare professionals from the Stroke Council of the American Heart Association. *Stroke.* 1999;30:1991-1994.

6. Williams MA, Fleg JL, Ades PA, et al. Secondary prevention of coronary heart disease in the elderly (with emphasis on patients >=75 years of age): an American Heart Association scientific statement from the Council on Clinical Cardiology Subcommittee on Exercise, Cardiac Rehabilitation, and Prevention. *Circulation.* 2002;105(14):1735-1743. Available from: http://circ.ahajournals.org.

7. Hu FB, Stampfer MJ, Colditz GA, et al. Physical activity and risk of stroke in women. *JAMA.* 2000;283(22):2961-2967. Available from: http://jama.ama-assn.org/cgi/content/abstract/283/22/2961.

8. Lee CD, Folsom AR, Blair SN. Physical activity and stroke risk: a meta-analysis. *Stroke.* 2003;34(10):2475-2481. Available from: http://stroke.ahajournals.org/cgi/content/abstract/34/10/2475.

9. Lee IM, Hennekens CH, Berger K, Buring JE, Manson JE. Exercise and risk of stroke in male physicians. *Stroke.* 1999;30(1):1-6. Available from: http://stroke.ahajournals.org/cgi/content/abstract/30/1/1.

10. Pearson TA, Blair SN, Daniels SR, et al. AHA guidelines for primary prevention of cardiovascular disease and stroke: 2002 update: consensus panel guide to comprehensive risk reduction for adult patients without coronary or other atherosclerotic vascular diseases. *Circulation.* 2002;106:388-391.

11. Thompson PD, Buchner D, Pina IL, et al. AHA scientific statement. Exercise and physical activity in the prevention and treatment of atherosclerotic cardiovascular disease. A statement from the Council on Clinical Cardiology (Subcommittee on Exercise, Rehabilitation, and Prevention) and the Council on Nutrition, Physical Activity, and Metabolism (Subcommittee on Physical Activity). *Circulation.* 2003;107:3109.

12. Hambrecht R, Wolf A, Gielen S, et al. Effect of exercise on coronary endothelial function in patients with coronary artery disease. *N Engl J Med.* 2000;342(7):454-460.

13. Paffenbarger RS, Hyde RT, Wing AL, Hsieh CC. Physical activity, all-cause mortality, and longevity of college alumni. *N Engl J Med.* 1986;314(10):605-613. Available from: http://content.nejm.org/cgi/content/abstract/314/10/605.

14. Endres M, Gertz K, Lindauer U, et al. Mechanisms of stroke protection by physical activity. *Ann Neurol.* 2003;54(5):582-590.

15. Dylewicz P, Bienkowska S, Szczesniak L, et al. Beneficial effect of short-term endurance training on glucose metabolism during rehabilitation after coronary bypass surgery. *Chest.* 2000;117(1):47-51.

16. Dylewicz P, Przywarska I, Szcześniak L, Rychlewski T, Bieńkowska S, Długiewicz I, Wilk M. The influence of short-term endurance training on the insulin bloodlevel, binding, and degradation of 125I-insulin by erythrocyte receptors in patients after myocardial infarction. *J Cardiopulm Rehabil.* 1999;19(2):98-105.

17. Sacco RL, Gan R, Boden-Albala B, et al. Leisure-time physical activity and ischemic stroke risk: the Northern Manhattan Stroke Study. *Stroke.* 1998;29(2):380-387.

18. Lee CD, Blair SN. Cardiorespiratory fitness and stroke mortality in men. *Med Sci Sports Exerc.* 2002;34:592-595.

19. Mostofsky E, Laier E, Levitan EB, Rosamond WD, Schlaug G, Mittleman MA. Physical activity and onset of acute ischemic stroke. *Am J Epidemiol.* 2011;173(3):330-336.

20. Franklin BA, Kahn JK. Delayed progression or regression of coronary atherosclerosis with intensive risk factor modification. Effects of diet, drugs, and exercise. *Sports Med.* 1996;22(5):306-320.

21. Haskell WL, Alderman EL, Fair JM, et al. Effects of intensive multiple risk factor reduction on coronary atherosclerosis and clinical cardiac events in men and women with coronary artery disease. The Stanford Coronary Risk Intervention Project (SCRIP). *Circulation.* 1994;89(3):975-990.

22. Suskin N, Arthur HM, Swabey T, Ross J. The Ontario Cardiac Rehabilitation Pilot Project—report and recommendations. Cardiac Care Network of Ontario; 2002.

23. Arthur HM, Swabey T, Suskin N, Ross J. The Ontario Cardiac Rehabilitation Pilot Project: recommendations for health planning and policy. *Can J Cardiol.* 2004;20(12):1251-1255.

24. Suskin NG, Heigenhauser G, Afzal R, Finegood D, Gerstein HC, McKelvie RS. The effects of exercise training on insulin resistance in patients with coronary artery disease. *Eur J Cardiovasc Prev Rehabil.* 2007;14(6):803-808.

25. Gordon NF, Gulanick M, Costa F, et al. Physical activity and exercise recommendations for stroke survivors: an American Heart Association scientific statement from the Council on Clinical Cardiology,

Subcommittee on Exercise, Cardiac Rehabilitation, and Prevention; the Council on Cardiovascular Nursing; the Council on Nutrition, Physical Activity, and Metabolism; and the Stroke Council. *Circulation.* 2004;109(16):2031-2041. Available from: http://circ.ahajournals.org.

26. Potempa K, Lopez M, Braun LT, Szidon JP, Fogg L, Tincknell T. Physiological outcomes of aerobic exercise training in hemiparetic stroke patients. *Stroke.* 1995;26(1):101-105.

27. Fletcher BJ, Dunbar SB, Felner JM, et al. Exercise testing and training in physically disabled men with clinical evidence of coronary artery disease. *Am J Cardiol.* 1994;73(2):170-174.

28. Duncan P, Studenski S, Richards L, et al. Randomized clinical trial of therapeutic exercise in subacute stroke. *Stroke.* 2003;34(9):2173-2180. Available from: http://stroke.ahajournals.org/cgi/content/abstract/34/9/2173.

29. Mackay-Lyons M, Gubitz G, Giacomantonio N, et al. Program of rehabilitative exercise and education to avert vascular events after non-disabling stroke or transient ischemic attack (PREVENT trial): a multi-centred, randomised controlled trial. *BMC Neurol.* 2010;10:122.

30. Furie KL, Kasner SE, Adams RJ, et al. Guidelines for the prevention of stroke in patients with stroke or transient ischemic attack: a guideline for healthcare professionals from the American Heart Association/American Stroke Association. *Stroke.* 2011;42(1):227-276. Available from: http://stroke.ahajournals.org/cgi/content/abstract/42/1/227.

31. Greenlund KJ, Giles WH, Keenan NL, Croft JB, Mensah GA. Physician advice, patient actions, and health-related quality of life in secondary prevention of stroke through diet and exercise. *Stroke.* 2002;33(2):565-570.

32. Lennon O, Carey A, Gaffney N, Stephenson J, Blake C. A pilot randomized controlled trial to evaluate the benefit of the cardiac rehabilitation paradigm for the non-acute ischaemic stroke population. *Clin Rehabil.* 2008;22(2):125-133.

33. Lennon O, Blake C. Cardiac rehabilitation adapted to transient ischaemic attack and stroke (CRAFTS): a randomised controlled trial. *BMC Neurol.* 2009;9(1):9. Available from: http://www.biomedcentral.com/1471-2377/9/9.

34. Hackam DG, Spence JD. Combining multiple approaches for the secondary prevention of vascular events after stroke: a quantitative modeling study. *Stroke.* 2007;38(6):1881-1885.

35. Tanne D, Tsabari R, Chechik O, et al. Improved exercise capacity in patients after minor ischemic stroke undergoing a supervised exercise training program. *Isr Med Assoc J.* 2008;10(2):113-116.

36. Gibbons RJ, Balady GJ, Bricker JT, et al. ACC/AHA 2002 guideline update for exercise testing: summary article. A report of the American College of Cardiology/American Heart Association Task Force on Practice Guidelines (Committee to Update the 1997 Exercise Testing Guidelines). *J Am Coll Cardiol.* 2002;40(8):1531-1540.

37. In collaboration with the American College of Sports Medicine, Thompson PD, Franklin BA, et al. Exercise and acute cardiovascular events: placing the risks into perspective: a scientific statement from the American Heart Association Council on Nutrition, Physical Activity, and Metabolism and the Council on Clinical Cardiology. *Circulation.* 2007;115(17):2358-2368. Available from: http://circ.ahajournals.org/cgi/content/abstract/115/17/2358.

38. Adams HP Jr, Adams RJ, Brott T, et al. Guidelines for the early management of patients with ischemic stroke: a scientific statement from the Stroke Council of the American Stroke Association. *Stroke.* 2003;34(4):1056-1083.

39. Balady GJ, Williams MA, Ades PA, et al. Core components of cardiac rehabilitation/secondary prevention programs: 2007 update: a scientific statement from the American Heart Association Exercise, Cardiac Rehabilitation, and Prevention Committee, the Council on Clinical Cardiology; the Councils on Cardiovascular Nursing, Epidemiology and Prevention, and Nutrition, Physical Activity, and Metabolism; and the American Association of Cardiovascular and Pulmonary Rehabilitation. *Circulation.* 2007;115(20):2675-2682. Available from: http://circ.ahajournals.org/cgi/content/abstract/115/20/2675.

40. American College of Sports Medicine. *Guidelines for Exercise Testing and Prescription.* 6th ed. Philadelphia: Lippincott Williams & Wilkins; 2000.

41. Borg GAV. Psychophysical basis of perceived exertion. *Med Sci Sports Exerc.* 1982(14):377-381.

42. Keteyian SJ, Isaac D, Thadani U, et al. Safety of symptom-limited cardiopulmonary exercise testing in patients with chronic heart failure due to severe left ventricular systolic dysfunction. *Am Heart J.* 2009;158(4):S72-S77.

43. Gordon N, Kohl HW. Exercise testing and sudden cardiac death. *J Cardiopulm Rehabil.* 1993; 13(6):381-6.

44. Bernhardt J, Dewey H, Thrift A, Collier J, Donnan G. A very early rehabilitation trial for stroke (AVERT): phase II safety and feasibility. *Stroke.* 2008;39(2):390-396. Available from: http://stroke. ahajournals.org/cgi/content/abstract/39/2/390.

45. Katz-Leurer M, Carmeli E, Shochina M. The effect of early aerobic training on independence six months post stroke. *Clin Rehabil.* 2003;17(7):735-741. Available from: http://cre.sagepub.com/ content/17/7/735.abstract.

Hypertension

J. David Spence
Ross Feldman

6

TOPICS

INTRODUCTION

After smoking cessation and diet, blood pressure control is probably the next most important intervention for stroke prevention.[1] Among patients on treatment for hypertension, more than 90% of strokes occur in those whose blood pressure is not controlled.[2] Collins et al[3] estimated that if blood pressure were controlled, 40% of strokes could be prevented, compared with only 20% of myocardial infarctions. The difference between those estimates is instructive; the difference between stroke and myocardial infarction is that virtually all myocardial infarctions are due to atherosclerosis, whereas there are many causes of stroke.[4] Hypertension is only indirectly related to atherosclerosis,[5] but it directly causes hypertensive small vessel disease, leading to lacunar infarction or intracerebral hemorrhage.[6]

The potential for stroke prevention by blood pressure control was illustrated by an experiment of nature in London, Canada, in the late 1970s. We obtained our first computed tomography (CT) scanner at Victoria Hospital in 1976, so by 1977, the year in which our hypertension clinic was established, it was possible to clearly distinguish hypertensive intracerebral hemorrhage and lacunar infarction from other causes of stroke. In 1978, the Department of Family Medicine at our university mounted a large study to increase detection and treatment of hypertension.[7]

They were able to refer patients with uncontrolled hypertension to our clinic for control, using the principles described below. By 1983, a population survey in the area showed that 94% of hypertensives were detected, 92% were on treatment, and 72% were controlled to levels below 140/90 mm Hg.[8] This remarkable result was thought to be due in large part to the Hawthorne effect (measurement of performance improves performance). What this achieved with regard to stroke prevention was even more than predicted: strokes were reduced by half between 1978 and 1984.[9] The strokes that were prevented were those due to hypertensive small vessel disease; strokes from large artery disease remained unchanged. Hypertensive strokes occur at the base of the brain, in a vascular territory that Hachinski called the "vascular centrencephalon." There, short arteries with few branches transmit pressure right through from large arteries to small resistance vessels; the cortex is perfused by long arteries with many branches that act like step-down transformers. Hemorrhages in the cortex and subcortical regions are due to causes other than hypertension, such as amyloid angiopathy, mycotic aneurysm, and vascular malformations.

Blood pressure control is a major missed opportunity. In most countries, less than a quarter of hypertensives are controlled to target levels, and although surveys now suggest better control among respondents,[10] practice-based surveys (which are free of selection bias) reveal[11] that fewer than 20% of patients are well controlled.

ACHIEVING CONTROL OF BLOOD PRESSURE

Although blood pressure can be controlled readily in most patients, there are many barriers to control that require attention. Hypertension must first be detected; many "healthy" young people do not attend physicians on a regular basis, and even when they do, for minor problems such as a sprained ankle, the blood pressure may not be checked. If a blood pressure elevation is detected, it might be attributed either by the patient or the physician to the "white coat" effect (usually a mistake[12]) and neglected. Even if treatment is initiated, many patients do not respond adequately. There are three main categories of reasons for resistant hypertension (Table 6–1): noncompliance, consumption of substances that aggravate hypertension, and a missed cause of secondary hypertension.

RESISTANT HYPERTENSION

Noncompliance

Noncompliance is common and difficult to deal with. About half of patients will admit they are not taking their medication.[13] Pharmacies can report the purchase record, and blood levels of some drugs can be measured. In some cases, however, noncompliance can be very difficult to detect. Among patients that JDS has had to admit to the hospital for control of resistant hypertension that could not be controlled on an outpatient basis, even using the approaches described below, noncompliance has explained most cases that were not due to causes such as

Table 6–1. Causes of Resistant Hypertension

1. Noncompliance Cost of medication Adverse drug effects Health beliefs About half of patients will admit noncompliance when asked in a nonjudgmental way[13]
2. Consumption of substances that aggravate hypertension Salt Licorice Oral contraceptives Decongestants Alcohol Nonsteroidal anti-inflammatory drugs (except sulindac[20])
3. Secondary hypertension Pheochromocytoma Primary aldosteronism[a] (usually due to bilateral adrenocortical hyperplasia) Renovascular hypertension Renal tumor Liddle syndrome and variants[a] Kuchel/Page syndrome (pseudopheochromocytoma)

[a]More common in people of African origin.

pheochromocytoma, primary aldosteronism, or severe renovascular hypertension. However, actual observation of the swallowing of pills, and observation for self-induced vomiting, or consumption of vasopressor agents may be necessary in cases of Munchausen syndrome.

Reasons for noncompliance include cost of medication, therapeutic burden (number of pills, number of doses per day), adverse drug effects, and health beliefs. Some of these problems can be dealt with by using combination drugs, using split tablets of high doses of drugs, providing drug samples to indigent patients, and by using simplified regimens. Feldman et al[14] showed that a simplified regimen in which all patients received a combination of diuretic and angiotensin receptor antagonist improved control rates from 50% to 65% (the high rate in the control group was attributable to the Hawthorne effect). Long-term persistence with medication is better with drugs that have fewer adverse effects, such as angiotensin receptor antagonists.[15] A particularly difficult problem is fallacious attribution of symptoms to drugs.[16] This problem, and approaches to minimizing the adverse effects of cardiovascular drugs, is discussed in Chapter 15.

CONSUMPTION OF SUBSTANCES THAT AGGRAVATE HYPERTENSION

Patients with resistant hypertension should be questioned carefully about their consumption of sodium, licorice, alcohol, decongestants, oral contraceptives, and nonsteroidal anti-inflammatory drugs. Reduction of such substances is an important part of blood pressure management.[17] The body only requires approximately half a gram of salt (sodium chloride) per day. The average North American eats much more; people who salt their food before tasting are averaging 10 g per day or more; those who salt their food after tasting are consuming 5 g per day or more. A daily intake of 2 to 3 g per day of salt (or less) should be the target for hypertensive patients, and this can be difficult to achieve without careful attention to salt added in the manufacture of prepared foods. Salty foods such as pickles (a gram in a normal-sized dill pickle), canned soup (a gram in a serving of soup), potato chips (crisps), popcorn, salami, etc, are obvious sources. However, many packaged foods have surprisingly high quantities of added salt; this is currently the subject of regulatory efforts in many countries. Joffres et al have estimated that an effective population-based approach to reducing sodium intake could reduce the prevalence of hypertension by 30%, doubling control rates.[18] The Dietary Approaches to Stop Hypertension (DASH) diet study[19] showed that a low-sodium diet high in fruits and vegetables lowers blood pressure; however, a low-sodium version of the Cretan Mediterranean diet is preferred for reasons explained in Chapter 3.

Alcohol aggravates hypertension in some patients; this may be related to catecholamine release, and may be more common in patients with low-renin hypertension. The recommended upper limit of alcohol intake is 14 standard drinks per week for men, and nine for women.[17] (Patients should be reminded of the definition of a standard drink; two generous doubles would be equivalent to four to six standard drinks, depending on how generous.) Many over-the-counter cold remedies and nasal sprays contain sympathomimetics that can aggravate hypertension. Rebound nasal congestion on stopping decongestant nasal sprays can be difficult; steroid nose sprays such as beclomethasone may be somewhat helpful with this problem. The only nonsteroidal anti-inflammatory drug that does not aggravate hypertension is sulindac.[20]

SECONDARY HYPERTENSION

Patients with resistant hypertension should be investigated for underlying causes that require specific treatment. Guidelines that assume that all patients are the same can be likened to a camel, that is, a horse designed by a committee. Even the best guidelines only mention in fine print the measurement of plasma renin and aldosterone, which are key tools in the management of resistant hypertension, as discussed below.

Pheochromocytoma

Perhaps the most important cause of secondary hypertension is pheochromocytoma, because it is fatal if missed, is curable with surgery, and is a fine teacher of pharmacology. Although it is important to ask about symptoms such as episodes of shaking, sweating, and pounding in the head and chest, it must be remembered that about half of patients with pheochromocytoma do not have such symptoms. The episodic nature of blood pressure elevation is not due to fluctuation in the production of catecholamine by the tumor(s), which after all are autonomous, and make catechols as fast as they can. Attacks of hypertension, shaking, pallor, and sweating are due to the release of catecholamines from millions of sympathetic boutons throughout the body, during episodic sympathetic discharge. About 80% of norepinephrine in the body is stored in these boutons, and after a discharge about 80% is taken back up into the boutons. A consequence of this is that it takes a week after removal of a pheo for plasma catecholamines to return to normal. Suppression of sympathetic discharge by a deep general anesthetic during surgery is followed by return of sympathetic function postoperatively; patients in the recovery room should be watched for surges of blood pressure after the removal of the tumor; this may be heralded by piloerection and commonly occurs during shivering.

Another consequence of this physiology is that episodes of severe hypertension may be triggered by an exaggerated baroreceptor reflex response to drugs that abruptly lower blood pressure. Vasodilation from histamine release during administration of radiographic contrast material is one example.

Treatment of hypertension in patients with pheo requires blockade of α-adrenergic receptors; β-blockers given alone can actually raise blood pressure because of unopposed blockade of β_2 receptors. Because very high levels of norepinephrine in the presynaptic space of boutons cannot be blocked adequately by doses of competitive α antagonists such as doxazosin, alpha blockade would best be done with the noncompetitive antagonist phenoxybenzamine,[21] but it can be difficult to obtain. Patients with pheo may be volume depleted because of long-standing vasoconstriction; they may require preoperative rehydration during intensive alpha blockade to minimize the risk of severe hypotension during or after surgery. As a principle of management, it is best to operate on the known abdominal pheochromocytoma via a laparotomy so that the abdomen can be explored for additional pheos—about 20% are bilateral and 10% are extra-adrenal. Meta-iodobenzylguanidine (MIBG) scans are probably the best way to detect pheos that are not in the adrenal glands, in particular those that are in locations such as the bladder, chest, neck, or head.

Pseudopheochromocytoma

As mentioned above, not all patients with pheochromocytoma present with classical symptoms; the other side of that coin is that not all patients with suggestive symptoms turn out to have a pheo. Some will turn out to have adrenomedullary hyperplasia, a precursor of pheo requiring surveillance lest they develop one. Conditions that can mimic a pheo include hypoglycemia, epilepsy (seizures from the insula, or deep seizures affecting the hypothalamus), strokes affecting the medulla or hypothalamus, neck surgery affecting the carotid baroreceptors, electroconvulsive therapy, and bladder stimulation in quadriplegia.[21]

In addition, there remains a poorly defined subset of patients who present with pheochromocytoma-like symptoms without any evidence of tumor being detectable either biochemically or radiologically. These patients represent a heterogeneous group, including patients with surreptitious intake of sympathomimetic drugs, panic attacks, and hypertension and those who demonstrate a syndrome of paroxysmal rises in blood pressure related to sympathetic nervous system hyper-activation. Some of these have Page syndrome, a term first coined by Kuchel and colleagues. This is seen in patients, mostly women, with primary hypertension and hypertensive episodes that mimic pheochromocytoma, excepting that the patients are more likely to be plethoric (instead of pale) and often have associated nausea and epigastric discomfort.[22] Patients with Page syndrome often present with stereotypical episodes often triggered by minor emotional upsets. It was suggested that biochemically these patients could be diagnosed by surges in conjugated dopamine levels in the course of their hyperadrenergic episodes.[23] However, these findings are not universal, and the sensitivity and/or specificity of this biochemical index were never validated. More recently it was suggested that the hyperadrenergic symptoms and signs in these patients were related to normal sympathetic noradrenergic outflow, adrenomedullary activation, and augmented blood pressure responses to changes in the sympathoneural release of norepinephrine.[24]

Management of these patients has typically relied on autonomic blockade strategies, including α_1-adrenergic antagonists, α_2-adrenergic agonists, and β-adrenergic antagonists. Notably, we have observed that this pattern is aggravated by even marginal decreases in fluid volume. Consequently, in some patients volume repletion is often the first (although counterintuitive) step in the management of abrupt elevations in blood pressure.

RENOVASCULAR HYPERTENSION

Renovascular hypertension is more common in patients with stroke, for at least two reasons: it is an important cause of uncontrolled hypertension leading to strokes from hypertensive small vessel disease, and it is more common in patients with carotid stenosis because such patients are severe arteriopaths and are more likely to also have renal artery stenosis. JDS reported that among patients with carotid stenosis followed in the ACAS and NASCET trials, 25% of those with resistant hypertension had renovascular hypertension.[25] Renal artery stenosis is also very common in patients with heart failure; as many as 34% of elderly patients with congestive heart failure (CHF) may have significant renal artery stenosis,[26] and this may aggravate the heart failure because of secondary hyperaldosteronism, as discussed below.

With severe stenosis of a renal artery, reduced pressure and perfusion distal to the stenosis causes the kidney to defend itself by making more and more renin and angiotensin; that kidney demands perfusion, never mind the cost to the rest of the body. JDS has called this the "renal barostat": the kidney simply takes charge of the blood pressure; each time a medication is added, the pressure falls transiently, and then returns to the same high set point required for that kidney to maintain perfusion.

Notwithstanding clinical trials that show limited benefit to revascularization, in some cases the blood pressure will only be controlled by restoring blood flow to the ischemic kidney.[27] Occasionally, nephrectomy of a kidney with very little perfusion, but high production of renin (which can be measured from the renal vein), may be necessary. A likely reason why clinical trials have not shown much benefit is that some or many of the cases randomized probably had incidental renal artery stenosis, rather than renovascular hypertension. Another reason was intention-to-treat analyses that included in the medical arm a high proportion of patients who crossed over to revascularization. Some patients with true renovascular hypertension, perhaps 10% or so, require intervention, either with angioplasty and stenting, or with renal artery bypass. The risk of angiography includes not only the effect of radiographic dye, but also the risk of embolization into the kidneys of atheromatous debris from the aorta. Renal bypass (hepatorenal on the right, splenorenal on the left, or autotransplantation lower in the abdomen with an anastomosis onto an iliac artery) is probably a better procedure than reimplanting a stenosed renal artery back into a severely atherosclerotic aorta; the aortic clamping itself is hazardous, and it can be difficult to find a segment of the abdominal aorta that is not severely diseased. In most cases, therefore, medical management is preferable if pressures can be controlled.

There is a mistaken tendency to avoid the very medications that will be most effective for renovascular hypertension, out of misplaced fear of precipitating renal failure. To be sure, in patients with severe bilateral renal artery stenosis or occlusion of one renal artery with severe stenosis of the other, addition of a drug that blocks the renin/angiotensin/aldosterone system (RAAS) may precipitate an acute illness, with a severe drop in blood pressure and acute renal failure. However, this event is transient and reversible in virtually all cases, and it is rare: in 30 years of seeing many patients with resistant hypertension, JDS has seen this problem fewer than 20 times. The mechanism has been called "kicking the back door out of the glomerulus"—the high resistance in the efferent arteriole of the glomerulus that maintains glomerular filtration in the face of low pressure in the afferent arteriole is lost, and filtration screeches to a halt (Figure 6–1).[28]

Because of this defense mechanism, the medications that are most effective in controlling blood pressure in renovascular hypertension are drugs that block the RAAS. Controlling blood pressure will help preserve renal function in the contralateral kidney, so in the long term, even if there is a transient mild drop in glomerular filtration rate (GFR), most patients with renovascular hypertension will do better with these drugs. Revascularization may be necessary if renal function is impaired too greatly by this approach.

Aortic coarctation can be thought of physiologically as a form of renovascular hypertension, aggravated by increased resistance in the upper part of the vasculature.[28]

PRIMARY ALDOSTERONISM

Primary aldosteronism is increasingly recognized as an important cause of secondary hypertension, accounting for approximately 20% of cases of resistant hypertension.[29] Much of the controversy about this condition is based on a reluctance to search for surgical causes of hypertension; however, the point of identifying this condition is that the right medical therapy depends on making the diagnosis.[30] It is also increasingly recognized that most cases of primary aldosteronism are due to bilateral adrenocortical hyperplasia,[31-33] so surgical therapy is a last option for most of these patients. Stowasser reviewed in 2009[34] the changing concepts in this condition,

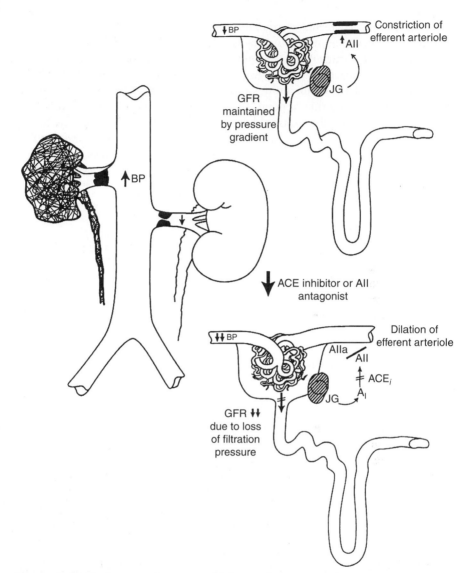

Figure 6–1. Mechanism of acute renal failure with angiotensin antagonists in renovascular hypertension. "Kicking the back door out of the glomerulus." With severe bilateral renal artery stenosis, pressure is low distal to the renal artery stenosis. To maintain filtration, the juxtaglomerular apparatus (JG) increases angiotensin II (AII) locally, constricting the efferent arteriole to maintain perfusion pressure. When this defense mechanism is lost because of drugs that block AII, filtration pressure collapses and glomerular filtration stops. (Permission was granted from Pulsus publications to reproduce from Hackam DG, Thain LMF, Abassakoor A, McKenzie FN, Spence JD. Trapped renal arteries: functional renal artery stenosis due to occlusion of the aorta in the arch and below the kidneys. *Can J Cardiol.* 2001;17:587-592.)

including the familial forms of primary aldosteronism. For most patients with primary aldosteronism, optimal therapy consists of aldosterone blockade with the specific aldosterone antagonists, spironolactone or eplerenone.[35] Unfortunately, aldosterone causes mastalgia and gynecomastia in most men, and eplerenone is costly and not available in all countries for the treatment of hypertension. A less ideal alternative is amiloride, a potassium- and magnesium-sparing diuretic; the disadvantage is that it will increase aldosterone levels without blocking them, and as discussed below, aldosterone has adverse effects on myocardium and the vasculature, independent of blood pressure effects. For purposes of selecting medical therapy (although not sufficient for planning surgical therapy), plasma levels of renin and aldosterone are very useful, as discussed below.

HYPERTENSION IN PATIENTS OF AFRICAN ORIGIN

It is well known that black patients with hypertension tend to have lower levels of plasma renin, and seem to respond better to diuretic therapy.[36] This accounts for the finding that diuretics were the best therapy in large US studies in which 40% of patients were black, whereas angiotensin-converting enzyme (ACE) inhibitors or calcium channel antagonists were more efficacious in studies carried out in Australia and Europe, in which fewer than 5% of patients were of African ancestry.[37] These are two clues to causes of secondary hypertension that are much more common in black, and indeed in patients of African origin, wherever they reside.[38,39] In the REGARDS study,[40] Howard et al documented that blacks were more likely to be diagnosed, more likely to be on treatment, and more likely to be on more intensive therapy for hypertension, but less likely to be controlled. This discrepancy probably accounts for much of the nearly two-fold excess of stroke among blacks,[41] which could be much reduced, or even eliminated, if blood pressure were well controlled.

Two causes of secondary hypertension that are much more common in patients of African origin are primary aldosteronism, mostly due to bilateral adrenocortical hyperplasia,[38] and variants of Liddle syndrome (abnormalities of the renal tubular sodium channel).[39,42] Both of these conditions cause retention of salt and water, with suppression of renin, but in primary aldosteronism the level of aldosterone is elevated, whereas with Liddle syndrome and its variants, the aldosterone level is also suppressed. Thus, as described below, the measurement of plasma renin and aldosterone is key to individualizing therapy for resistant hypertension.

PHYSIOLOGICALLY BASED INDIVIDUALIZED THERAPY BASED ON RENIN/ALDOSTERONE PHENOTYPING

After excluding noncompliance, ingestion of substances such as licorice, and rare causes of hypertension such as pheochromocytoma or aortic coarctation, most causes of resistant hypertension will be found in the RAAS, and their treatment should be based on that physiology (Figure 6–2).[35] Patients with primary aldosteronism will have low levels of renin with high aldosterone, and should be treated with aldosterone antagonists (discussed below); where eplerenone is not available, amiloride

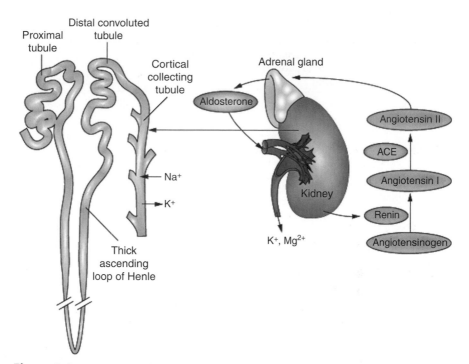

Figure 6–2. Treatment tailored to the renin/angiotensin/aldosterone system (RAAS). In normal physiology, if the blood pressure is too low or the body too dry, the kidney releases renin, an enzyme that converts angiotensinogen to angiotensin I. Angiotensin I (AI) is converted by angiotensin-converting enzyme (ACE) to its active form, angiotensin II (AII). This in turn causes the adrenal cortex to release aldosterone, which in the kidney causes salt and water retention, and excretion of potassium, magnesium, and other ions. When this system is disordered, it causes hypertension. Renal or renovascular causes of hypertension increase renin and angiotensin levels, with secondary hyperaldosteronism. Primary aldosteronism increases aldosterone and suppresses renin. Abnormalities of the renal tubule that cause salt and water retention suppress renin (this happens with variants of Liddle syndrome). Treatments for these conditions are different. Angiotensin receptor blockers (ARBs) block AII; ACE inhibitors block activation of AI to AII; aldosterone and eplerenone block aldosterone. Amiloride blocks the effects of aldosterone in the renal tubule, and is the specific treatment for Liddle variants. (Reproduced by permission of the publisher from Spence JD. Secondary Stroke Prevention. *Nat Rev Neurol* 2010;6:477-86.)

can be used in high doses for men (who get gynecomastia from spironolactone). Adrenalectomy is best reserved for patients who cannot be controlled medically. Patients with renal or renovascular hypertension will have a high renin with secondary hyperaldosteronism; they are best treated with angiotensin receptor blockers or aliskiren. (ACE inhibitors are less effective because of angiotensin escape pathways such as chymase and cathepsin.) Patients with variants of Liddle syndrome will have a low renin and low aldosterone, and the specific treatment is amiloride. This algorithm is shown in Table 6–2.

Table 6–2. Individualized Therapy Based on Renin/Aldosterone Profiling

	Primary Aldosteronism (mainly due to adrenocortical hyperplasia)	Liddle Syndrome and Variants	Renal or Renovascular
Renin	Low	Low	High
Aldosterone	High	Low	High
Primary treatment	Aldosterone antagonists (spironolactone, eplerenone) Amiloride where these are not available Rarely surgical	Amiloride	Angiotensin receptor blockers or aliskiren Sometimes surgery or angioplasty/stenting may be necessary

BLOCKADE OF ALDOSTERONE

Beyond primary hyperaldosteronism, the role of aldosterone in both the pathogenesis of the hypertensive state and in the development of hypertension-related cardiovascular complications has been underappreciated. However, following the RALES study,[43] a number of investigators began to re-examine the significance of aldosterone as a cardiovascular risk factor and the role of aldosterone blockade in the management of hypertension and hypertension-related complications. In this context, it was appreciated, on revisiting the results of the SHEP study,[44] that patients with persistent hypokalemia had an event rate almost identical to those in the placebo group. The mechanism underlying this finding was not clear, but the increased event rates suffered were not due to arrhythmias (as might be anticipated if this were directly related to hypokalemia). It was speculated that these adverse events might be related to hyperaldosteronemia, for which hypokalemia served as the index, independent of the degree of blood pressure control. These findings in aggregate triggered a concerted effort to identify potential pathological mechanisms mediated by aldosterone, beyond salt and water retention.

Over the past decade it has been appreciated that aldosterone has a range of extra-renal effects, all of which may be harmful. These include actions on smooth muscle contractility, cardiac fibrosis, inflammation, cardiac inotropy, and cardiovascular cell growth/death.[45] These effects probably aggravate left ventricular hypertrophy and heart failure, and inflammatory effects of aldosterone probably aggravate atherosclerosis.[46]

The signaling mechanisms underlying this range of processes have been a focus of intense interest. The effects of mineralocorticoids have traditionally been ascribed to mineralocorticoid receptor activation—primarily relating to triggering of transcriptional pathways by the actions of nuclear receptors. However, in studies dating from the 1950s, acute actions of mineralocorticoids on smooth muscle function were described—that is, over a time course much too rapid for transcriptional events.[47] These rapid (so-called nongenomic) actions of aldosterone have now been shown to be an important component of the vascular effects of aldosterone.[48] Additionally, recent studies have identified that these mechanisms of aldosterone effects are mediated not only by the classic mineralocorticoid receptor, but also by a recently appreciated G-protein coupled receptor, GPR30.[49]

In aggregate, these findings have rekindled interest in the blockade of aldosterone-mediated effects in the management of hypertension—especially in patients with refractory hypertension who have high levels of aldosterone, either because of diuretic therapy or from an underlying cause of primary or secondary hyperaldosteronism. In either setting the importance of aldosterone blockade in patients with resistant hypertension has been increasingly appreciated.[50,51] Interestingly, amiloride, a renal sodium channel blocker that would be expected to selectively mimic the renal actions of spironolactone or eplerenone, has been reported to be effective in patients with resistant hypertension (although perhaps to a lesser extent than spironolactone).[52]

TREATING HYPERTENSION IN ACUTE STROKE

Whether and how to treat hypertension in the setting of acute stroke is a long-standing controversy. Fear of lowering blood pressure and thus aggravating ischemia in the tissue at risk is in part due to excessive lowering of pressure with uncontrollable therapies such as "sublingual" nifedipine, which should never be used.[53] In some patients, for example, those whose stroke is due to dissection of the aorta or a recent myocardial infarction, the blood pressure must be lowered on account of the coexisting medical condition.[54] With the advent of thrombolytic therapy for acute stroke, it has become necessary to lower blood pressure in some patients so that they can be treated. Blood pressure should be lowered in this setting with therapies that can be controlled, such as short-acting intravenous therapies or nitrate patches.[55,56]

REFERENCES

1. Hackam DG, Spence JD. Combining multiple approaches for the secondary prevention of vascular events after stroke: a quantitative modeling study. *Stroke.* 2007;38:1881-1885.
2. Li C, Engström G, Hedblad B, Berglund G, Janzon L. Blood pressure control and risk of stroke: a population-based prospective cohort study. *Stroke.* 2005;36:725-730.
3. Collins R, Peto R, MacMahon S, et al. Blood pressure, stroke, and coronary heart disease. Part 2, short-term reductions in blood pressure: overview of randomised drug trials in their epidemiological context. *Lancet.* 1990;335:827-838.
4. Spence JD. Homocysteine-lowering therapy: a role in stroke prevention? *Lancet Neurol.* 2007;7: 830-838.
5. Spence JD. Cerebral consequences of hypertension: where do they lead? *J Hypertens Suppl.* 1996;14:S139-S145.
6. Spence JD. Cerebral consequences of hypertension. In: Laragh JH, Brenner BM, eds. *Hypertension: Pathophysiology, Diagnosis, and Management.* 2nd ed. New York: Raven Press; 1995:745-753.
7. Bass MJ, McWhinney IR, Donner A. Do family physicians need medical assistants to detect and manage hypertension? *Can Med Assoc J.* 1986;134:1247-1255.
8. Birkett NJ, Donner AP, Maynard M. Prevalence and control of hypertension in an Ontario county. *Can Med Assoc J.* 1985;132:1019-1024.
9. Spence JD. Antihypertensive drugs and prevention of atherosclerotic stroke. *Stroke.* 1986;17:808-810.
10. Wilkins K, Campbell NR, Joffres MR, et al. Blood pressure in Canadian adults. *Health Rep.* 2010;21:37-46.

11. Petrella RJ, Merikle EP, Jones J. Prevalence, treatment, and control of hypertension in primary care: gaps, trends, and opportunities. *J Clin Hypertens (Greenwich)*. 2007;9:28-35.

12. Spence JD. White-coat hypertension is hypertension. *Hypertension*. 2008;51:1272.

13. Haynes RB, Taylor DW, Sackett DL, Gibson ES, Bernholz CD, Mukherjee J. Can simple clinical measurements detect patient noncompliance? *Hypertension*. 1980;2:757-764.

14. Feldman RD, Zou GY, Vandervoort MK, Wong CJ, Nelson SA, Feagan BG. A simplified approach to the treatment of uncomplicated hypertension. A cluster randomized, controlled trial. *Hypertension*. 2009;53(4):646-653.

15. Marentette MA, Gerth WC, Billings DK, Zarnke KB. Antihypertensive persistence and drug class. *Can J Cardiol*. 2002;18:649-656.

16. Spence JD. *How to Prevent Your Stroke*. Nashville: Vanderbilt University Press; 2006.

17. Hackam DG, Khan NA, Hemmelgarn BR, et al. The 2010 Canadian Hypertension Education Program recommendations for the management of hypertension: part 2—therapy. *Can J Cardiol*. 2010;26: 249-258.

18. Joffres MR, Campbell NR, Manns B, Tu K. Estimate of the benefits of a population-based reduction in dietary sodium additives on hypertension and its related health care costs in Canada. *Can J Cardiol*. 2007;23:437-443.

19. Sacks FM, Svetkey LP, Vollmer WM, et al. Effects on blood pressure of reduced dietary sodium and the Dietary Approaches to Stop Hypertension (DASH) diet. DASH-Sodium Collaborative Research Group. *N Engl J Med*. 2001;344:3-10.

20. Wong DG, Spence JD, Lamki L, McDonald JWD. Effect of non-steroidal anti-inflammatory drugs on control of hypertension by beta-blockers and diuretics. *Lancet*. 1986;1(8488):997-1001.

21. Spence JD. Hypertension and the central nervous system. In: Hall HE, Lip GY, eds. *Comprehensive Hypertension*. New York: Elsevier; 2007:931-938.

22. Kuchel O, Buu NT, Larochelle P, Hamet P, Genest J Jr. Episodic dopamine discharge in paroxysmal hypertension. Page's syndrome revisited. *Arch Intern Med*. 1986;146:1315-1320.

23. Kuchel O, Buu NT, Hamet P, Larochelle P, Bourque M, Genest J. Dopamine surges in hyperadrenergic essential hypertension. *Hypertension*. 1982;4:845-852.

24. Sharabi Y, Goldstein DS, Bentho O, et al. Sympathoadrenal function in patients with paroxysmal hypertension: pseudopheochromocytoma. *J Hypertens*. 2007;25:2286-2295.

25. Spence JD. Management of resistant hypertension in patients with carotid stenosis: high prevalence of renovascular hypertension. *Cerebrovasc Dis*. 2000;10:249-254.

26. MacDowall P, Kalra PA, O'Donoghue DJ, Waldek S, Mamtora H, Brown K. Risk of morbidity from renovascular disease in elderly patients with congestive cardiac failure. *Lancet*. 1998;352:13-16.

27. Spence JD. Treatment options for renovascular hypertension. *Exp Opin Pharmacother*. 2002;3: 411-416.

28. Hackam DG, Thain LMF, Abassakoor A, McKenzie FN, Spence JD. Trapped renal arteries: functional renal artery stenosis due to occlusion of the aorta in the arch and below the kidneys. *Can J Cardiol*. 2001;17:587-592.

29. Calhoun DA, Jones D, Textor S, et al. Resistant hypertension: diagnosis, evaluation, and treatment. A scientific statement from the American Heart Association Professional Education Committee of the Council for High Blood Pressure Research. *Hypertension*. 2008;51:1403-1419.

30. Spence JD. Diagnosis of primary aldosteronism: for medical management, not just surgery. *J Hypertens*. 2009;27:204-205.

31. Biglieri EG, Kater CE, Arteaga EE. Primary aldosteronism is composed of primary adrenal hyperplasia and adenoma. *J Hypertens*. 1984;2(Suppl):S259-S261.

32. Spence JD. The current epidemic of primary aldosteronism: causes and consequences. *J Hypertens*. 2004;22:2038-2039.

33. Rayner B. Primary aldosteronism and aldosterone-associated hypertension. *J Clin Pathol*. 2008;61:825-831.

34. Stowasser M. Update in primary aldosteronism. *J Clin Endocrinol Metab*. 2009;94:3623-3630.

35. Spence JD. Physiologic tailoring of treatment in resistant hypertension. *Curr Cardiol Rev*. 2010;6: 213-219.

36. Lindhorst J, Alexander N, Blignaut J, Rayner B. Differences in hypertension between blacks and whites: an overview. *Cardiovasc J Afr*. 2007;18:241-247.

37. Spence JD. Individualized therapy for hypertension. *Hypertension.* 2006;47:e11.

38. Russell RP, Masi AT. The prevalence of adrenal cortical hyperplasia at autopsy and its association with hypertension. *Ann Intern Med.* 1970;73:195-205.

39. Rayner BL, Owen EP, King JA, et al. A new mutation, R563Q, of the beta subunit of the epithelial sodium channel associated with low-renin, low-aldosterone hypertension. *J Hypertens.* 2003;21: 921-926.

40. Howard G, Prineas R, Moy C, et al. Racial and geographic differences in awareness, treatment, and control of hypertension: the REasons for Geographic And Racial Differences in Stroke study. *Stroke.* 2006;37:1171-1178.

41. Roger VL, Go AS, Lloyd-Jones DM, et al. Heart disease and stroke statistics—2011 update: a report from the American Heart Association. *Circulation.* 2011;123(4):e18-e209.

42. Baker EH, Duggal A, Dong Y, et al. Amiloride, a specific drug for hypertension in black people with T594M variant? *Hypertension.* 2002;40:13-17.

43. Pitt B, Zannad F, Remme WJ, et al. The effect of spironolactone on morbidity and mortality in patients with severe heart failure. Randomized Aldactone Evaluation Study Investigators. *N Engl J Med.* 1999;341:709-717.

44. Franse LV, Pahor M, Di BM, Somes GW, Cushman WC, Applegate WB. Hypokalemia associated with diuretic use and cardiovascular events in the Systolic Hypertension in the Elderly Program. *Hypertension.* 2000;35:1025-1030.

45. Feldman RD, Gros R. Rapid vascular effects of steroids—a question of balance? *Can J Cardiol.* 2010;26(Suppl A):22A-26A.

46. Brown NJ. Aldosterone and vascular inflammation. *Hypertension.* 2008;51:161-167.

47. Streeten DH, Hirschowitz BI, Henley KS, Pollard HM. Effects of adrenocortical steroids on the propulsive motility of small intestine. *Am J Physiol.* 1957;189:108-112.

48. Feldman RD, Gros R. Unraveling the mechanisms underlying the rapid vascular effects of steroids: sorting out the receptors and the pathways. *Br J Pharmacol.* 2011;163(6):1163-1169.

49. Gros R, Ding Q, Sklar LA, et al. GPR30 expression is required for the mineralocorticoid receptor-independent rapid vascular effects of aldosterone. *Hypertension.* 2011;57:442-451.

50. Alvarez-Alvarez B, Abad-Cardiel M, Fernandez-Cruz A, Martell-Claros N. Management of resistant arterial hypertension: role of spironolactone versus double blockade of the renin-angiotensin-aldosterone system. *J Hypertens.* 2010;28:2329-2335.

51. Calhoun DA, White WB. Effectiveness of the selective aldosterone blocker, eplerenone, in patients with resistant hypertension. *J Am Soc Hypertens.* 2008;2:462-468.

52. Lane DA, Beevers DG. Amiloride 10 mg is less effective than spironolactone 25 mg in patients with hypertension resistant to a multidrug regime including an angiotensin-blocking agent. *J Hypertens.* 2007;25:2515-2516.

53. Spence JD, Paulson OB, Strandgaard S. Hypertension and stroke. In: Messerli FH, ed. *The ABCs of Antihypertensive Therapy.* 2nd ed. New York: Lippincott Williams & Wilkins; 2000:279-296.

54. Spence JD, Del Maestro RF. Hypertension in acute ischemic strokes. *Treat Arch Neurol.* 1985;42: 1000-1002.

55. Spence JD. New treatment options for hypertension during acute ischemic or hemorrhagic stroke. *Curr Treat Options Cardiovasc Med.* 2007;9:242-246.

56. Spence JD. Treating hypertension in acute ischemic stroke. *Hypertension.* 2009;54:702-703.

Antiplatelet Therapy

7

Aurauma Chutinet
Karen L. Furie
Henry J. M. Barnett

TOPICS

Antiplatelet therapy is an essential component of a secondary noncardioembolic stroke prevention regimen. A meta-analysis among 18,270 patients in 21 trials showed that the use of antiplatelet therapy could prevent 36 serious vascular events for every 1000 stroke or transient ischemic attack (TIA) patients treated with an antiplatelet agent for two years.[1] This chapter summarizes the mechanism of action, drug resistance, and evidence for the efficacy of antiplatelet agents for secondary stroke prevention.

Aspirin

MECHANISM OF ACTION

The pharmacokinetics and pharmacodynamics of aspirin are described in Table 7–1.[2-4] Arachidonic acid is metabolized to cyclic prostanoids, including thromboxane A_2 (TXA_2), prostaglandin I_2 (prostacyclin, PGI_2), prostaglandin E_2 (PGE_2), prostaglandin D_2 (PGD_2), and prostaglandin $F_{2\alpha}$ ($PGF_{2\alpha}$) by the enzyme prostaglandin (PG) H-synthase/cyclooxygenase (COX) and specific synthases.[5] TXA_2 and PGI_2 play important roles in platelet aggregation. TXA_2, the principal cyclooxygenase product of arachidonic acid in the platelet, increases platelet aggregation and causes vasoconstriction, whereas PGI_2, the predominant cyclooxygenase metabolite formed in the vascular endothelium, decreases platelet aggregation and induces vasodilatation.[6]

Aspirin reduces platelet aggregation mainly by irreversibly acetylating cyclooxygenase-1 (COX-1) enzyme at specific residue ser529, and cyclooxygenase-2 (COX-2) enzyme at specific residue ser516.[7] The inhibition of COX-1 is 170-fold more potent than the inhibition of COX-2.[8] The irreversible acetylation of COX-1 enzyme results in inhibition of TXA_2 and PGI_2 and affects homeostasis. The antithrombotic effects of TXA_2 inhibition are more prominent and clinically

Table 7–1. Summary of Pharmacokinetics and Pharmacodynamics of Antiplatelet Agents

Drugs	Structure	Absorption	Excretion	Peak Plasma Level	Time to Inhibit Platelet Function	Plasma Half-Life	Effect Persist	Frequency	References
Aspirin	—	Stomach, duodenum	—	30-40 min; 3-8 h (enteric coated)	1 h	15-20 min	10 d	Daily	2,3,4
Ticlopidine	Thienopyridine	—	60% urine, 20% feces	1-3 h	5-14 d	—	—	bid	—
Clopidogrel	Thienopyridine	—	50% urine, 50% feces	45 min	6 d; 2 h (loading dose 300-400 mg)	—	7-10 d	Daily	32,33
Prasugrel	Thienopyridine	—	75% urine	30 min	1 h	—	72 h	Daily	47,48,49
Ticagrelor	Cyclopentyl triazolopyrimidine	—	—	2-3 h	2 h	—	—	bid	47
Extended-release dipyridamole	Phosphodiesterase inhibitor	—	95% feces	1-6 h	24 h	—	—	bid	56
Terutroban	Selective TP receptor	—	—	30 min-2 h	1 h	5.8-10 h	12 h	Daily	68
Cilostazol	Selective phosphodiesterase inhibitor	—	—	—	6 h	10 h	48 h	bid	74,75
Triflusal	—	Small intestine	Urine	0.88 h; 4.96 h (active metabolite)	8-10 d	0.53 h; 34.29 h (active metabolite)	—	bid	82,83

b.i.d., twice a day; t.i.d., three times a day.

relevant than PGI_2 inhibition.[9] Inhibition of TXA_2 formation requires lower doses of aspirin than blockade of PGI_2 synthesis.[10]

DOSE OF ASA: INHIBITION OF PLATELET THROMBOXANE VERSUS ENDOTHELIAL PROSTACYCLIN

There are many studies measuring platelet aggregation with variable doses of aspirin. A single dose of 20 to 650 mg aspirin results in 34% to greater than 95% inhibition of platelet cyclooxygenase after 24 hours, and a single 325-mg aspirin dose inactivates 89% of platelet cyclooxygenase. Daily doses of 20 to 325 mg aspirin for 5 to 7 days produced 61% to greater than 95% inactivation of platelet cyclooxygenase after 24-hour cessation of the drug.[4] A daily dose of 0.45 mg/kg (30 mg) suppresses more than 95% of TXA_2 within five days and maintains suppression with long-term daily dosing.[10] The Dutch TIA trial found that 30 mg of aspirin daily was slightly more effective than 283 mg of aspirin in the prevention of vascular events and had fewer side effects.[11] The benefits of high-dose aspirin remain unproven.

INHIBITION OF PLATELET THROMBOXANE VERSUS ENDOTHELIAL PROSTACYCLIN

TXA_2 induces irreversible platelet aggregation, and vessel walls generate PGI_2 that inhibits human platelet aggregation.[12] Therefore, changing TXA_2 and PGI_2 levels has the potential to significantly affect platelet aggregation. The selection of the optimal dose of aspirin required to inhibit platelet thromboxane without having deleterious effects on endothelial prostacyclin production remains controversial.

A 75-mg controlled-release aspirin, designed to release 10 mg/h, selectively blocked TXA_2 but preserved prostacyclin during platelet inhibition in humans.[13]

COX-1 catalyzes the synthesis of TXA_2, whereas COX-2 is primarily responsible for the biosynthesis of prostacyclin (PGI_2). Aspirin is a more potent inhibitor of COX-1 than COX-2.[14]

ASPIRIN RESISTANCE: IS IT REAL, DOES IT MATTER?

The term "aspirin resistance" has been used extensively in the literature and defined in various ways. A standard definition of aspirin resistance has not been established. In general, there are two commonly used definitions: clinical resistance and laboratory resistance. "Clinical aspirin resistance" or "treatment failure" refers to the failure of aspirin to protect individuals from recurrent thrombotic vascular events such as acute myocardial infarction or acute ischemic stroke despite long-term regular aspirin therapy.[2,15] "Laboratory aspirin resistance" has been defined as the inability of aspirin to prolong the bleeding time, inhibit COX-1 and TXA_2 production, or prevent platelet aggregation as measured by platelet function assays.[16]

A study in Germany classified aspirin resistance based on the in vitro response to collagen. Aspirin responders showed complete (>95%) inhibition of platelet aggregation and thromboxane formation by oral aspirin treatment (100 mg/d). In type I resistance (pharmacokinetic type), oral aspirin was ineffective but the addition of aspirin (100 μM) in vitro resulted in complete inhibition of collagen-induced platelet aggregation and thromboxane formation. In type II resistance (pharmacodynamic type), either oral aspirin or the addition of aspirin in vitro could not inhibit platelet aggregation and thromboxane formation. In type III resistance (pseudoresistance), oral aspirin completely inhibited thromboxane formation, but platelet aggregation was induced by a low concentration of collagen (1 μg/mL) in vitro.[17] This classification may be useful in elucidating the cause of aspirin resistance. Another study in German patients with ischemic stroke defined aspirin nonresponders as having TXB_2 concentration greater than 25 ng/mL after oral or in vitro administration of aspirin.[18] A study in Japanese stroke or TIA patients defined aspirin resistance (biological aspirin resistance) as a failure in the inhibition of platelet aggregation induced by arachidonic acid, which is totally dependent on TXA_2. Complete resistance was defined as full aggregation induced by 1 mM arachidonic acid despite taking aspirin. Trace aggregation induced by 1 mM arachidonic acid, but no aggregation induced by less than 1 mM arachidonic acid, was considered partial resistance.[19]

The prevalence of aspirin resistance is estimated to vary widely from 0% to 57%. The variability is due to the application of different criteria to define aspirin resistance, heterogeneous populations, and disparate laboratory methods.[20] A systemic review of 42 studies showed that the mean prevalence was 24%. Populations taking aspirin doses of 100 mg or less had a significantly higher prevalence than those using doses of 300 mg or more.[20] In a meta-analysis, the prevalence of aspirin resistance was 28% in patients taking 75 to 325 mg/d and was significantly higher in women than men.[21]

Aspirin resistance has been studied specifically in stroke and TIA patients. In a two-year follow-up of 180 poststroke patients who received aspirin 1500 mg/d, 33% of patients were aspirin nonresponders.[22] The prevalence of aspirin resistance in 50 Australian stroke patients receiving aspirin 100 mg/d was 30% using the Ultegra Rapid Platelet Function Assay.[23] A cohort study in 129 ischemic stroke patients who were taking aspirin showed that 37% of patients had normal platelet function as measured by a platelet function analyzer (PFA-100). Normal platelet function was found in 56% and 28% of patients who were taking low-dose (≤162 mg/d) and high-dose (≥325 mg/d) aspirin, respectively. Older patients and women were more likely to have aspirin resistance.[24] The prevalence of aspirin resistance in 857 Japanese stroke and TIA patients was 25.6% and 11.2% in patients taking low-dose (<80 mg/d) and high-dose (>80 mg/d) aspirin, respectively.[19] The proportion of aspirin resistance tends to be higher with lower doses of aspirin.[25]

Based on existing evidence, aspirin resistance appears to be a clinically relevant phenomenon.[25] In a meta-analysis, patients with aspirin resistance had a greater risk of suffering a cardiovascular event than aspirin-sensitive patients (odds ratio [OR] 3.85).[21] In a high-risk population, there was a correlation between ischemic stroke or TIA and aspirin resistance.[23]

There are many causes of aspirin resistance, including reduced bioavailability of aspirin such as inadequate intake of aspirin (poor compliance), inadequate dose of aspirin, reduced absorption or increased metabolism of aspirin, altered binding to COX-1 (such as drug interaction from ibuprofen, indomethacin), nonplatelet sources of thromboxane production such as COX-2 in monocytes and macrophages, vascular endothelial cells, alternative pathways of platelet activation such as pathways that are not blocked by aspirin (eg, red blood cell–induced platelet activation), increased platelet sensitivity to collagen and adenosine 5′-diphosphate (ADP), increased turnover of platelets such as response to stress (eg, after coronary artery bypass surgery, carotid endarterectomy), and genetic polymorphisms such as polymorphisms of COX-1, COX-2, and glycoprotein Ia/IIa.[15]

ASPIRIN IN SECONDARY PREVENTION OF STROKE AND TIA

Aspirin has been widely used in secondary prevention of atherothrombotic diseases, including ischemic stroke and TIA, due to its efficacy, safety, and low cost. Many studies showed the efficacy of aspirin for preventing recurrent stroke/TIA in patients. The Canadian Cooperative Study Group found that aspirin (1300 mg/d) during an average of 26 months reduced the risk of stroke or death by 31%.[26] The SALT study (aspirin 75 mg/d vs placebo) in Sweden showed a reduction of 18% in the risk of stroke or death in the aspirin group during mean follow-up of 32 months.[27] The overview of randomized trials of antiplatelet therapy showed that antiplatelet therapy, mostly aspirin, in patients with prior stroke/TIA resulted in a 23% reduction in nonfatal stroke.[28]

The efficacy of aspirin is similar for doses ranging from 30 to 1500 mg/d. For example, the Dutch TIA Trial Study found that 30 mg of aspirin daily was no less effective in the prevention of vascular events than a 283-mg dose in patients with minor stroke/TIA and resulted in fewer adverse effects.[18] The UK-TIA aspirin trial showed no difference in efficacy between 300- and 1200-mg daily doses of aspirin, and the lower dose had fewer gastrointestinal side effects.[29] The overview of randomized trials of antiplatelet therapy showed that aspirin ranging from 75 to 1500 mg/d was similarly effective in decreasing myocardial infarction, stroke, or vascular death,[28] and a meta-regression analysis of aspirin compared with placebo in stroke/TIA patients showed that aspirin reduced the risk of stroke 15% across aspirin doses of 50 to 1500 mg/d.[30] A meta-analysis showed that aspirin therapy increased the risk of hemorrhagic stroke (12 events per 10,000 persons, $P < .001$), but the overall benefit of aspirin in secondary prevention of stroke/TIA greatly exceeded the potential for adverse effects.[31]

THIENOPYRIDINES

Ticlopidine

Ticlopidine is not recommended because of its adverse effects (most importantly, neutropenia).

Clopidogrel

MECHANISM OF ACTION

The pharmacokinetics and pharmacodynamics of clopidogrel are described in Table 7–1.[32,33] Clopidogrel is a second-generation thienopyridine derivative and inhibits ADP-induced platelet aggregation by selectively binding to P2Y12 receptors on the platelet surface.[34,35] Clopidogrel is rapidly absorbed from the intestine and 85% of pro-drug is transformed into inactive carboxylic acid metabolite, whereas 15% is transformed by hepatic cytochrome isoenzymes P450 (CYP3A4, CYP3A5, CYP2C19) in the liver by a two-step oxidation into an active thiol metabolite.[34,35] This short-lived active thiol metabolite binds to the P2Y12 receptor at two cysteine residues (cys17 and cys270) via the disulfide bridge, irreversibly inhibiting the binding of ADP to the P2Y12 receptor and blocking the activation of the glycoprotein IIb/IIIa pathway. Clopidogrel also reduces platelet–leukocyte aggregation formation and the rate of thrombin formation, and indirectly inhibits collagen-induced aggregation and thrombin-induced aggregation.[2,34]

The adverse effects of clopidogrel such as gastrointestinal symptoms, rash, and neutropenia are less common than with ticlopidine, and fatal complications are rare. In the CAPRIE study, rash and diarrhea occurred in the clopidogrel group more than the aspirin group, whereas upper gastrointestinal discomfort, intracranial hemorrhage, and gastrointestinal hemorrhage were more common in the aspirin group.[36] Thrombotic thrombocytopenic purpura has been reported with clopidogrel, often within the first two weeks of treatment.

CLOPIDOGREL RESISTANCE

Clopidogrel resistance, as defined by "laboratory resistance," is the failure of clopidogrel to inhibit platelet function in vitro, measured by one or more laboratory tests of platelet activation and aggregation.[35,37] One study defined clopidogrel nonresponsiveness as an absolute change between pre- and post-treatment in aggregation inhibition of 10% or less.[38] Many tests can be used to assess platelet function in response to clopidogrel.[35] Light transmission aggregometry is historically the gold standard, but is time-consuming and uses a high sample volume; VerifyNow is a simple to use, point-of-care device that uses a low sample volume but has a limited hematocrit and platelet count range; Plateletworks requires minimal sample preparation, is a whole-blood assay, but has limited studies to endorse its utility. Vasodilator-stimulated phosphoprotein (VASP) measures the effect of P2Y12 inhibitors and uses a low sample volume, whole-blood assay, but requires flow cytometry and an experienced technician. Like aspirin resistance, defining clopidogrel resistance is difficult, varies across studies and is not standardized.

The prevalence of clopidogrel resistance varies from 4% to 30%.[37] Mechanisms of clopidogrel resistance are divided into extrinsic and intrinsic mechanisms.[37] Extrinsic mechanisms are patient noncompliance, underdosing or inappropriate dosing of clopidogrel, and drug-drug interactions involving hepatic cytochrome P450 (CYP) enzymes such as CYP3A4, CYP3A5, CYP2C19. Intrinsic mechanisms are genetic variables such as polymorphisms of CYP3As, CYP2C19, or the P2Y12 receptor; increased ADP release; and alternative pathways of platelet activation (eg, failure to inhibit catecholamine-mediated platelet activation [epinephrine], greater extent of P2Y1-dependent platelet aggregation, upregulation of P2Y12-independent pathways [thrombin, thromboxane A2, collagen]).

Current evidence suggests that statins can be safely used with clopidogrel.[35]

CYP2C19 VARIANTS

CYP2C19 plays an important role in converting clopidogrel pro-drug into its active thiol metabolite. There are genetic polymorphisms in several CYP450 enzymes including CYP2C19, and variants in CYP2C19 can affect platelet aggregation and clinical outcomes.[39] The CYP2C19*1 allele is responsible for the full functional metabolism of clopidogrel; the CYP2C19*2 and *3 allele have no functional metabolism of clopidogrel.[39] The loss of two functional alleles conveys a poor metabolizer status.[39] A study in 162 healthy subjects who were treated with clopidogrel showed that carriers of at least one CYP2C19 reduced-function allele had significantly lower levels of the active metabolite of clopidogrel and decreased platelet inhibition compared with noncarriers ($P < .001$ and $P < .001$, respectively).[40] In the TRITON-TIMI 38 trial, 1477 subjects with acute coronary syndrome were treated with clopidogrel. Carriers of a reduced-function CYP2C19 allele had a significantly higher rate of major adverse cardiovascular events than noncarriers (2.6% vs 0.8%; hazard ratio [HR] 3.09; 95% confidence interval [CI], 1.19-8.00; $P = .02$).[40] In 2208 patients with acute myocardial infarction receiving clopidogrel in the FAST-MI trial, subjects carrying any two of the CYP2C19 loss-of-function alleles (*2, *3, *4, or *5) had a higher rate of cardiovascular events than noncarriers (21.5% vs 13.3%; adjusted HR 1.98; 95% CI,1.10-3.58).[41]

A recent meta-analysis of 8043 clopidogrel-treated patients with coronary artery disease from seven prospective cohort studies showed that the CYP2C19*2 polymorphism is associated with an increased risk of major adverse cardiovascular events (relative risk [RR] 1.96; 95% CI, 1.14-3.37; $P = .02$) and stent thrombosis (RR 3.82; 95% CI, 2.23-6.54; $P = .0001$).[42]

However, a genetic study in 5059 patients with acute coronary syndrome or atrial fibrillation from two large, randomized trials that compared clopidogrel with placebo showed that the effect of clopidogrel remained superior to placebo in reducing the rate of the primary outcome irrespective of CYP2C19 genotype.[43]

In summary, current evidence shows a compelling association between CYP2C19 variants and clinical outcomes, but the optimal management strategy remains controversial. There are several ongoing studies evaluating the effect of CYP2C19 variants on the antiplatelet function of clopidogrel therapy.[39]

PROTON PUMP INHIBITORS (PPIs)

Most PPIs are metabolized by the hepatic cytochrome P450, principally by the isozymes, predominantly CYP2C19 and CYP3A4. PPIs may competitively inhibit CYP2C19, thereby inhibiting the conversion of clopidogrel to its active metabolite. An important exception is pantoprazole, which is probably the PPI of choice in patients taking clopidogrel.[44]

CLOPIDOGREL IN SECONDARY PREVENTION OF STROKE OR TIA

Clopidogrel has been compared to aspirin and extended-release dipyridamole-aspirin in large clinical trials. A randomized, blinded trial of clopidogrel (75 mg/d) versus aspirin (325 mg/d) in patients at risk of ischemic events (CAPRIE) enrolled 19,185 patients with recent ischemic stroke, recent myocardial infarction, or symptomatic peripheral arterial disease, with a mean follow-up 1.91 years. This trial showed that patients taking clopidogrel had a modest but statistically significant lower annual risk of ischemic stroke, myocardial infarction, or vascular death as compared to subjects treated with aspirin (5.32% vs 5.83%; relative risk reduction [RRR] 8.7%; 95% CI, 0.3-16.5; $P = .043$). However, subgroup analysis restricted to the stroke patients found that subjects on clopidogrel did not have a lower annual risk of ischemic stroke, myocardial infarction, or vascular death than those treated with aspirin (7.15% vs 7.71%; RRR 7.3%; 95% CI, −5.7-18.7; $P = .26$). Patients assigned to the clopidogrel arm had more rash and diarrhea but fewer reports of upper gastrointestinal discomfort, intracranial hemorrhage, and gastrointestinal hemorrhage than those assigned to aspirin.[36] The Prevention Regimen for Effectively Avoiding Second Strokes (PROFESS) trial, a double-blind, 2-by-2 factorial trial, compared the efficacy and safety of aspirin (25 mg) plus extended-release dipyridamole (200 mg) twice daily (ASA-ERDP) versus clopidogrel (75 mg daily). A total of 20,332 patients with recent ischemic stroke were enrolled and followed for a mean of two and a half years. There was no significant difference in the recurrent stroke rate between the ASA-ERDP and clopidogrel arms (9.0% vs 8.8%; HR 1.01; 95% CI, 0.92-1.11). The composite of stroke, myocardial infarction, or death from vascular causes were the same in both groups (13.1%) (HR 0.99; 95% CI, 0.92-1.07). The rate of major hemorrhagic events was higher in the ASA-ERDP group (4.1% vs 3.6%; HR 1.15; 95% CI, 1.00-1.32).[45,46] See Chapter 13 for a discussion of Dr. Barnett's concerns about the CAPRIE study.

Prasugrel

MECHANISM OF ACTION

The pharmacokinetics and pharmacodynamics of prasugrel are described in Table 7–1.[47-49]

Prasugrel is a third-generation thienopyridine derivative. Prasugrel is a prodrug, and after oral administration, it is metabolized via hepatic CYP450.[47] The active metabolite of prasugrel irreversibly inhibits the platelet P2Y12 receptor and results in inhibition of ADP-mediated platelet activation and aggregation.[48] The mechanism of action is similar to clopidogrel. However, the active metabolite of prasugrel has greater efficacy in vivo than the active metabolite of clopidogrel.

PRASUGREL IN SECONDARY PREVENTION OF STROKE OR TIA

TRITON TIMI 38 trial, a double-blind, randomized trial comparing prasugrel (60-mg loading dose followed by 10 mg daily) and clopidogrel (300-mg loading dose followed by 75 mg daily) in 13,608 high-risk patients with acute coronary syndrome who required percutaneous coronary intervention (PCI) showed that prasugrel was effective at reducing ischemic events but had a higher rate of major and fatal bleeding complications than clopidogrel.[50] A post-hoc analysis of the TRITON TIMI 38 trial in 518 patients with previous ischemic stroke or TIA found no benefit and an increased risk of major bleeding in the prasugrel group.[51]

To date, there is no evidence to support the use of prasugrel for secondary stroke prevention.

Ticagrelor

MECHANISM OF ACTION

The pharmacokinetics and pharmacodynamics of ticagrelor are described in Table 7–1.[47]

Ticagrelor is a cyclopentyl triazolopyrimidine derivative, is orally active, and is a reversible and direct P2Y12 receptor antagonist. Ticagrelor does not require hepatic conversion, but does have biologically active metabolites.[47]

Its reversibility, rapid onset, and short half-life may be advantageous to patients requiring surgery.[47] A double-blind study comparing ticagrelor with aspirin and clopidogrel with aspirin in 200 patients with atherosclerotic disease showed that different doses of ticagrelor did not significantly alter platelet inhibition. Ticagrelor 100 mg and 200 mg twice daily were well tolerated and superior to ticagrelor 50 mg twice daily and clopidogrel 75 mg daily.[52] There was no difference in the rate of major bleeding between the ticagrelor and clopidogrel groups. However, ticagrelor was associated with dose-related dyspnea (10%-20%).[52]

TICAGRELOR IN SECONDARY PREVENTION OF STROKE OR TIA

Further studies are needed to determine the efficacy of ticagrelor for secondary stroke prevention.

Dipyridamole

MECHANISM OF ACTION

Dipyridamole inhibits platelet activation through two major pathways. Dipyridamole inhibits adenosine uptake by red blood cells by more than 90% and increases plasma adenosine levels by 60%, leading to decreased platelet reactivity and inhibition of platelet aggregation.[53] In addition, dipyridamole is a phosphodiesterase inhibitor and prevents the conversion of cyclic adenosine monophosphate (cAMP) to AMP and cyclic guanine monophosphate (cGMP) to GMP. High levels of cAMP and cGMP in platelets result in reversibly inhibited platelet aggregation and platelet-mediated thrombotic disease.[54]

Besides the antiplatelet effect, dipyridamole also has other vascular effects: vasodilatation through increased local adenosine levels, increased prostacyclin production and enhanced cGMP-dependent downstream vasodilatory effects, and antioxidative and anti-inflammatory effects and impact on the nitric oxide pathway.[54,55]

The pharmacokinetics and pharmacodynamics are described in Table 7–1.[56] There are two formulations of dipyridamole. The immediate-release (IR) formulation requires administration four times daily, whereas the extended-release (ER) formulation is twice daily administration and was developed to optimize antiplatelet efficacy. The pharmacokinetics of both formulations are linear and nearly identical. The ER formulation has more consistent, reproducible absorption and has the advantage less frequency of administration.

Dipyridamole Monotherapy in Secondary Prevention of Stroke or TIA

Dipyridamole monotherapy has not been shown to be effective in the treatment of ischemic heart disease.[56] Dipyridamole monotherapy is not recommended for secondary stroke prevention.

Aspirin/Immediate-Release Dipyridamole Combination in Secondary Prevention of Stroke or TIA

There have been three studies comparing aspirin/IR dipyridamole with aspirin or placebo.[57-59] These studies did not demonstrate the superiority of IR dipyridamole plus aspirin over aspirin alone.

Aspirin/Extended-Release Dipyridamole Combination in Secondary Prevention of Stroke or TIA

Three large studies compared aspirin plus ER-dipyridamole to an alternative antiplatelet agent. The European Stroke Prevention Study 2 (ESPS-2) was a randomized, placebo-controlled, double-blind study that compared four treatment groups: aspirin alone (25 mg twice daily), ER-dipyridamole alone (200 mg twice daily), the combination of two agents (aspirin plus ER-dipyridamole, 25/200 mg twice daily), and placebo in 6602 patients with previous stroke or TIA. The follow-up was two years. Factorial analysis showed that aspirin and dipyridamole significantly reduced the risk of stroke (RRR 21% and 19.3%, respectively; $P \leq .001$) and stroke or death combined (RRR 12%, $P < .003$, and RRR 14.2%, $P < .002$, respectively). In pairwise comparisons, the risk of stroke was reduced by 18.1% with aspirin alone ($P = .013$), 16.3% with ER-dipyridamole alone ($P = .039$), and 37% with aspirin plus ER-dipyridamole ($P < .001$) when each group was compared with placebo. The risk of stroke was also reduced by 23.1% with aspirin plus ER-dipyridamole compared with aspirin alone ($P = .006$) and 24.7% with aspirin plus ER-dipyridamole compared with ER-dipyridamole alone ($P = .002$). The risk of stroke or death was reduced by 13.2% with aspirin alone ($P = .016$), 15.4% with dipyridamole alone ($P = .015$), and 24.4% with aspirin plus ER-dipyridamole ($P < .001$) relative to placebo. Headache was the most common adverse event across all treatment groups, including placebo, and occurred more frequently in dipyridamole-treated patients. ESPS-2 showed that aspirin alone (25 mg twice daily) and ER-dipyridamole alone (200 mg twice daily) were similarly effective for the secondary prevention of ischemic stroke, and combination of these drugs was additively effective.[60] The European/Australasian Stroke Prevention in Reversible Ischemic Trial (ESPRIT) study group performed a prospective, open-label, randomized controlled trial in 2749 patients with TIA or minor ischemic stroke within six months. The primary outcome event was prevention of death from all vascular causes, nonfatal stroke, nonfatal myocardial infarction, or major bleeding complication during mean follow-up of three and a half years. The dose of aspirin varied from 30 to 325 mg daily. However, the mean aspirin dose in each group was 75 mg. The dose of dipyridamole was 200 mg twice daily, and ER-dipyridamole was used by 83% of those assigned to the combination regimen.

Primary outcome events occurred in 13% of the aspirin-plus-dipyridamole group and 16% in patients on aspirin alone (HR 0.80, 95% CI, 0.66-0.98; absolute risk reduction 1.0% per year, 95% CI, 0.1-1.8).[61] The meta-analysis of previous studies including the ESPRIT trial showed an overall risk ratio for the composite of death, stroke, or myocardial infarction of 0.82 (95% CI, 0.74-0.91) for aspirin plus dipyridamole.[61] The PROFESS study, described earlier, failed to demonstrate the noninferiority of ER-dipyridamole and aspirin over clopidogrel. Adverse events leading to permanent discontinuation of the study drug were more common in the aspirin-plus-ER-dipyridamole group as compared to the clopidogrel group (16.4% vs 10.6%).[45]

Terutroban

MECHANISM OF ACTION

Terutroban is a selective TP receptor (thromboxane and prostaglandin endoperoxide PGG_2-PGH_2 receptors) antagonist. TP receptors are specific membrane-bound G-coupled receptors found on platelets, macrophages, monocytes, vascular endothelial cells, and smooth muscle cells, and are increased in atherosclerotic plaque.[62] Terutroban reversibly inhibits TP receptors on platelets and monocytes/macrophages in the vessel wall, and in smooth muscle cells and atherosclerotic plaque.[63] A TP receptor antagonist has an advantage over aspirin because it can block the effect of TXA_2 on platelets and also inhibits all ligands of TP receptors at other sites, such as prostaglandin endoperoxides and isoprostanes. Because of the broad distribution of TP receptors, terutroban has a theoretical superiority over previous antiplatelet agents such as aspirin, ticlopidine, and clopidogrel.[62]

Terutroban has three principal effects: antithrombotic, anti-vasoconstrictive, and anti-atherosclerotic. Terutroban has a dose-dependent antithrombotic effect that is reversible within 96 hours. A dose of 100 µg/kg/d displayed antithrombotic effects similar to those of clopidogrel and superior to those of aspirin.[64] The TAIPAD study group compared five oral dosages of terutroban (1, 2.5, 5, 10, or 30 mg daily) versus aspirin 75 mg daily in 435 patients with peripheral arterial disease and showed that terutroban (range 5-30 mg daily) was safe and as effective as aspirin 75 mg/d in inhibiting platelet aggregation in patients with peripheral arterial disease.[62] A double-blind, parallel-group, 10-day study in 48 patients with ischemic stroke and/or carotid stenosis compared four groups: terutroban 10 mg/d, aspirin 300 mg/d, terutroban 10 mg/d plus aspirin 300 mg/d, and clopidogrel 75 mg/d plus aspirin 300 mg/d. This study measured parameters from an ex vivo model of thrombosis, platelet aggregation in platelet-rich plasma, and plasma biomarkers of endothelial/platelet activation. The mean cross-sectional surface of dense thrombus between days 0 and 10 significantly decreased with terutroban (58%, $P = .001$), terutroban plus aspirin (63%, $P = .005$), and clopidogrel plus aspirin (61%, $P < .05$). Similar results were demonstrated in total thrombus surface and platelet aggregation. There was almost complete platelet inhibition by day 10 in both terutroban groups, but not in the others. By day 10, levels of thrombomodulin significantly increased and plasma soluble P selectin significantly decreased in both terutroban groups. The authors concluded that terutroban had an antiplatelet effect superior to aspirin and similar to clopidogrel plus aspirin.[63] A study in 20 patients with stable coronary artery disease showed that terutroban 10 mg daily significantly improved endothelium-dependent vasodilatation in the peripheral arteries compared with placebo.[65] In an animal model, terutroban prevented atherogenesis and reduced advanced atherosclerosis.[66] PERFORM is an ongoing study comparing change in carotid intima-media thickness (CIMT) in 1141 patients with ischemic stroke or TIA between those treated with terutroban 30 mg/d versus aspirin 100 mg/d.[67]

A study in 30 patients with peripheral artery disease receiving five different oral dosages of terutroban (1, 2.5, 5, 10, or 30 mg daily) for 12 weeks showed that the pharmacokinetics of terutroban was linear, with peak plasma levels being reached from 30 minutes to two hours and a terminal half-life of 5.8 to 10 hours. Maximal inhibition of platelet-induced aggregation was achieved within one hour with all doses and persisted for at least 12 hours.[68]

TERUTROBAN IN SECONDARY PREVENTION OF STROKE OR TIA

The Prevention of cerebrovascular and cardiovascular Events of ischemic origin with teRutroban in patients with a history oF ischemic strOke or tRansient ischeMic attack (PERFORM) study randomized 19,119 patients aged 55 years or older with recent ischemic stroke (≤3 months) or TIA (≤8 days) to terutroban (30 mg/d) or aspirin (100 mg/d). Of these patients, 90% had ischemic stroke and 67% had large vessel disease.[69] The primary efficacy endpoint was a composite of ischemic stroke (fatal or nonfatal), myocardial infarction (fatal or nonfatal), or other vascular death (excluding hemorrhagic death of any origin). The trial was stopped early for futility.[70] Terutroban is therefore not recommended for the secondary prevention of ischemic stroke or TIA.

Cilostazol

MECHANISM OF ACTION

Cilostazol is a selective inhibitor of phosphodiesterase 3 (PDE 3) that increases the cyclic adenosine monophosphate (cAMP) levels via suppression of cAMP phosphodiesterase, leading to inhibition of platelet aggregation and proliferation of vascular smooth muscle cells.[71] Cilostazol also inhibits shear stress-induced platelet aggregation and induces antiplatelet effects of endothelium-derived prostacyclin (PGI_2).[72] Cilostazol can inhibit monocyte chemoattractant protein-1 (MCP-1) and retard atherogenesis. A study in 10 healthy men demonstrated that cilostazol had less effect on bleeding time than aspirin or ticlopidine ($P < .01$), and no significant prolongation of bleeding time was observed with cilostazol monotherapy.[73] cilostazol did not prolong bleeding time when added to aspirin, clopidogrel, or aspirin plus clopidogrel.

Cilostazol is metabolized via the CYP450 system with potential for interaction with drugs such as erythromycin and omeprazole.[74] Cilostazol has an acute onset of action and rapid reversal on discontinuation.[71] A study in 24 patients with prior stroke showed that cilostazol 100 mg reduced platelet aggregation within six hours of the first oral dose and reversed without rebound 48 hours after discontinuation.[75]

The half-life is approximately 10 hours.[74] Cilostazol is extensively protein bound (95%).

CILOSTAZOL IN SECONDARY PREVENTION OF STROKE OR TIA

The Cilostazol Stroke Prevention Study (CSPS), a randomized, placebo-controlled, double-blind trial, included 1052 Japanese patients with recent ischemic stroke (one to six months). Cilostazol (100 mg twice daily) was compared with placebo over nearly two years follow-up. CSPS showed that the cilostazol group had a significant relative risk reduction of 41.7% (95% CI, 9.2-62.5; $P = .015$) in the recurrence of ischemic stroke compared to placebo group. The greatest risk reduction of cilostazol over placebo was found in patients with lacunar infarction (RRR 43.4%; 95% CI, 3-67; $P = .0373$), suggesting that cilostazol might have a specific benefit in small vessel disease. Patients in the cilostazol group had significantly more headache and palpitations, increase in pulse rate, and increase in serum high-density lipoprotein (HDL) than those in the placebo group.[76,77] A subgroup analysis of CSPS showed that cilostazol was superior to placebo in reducing rates of cerebral infarction in high-risk patients with diabetes and/or hypertension.[78] The Cilostazol versus Aspirin for Secondary Ischemic Stroke Prevention (CASISP) study, a prospective, double-blind, randomized trial, compared cilostazol (100 mg twice daily) with aspirin (100 mg/d) in 719 patients with ischemic stroke within one to six months. The follow-up period was 12 to 18 months. The primary endpoint was any recurrence of stroke (ischemic stroke, hemorrhagic stroke, or subarachnoid hemorrhage). The study showed no significant difference in the rate of recurrent stroke between the cilostazol and aspirin groups, but trended to a higher rate of recurrent stroke in the cilostazol group (HR 0.62; 95% CI. 0.30-1.26; $P = .185$). Subjects treated with cilostazol had a higher incidence of headache, dizziness, and tachycardia.[79] The second Cilostazol Stroke Prevention Study (CSPS 2), an aspirin-controlled, double-blind, randomized noninferiority trial, established the noninferiority of cilostazol (100 mg twice daily) versus aspirin (81 mg once daily) for the prevention of stroke and compared the efficacy and safety of both drugs in 2757 patients with noncardioembolic ischemic stroke. The mean follow-up was 29 months and the primary endpoint was the first occurrence of stroke (cerebral infarction, cerebral hemorrhage, or subarachnoid hemorrhage). The primary endpoint occurred in 2.76% of the cilostazol group and 3.71% of the aspirin group (HR 0.734; 95% CI, 0.564-0.981; $P = .03$). This study showed no significant difference in the occurrence of ischemic stroke and ischemic stroke or TIA between the groups ($P = .4189$ and $P = .4582$, respectively). Patients on cilostazol had significantly fewer hemorrhagic events but more headache, diarrhea, palpitation, dizziness, and tachycardia.[80]

In addition to its role in secondary stroke prevention, one study demonstrated that cilostazol was superior to placebo in preventing the progression of symptomatic intracranial arterial stenosis.[81] This finding is being pursued in an ongoing study (CATHARSIS). Cilostazol appears to be noninferior and safe relative to aspirin. However, larger trials comparing cilostazol with standard antiplatelet therapies in broad ethnic groups are needed.

Triflusal

MECHANISM OF ACTION

The pharmacokinetics and pharmacodynamics of triflusal are described in Table 7-1.[82,83]

Triflusal inhibits platelet aggregation and interaction with subendothelium. The primary mechanism is selective inhibition of arachidonic acid metabolism in platelets through irreversible COX-1 inhibition and reduced thromboxane B_2 (TXB_2) production, sparing the metabolic function of vascular endothelial cells.[84] This mechanism differs from that of aspirin because aspirin inhibits both platelet and vascular endothelial arachidonic acid metabolism. Triflusal has an active metabolite, 3-hydroxy-4-trifluoro-methylbenzoic acid (HTB), which is less potent in inhibiting COX-1 and reducing TXB_2 than triflusal. Triflusal is also less potent in inhibiting COX-1 and reducing TXB_2 than aspirin. However, HTB potentiates the effect of triflusal on COX-1 inhibition.[84] Triflusal can increase levels of cGMP and inhibit cAMP phosphodiesterase, leading to an increase in cAMP, a decrease in calcium mobilization, and ultimately decreased platelet aggregation.[82,83] Triflusal also enhances the production of nitric oxide (NO) by neutrophils by as much as 150%.[82,83] Moreover, triflusal has a potential neuroprotective effect based on multiple mechanisms including decreased oxidative stress and decreased prostaglandin accumulation.[83]

TRIFLUSAL IN SECONDARY PREVENTION OF STROKE OR TIA

A pilot study compared triflusal (300 mg thrice daily) to aspirin (330 mg daily) in 217 patients with ischemic stroke. After four years of follow-up, the combined incidence of cerebral infarcts, ischemic cardiomyopathy, and vascular death was not significantly different between the two drugs but triflusal reduced hemorrhagic complications by 76% compared with aspirin.[85] The Triflusal versus Aspirin in Cerebral Infarction Prevention (TACIP) study was a randomized, double-blind trial comparing triflusal (600 mg/d) to aspirin (325 mg/d) in 2113 patients with ischemic stroke or TIA. The mean follow-up period was 30.1 months. The study showed no significant difference between the two arms in both a composite endpoint (the incidence of nonfatal ischemic stroke, nonfatal acute myocardial infarction, or vascular death; 13.1% for triflusal, 12.4% for aspirin [HR 1.09; 95% CI, 0.85-1.38; $P = .647$]) and the incidence of these events separately. However, the overall incidence of hemorrhage was significantly lower in the triflusal group (16.7% vs 25.2%; OR 0.76; 95% CI, 0.67-0.86; $P < .001$).[86] TAPIRSS (Triflusal versus Aspirin for Prevention of Infarction: a Randomized Stroke Study) compared aspirin (325 mg daily) with triflusal (600 mg daily) in 429 patients with ischemic stroke or TIA. The mean follow-up was 586 days. The results were similar to those of the TACIP study. No differences were found in the primary combined endpoint (the incidence of vascular death, cerebral ischemic infarction, nonfatal myocardial infarction, or major hemorrhage; aspirin 13.9%, triflusal 12.7% [OR 1.11; 95% CI, 0.64-1.94; $P = .711$]) and each event separately. The overall rate of hemorrhagic events was significantly lower in the triflusal group.[87]

Triflusal is effective in the prevention of vascular complications after ischemic stroke or TIA and has a lower risk of hemorrhagic complications. However, larger phase three studies in disparate ethnic groups are needed.

Sarpogrelate

MECHANISM OF ACTION

Sarpogrelate is a selective 5-hydroxytryptamine (5-HT) receptor antagonist that inhibits responses to 5-HT mediated by 5-HT$_{2A}$ receptors, including platelet aggregation and vasoconstriction.[88] 5-HT has a role in the pathogenesis of athero-thrombosis and induces platelet activation.[89] 5-HT released from intracellular storage sites in activated platelets stimulates smooth muscle cell proliferation, inducing thrombus formation and vessel occlusion.[90] Previous studies found that 5-HT concentration was higher in patients with stroke.[89] A double-blind, controlled clinical-pharmacological study of three different dosages of sarpogrelate (25 mg, 50 mg, or 100 mg three times daily for seven days) in 47 patients with ischemic stroke showed that sarpogrelate treatment inhibited platelet aggregation in a dose-dependent fashion.[91]

SARPOGRELATE IN SECONDARY PREVENTION OF STROKE OR TIA

The Sarpogrelate-Aspirin Comparative Clinical Study for Efficacy and Safety in Secondary Prevention of Cerebral Infarction (S-ACCESS), a randomized, double-blind study, compared sarpogrelate (100 mg three times per day) with aspirin (81 mg/d) in 1510 patients with recent ischemic stroke. Mean follow-up was 1.59 years. The rate of recurrence of cerebral infarction was not significantly different between sarpogrelate and aspirin (6.09%/year vs 4.86%/year; HR 1.25; 95% CI, 0.89-1.77; $P = .19$). The overall rate of bleeding was lower in the sarpogrelate arm as compared to the aspirin arm (11.9% and 17.3%, respectively; $P < .01$).[92] Additional clinical studies are needed.

ASPIRIN PLUS CLOPIDOGREL IN SECONDARY PREVENTION OF STROKE OR TIA

Several trials have tested combination clopidogrel and aspirin versus monotherapy for early and late stroke recurrence. MATCH (Management of ATherothrombosis with Clopidogrel in High-risk patients), a randomized, double-blind, placebo-controlled trial, compared aspirin (75 mg/d) with placebo in 7599 high-risk patients with recent ischemic stroke or transient ischemic attack and at least one additional vascular risk factor. The follow-up was 18 months. There was no significant difference between the rate of the composite endpoint of ischemic stroke, myocardial infarction, vascular death, or rehospitalization in aspirin plus clopidogrel treated subjects compared to clopidogrel therapy alone (15.7% vs 16.7%; RRR 6.4%; 95% CI, -4.6-16.3; $P = .244$). However, the risk of life-threatening or major bleeding is significantly increased by the addition of aspirin to clopidogrel (2.6% vs 1.3%; $P < .0001$).[93]

The Clopidogrel for High Atherothrombotic Risk and Ischemic Stabilization, Management, and Avoidance (CHARISMA) trial enrolled 15,603 patients with either clinically evident cardiovascular disease or multiple risk factors to receive clopidogrel (75 mg per day) plus low-dose aspirin (75-162 mg per day) or placebo plus low-dose aspirin. The median follow-up period was 28 months. The primary outcome (myocardial infarction, stroke, or death from cardiovascular causes) rate did not differ significantly in the clopidogrel plus aspirin (6.8%) and placebo plus aspirin (7.3%) (RR 0.93; 95% CI, 0.83-1.05; P = .22) groups. Subgroup analyses by the type of index atherothrombotic event, including ischemic stroke, were also negative.[94] Based on the results of the MATCH and CHARISMA studies, the combination of aspirin plus clopidogrel is not routinely recommended for secondary stroke prevention. There is an ongoing study sponsored by the National Institutes of Health (NIH). The Secondary Prevention of Small Subcortical Strokes trial (SPS3) will enroll 3000 patients with lacunar stroke confirmed by magnetic resonance imaging (MRI). This trial will compare the efficacy of aspirin (325-mg) plus clopidogrel (75 mg) with aspirin alone (325 mg) in preventing any recurrent stroke, the rate of cognitive decline, and major vascular events. The Fast Assessment of Stroke and Transient ischemic attack to prevent Early Recurrence (FASTER) trial was designed to evaluate the efficacy of combination therapy in preventing early recurrence. This trial enrolled 392 patients with TIA or minor stroke within 24 hours of symptom onset and compared the efficacy of clopidogrel (300 mg loading dose then 75 mg daily) plus aspirin (75 mg daily) with aspirin alone. The patients on clopidogrel plus aspirin trended to have fewer recurrent strokes but more hemorrhagic events than patients on aspirin alone. However, the trial was prematurely stopped due to slow recruitment.[95] There were two small studies (CARESS and CLAIR) in patients with symptomatic carotid or intracranial stenosis that used microembolic signals (MES) on transcranial Doppler ultrasound as a surrogate parameter of drug efficacy.[96,97] Both studies showed that clopidogrel plus aspirin was more effective than aspirin alone in reducing microembolic signals in patients with recently symptomatic large vessel atherosclerosis.

SELECTION OF ORAL ANTIPLATELET THERAPY

Each of the antiplatelet agents (aspirin, clopidogrel, or aspirin plus ER-dipyridamole) is effective in preventing ischemic stroke after stroke or TIA.[98,99] The selection should be individualized and based on patient risk factors, cost, tolerance, compliance, and other clinical factors. Patients who suffer recurrent stroke while taking an antiplatelet agent should undergo extensive exploration for the mechanism of recurrence. Changing antiplatelet agents in this situation may be reasonable but is an unproven strategy. As discussed in Chapter 12, if a patient has a TIA or stroke while on antiplatelet therapy, it is more important to consider other causes of the event than to focus on which antiplatelet agent to use. In the future, platelet functional assays and pharmacogenomics may be useful in individualizing the choice of agent and dose.

REFERENCES

1. Collaborative meta-analysis of randomised trials of antiplatelet therapy for prevention of death, myocardial infarction, and stroke in high risk patients. *BMJ.* 2002;324(7329):71-86.

2. Patrono C, Coller B, FitzGerald GA, Hirsh J, Roth G. Platelet-active drugs: the relationships among dose, effectiveness, and side effects: the Seventh ACCP Conference on Antithrombotic and Thrombolytic Therapy. *Chest.* 2004;126(3 Suppl):234S-264S.

3. Roth GJ, Majerus PW. The mechanism of the effect of aspirin on human platelets. I. Acetylation of a particulate fraction protein. *J Clin Invest.* 1975;56(3):624-632.

4. Burch JW, Stanford N, Majerus PW. Inhibition of platelet prostaglandin synthetase by oral aspirin. *J Clin Invest.* 1978;61(2):314-319.

5. Awtry EH, Loscalzo J. Aspirin. *Circulation.* 2000;101(10):1206-1218.

6. FitzGerald GA, Oates JA. Selective and nonselective inhibition of thromboxane formation. *Clin Pharmacol Ther.* 1984;35(5):633-640.

7. Loll PJ, Picot D, Garavito RM. The structural basis of aspirin activity inferred from the crystal structure of inactivated prostaglandin H2 synthase. *Nat Struct Biol.* 1995;2(8):637-643.

8. Vane JR, Bakhle YS, Botting RM. Cyclooxygenases 1 and 2. *Annu Rev Pharmacol Toxicol.* 1998;38: 97-120.

9. Patrono C, Coller B, Dalen JE, et al. Platelet-active drugs: the relationships among dose, effectiveness, and side effects. *Chest.* 1998;114(5 Suppl):470S-488S.

10. Patrignani P, Filabozzi P, Patrono C. Selective cumulative inhibition of platelet thromboxane production by low-dose aspirin in healthy subjects. *J Clin Invest.* 1982;69(6):1366-1372.

11. A comparison of two doses of aspirin (30 mg vs. 283 mg a day) in patients after a transient ischemic attack or minor ischemic stroke. The Dutch TIA Trial Study Group. *N Engl J Med.* 1991;325(18): 1261-1266.

12. Moncada S, Gryglewski R, Bunting S, Vane JR. An enzyme isolated from arteries transforms prostaglandin endoperoxides to an unstable substance that inhibits platelet aggregation. *Nature.* 1976;263(5579):663-665.

13. Clarke RJ, Mayo G, Price P, FitzGerald GA. Suppression of thromboxane A2 but not of systemic prostacyclin by controlled-release aspirin. *N Engl J Med.* 1991;325(16):1137-1141.

14. Catella-Lawson F. Vascular biology of thrombosis: platelet-vessel wall interactions and aspirin effects. *Neurology.* 2001;57(5 Suppl 2):S5-S7.

15. Tran HA, Anand SS, Hankey GJ, Eikelboom JW. Aspirin resistance. *Thromb Res.* 2007;120(3): 337-346.

16. Patrono C. Aspirin resistance: definition, mechanisms and clinical read-outs. *J Thromb Haemost.* 2003;1(8):1710-1713.

17. Weber AA, Przytulski B, Schanz A, Hohlfeld T, Schror K. Towards a definition of aspirin resistance: a typological approach. *Platelets.* 2002;13(1):37-40.

18. Hohlfeld T, Weber AA, Junghans U, et al. Variable platelet response to aspirin in patients with ischemic stroke. *Cerebrovasc Dis.* 2007;24(1):43-50.

19. Uchiyama S, Nakamura T, Yamazaki M, Kimura Y, Iwata M. New modalities and aspects of antiplatelet therapy for stroke prevention. *Cerebrovasc Dis.* 2006;21(Suppl 1):7-16.

20. Hovens MM, Snoep JD, Eikenboom JC, van der Bom JG, Mertens BJ, Huisman MV. Prevalence of persistent platelet reactivity despite use of aspirin: a systematic review. *Am Heart J.* 2007;153(2): 175-181.

21. Krasopoulos G, Brister SJ, Beattie WS, Buchanan MR. Aspirin "resistance" and risk of cardiovascular morbidity: systematic review and meta-analysis. *BMJ.* 2008;336(7637):195-198.

22. Grotemeyer KH, Scharafinski HW, Husstedt IW. Two-year follow-up of aspirin responder and aspirin non responder. A pilot-study including 180 post-stroke patients. *Thromb Res.* 1993;71(5):397-403.

23. Bennett D, Yan B, Macgregor L, Eccleston D, Davis SM. A pilot study of resistance to aspirin in stroke patients. *J Clin Neurosci.* 2008;15(11):1204-1209.

24. Alberts MJ, Bergman DL, Molner E, Jovanovic BD, Ushiwata I, Teruya J. Antiplatelet effect of aspirin in patients with cerebrovascular disease. *Stroke.* 2004;35(1):175-178.

25. Alberts MJ. Platelet function testing for aspirin resistance is reasonable to do: yes! *Stroke.* 2010;41(10): 2400-2401.

26. A randomized trial of aspirin and sulfinpyrazone in threatened stroke. The Canadian Cooperative Study Group. *N Engl J Med.* 1978;299(2):53-59.

27. Swedish Aspirin Low-Dose Trial (SALT) of 75 mg aspirin as secondary prophylaxis after cerebrovascular ischaemic events. The SALT Collaborative Group. *Lancet.* 1991;338(8779):1345-1349.

28. Collaborative overview of randomised trials of antiplatelet therapy—I: prevention of death, myocardial infarction, and stroke by prolonged antiplatelet therapy in various categories of patients. Antiplatelet Trialists' Collaboration. *BMJ.* 1994;308(6921):81-106.

29. Farrell B, Godwin J, Richards S, Warlow C. The United Kingdom transient ischaemic attack (UK-TIA) aspirin trial: final results. *J Neurol Neurosurg Psychiatry.* 1991;54(12):1044-1054.

30. Johnson ES, Lanes SF, Wentworth CE 3rd, Satterfield MH, Abebe BL, Dicker LW. A metaregression analysis of the dose-response effect of aspirin on stroke. *Arch Intern Med.* 1999;159(11):1248-1253.

31. He J, Whelton PK, Vu B, Klag MJ. Aspirin and risk of hemorrhagic stroke: a meta-analysis of randomized controlled trials. *JAMA.* 1998;280(22):1930-1935.

32. Thebault JJ, Kieffer G, Lowe GD, Nimmo WS, Cariou R. Repeated-dose pharmacodynamics of clopidogrel in healthy subjects. *Semin Thromb Hemost.* 1999;25(Suppl 2):9-14.

33. Savcic M, Hauert J, Bachmann F, Wyld PJ, Geudelin B, Cariou R. Clopidogrel loading dose regimens: kinetic profile of pharmacodynamic response in healthy subjects. *Semin Thromb Hemost.* 1999;25(Suppl 2):15-19.

34. Gurbel PA, Tantry US. Clopidogrel resistance? *Thromb Res.* 2007;120(3):311-321.

35. Ma TK, Lam YY, Tan VP, Kiernan TJ, Yan BP. Impact of genetic and acquired alteration in cytochrome P450 system on pharmacologic and clinical response to clopidogrel. *Pharmacol Ther.* 2010;125(2):249-259.

36. A randomised, blinded, trial of clopidogrel versus aspirin in patients at risk of ischaemic events (CAPRIE). CAPRIE Steering Committee. *Lancet.* 1996;348(9038):1329-1339.

37. Nguyen TA, Diodati JG, Pharand C. Resistance to clopidogrel: a review of the evidence. *J Am Coll Cardiol.* 2005;45(8):1157-1164.

38. Gurbel PA, Bliden KP, Hiatt BL, O'Connor CM. Clopidogrel for coronary stenting: response variability, drug resistance, and the effect of pretreatment platelet reactivity. *Circulation.* 2003;107(23):2908-2913.

39. Holmes DR Jr, Dehmer GJ, Kaul S, Leifer D, O'Gara PT, Stein CM. ACCF/AHA clopidogrel clinical alert: approaches to the FDA "boxed warning": a report of the American College of Cardiology Foundation Task Force on clinical expert consensus documents and the American Heart Association endorsed by the Society for Cardiovascular Angiography and Interventions and the Society of Thoracic Surgeons. *J Am Coll Cardiol.* 2010;56(4):321-341.

40. Mega JL, Close SL, Wiviott SD, et al. Cytochrome P-450 polymorphisms and response to clopidogrel. *N Engl J Med.* 2009;360(4):354-362.

41. Simon T, Verstuyft C, Mary-Krause M, et al. Genetic determinants of response to clopidogrel and cardiovascular events. *N Engl J Med.* 2009;360(4):363-375.

42. Sofi F, Giusti B, Marcucci R, Gori AM, Abbate R, Gensini GF. Cytochrome P450 2C19(*)2 polymorphism and cardiovascular recurrences in patients taking clopidogrel: a meta-analysis. *Pharmacogenomics J.* Mar 30 2010. [Epub ahead of print]

43. Pare G, Mehta SR, Yusuf S, et al. Effects of CYP2C19 genotype on outcomes of clopidogrel treatment. *N Engl J Med.* 2010;363(18):1704-1714.

44. Juurlink DN, Gomes T, Ko DT, et al. A population-based study of the drug interaction between proton pump inhibitors and clopidogrel. *CMAJ.* 2009;180(7):713-718.

45. Sacco RL, Diener HC, Yusuf S, et al. Aspirin and extended-release dipyridamole versus clopidogrel for recurrent stroke. *N Engl J Med.* 2008;359(12):1238-1251.

46. Bath PM, Cotton D, Martin RH, et al. Effect of combined aspirin and extended-release dipyridamole versus clopidogrel on functional outcome and recurrence in acute, mild ischemic stroke: PRoFESS subgroup analysis. *Stroke.* 2010;41(4):732-738.

47. Shalito I, Kopyleva O, Serebruany V. Novel antiplatelet agents in development: prasugrel, ticagrelor, and cangrelor and beyond. *Am J Ther.* 2009;16(5):451-458.

48. Cattaneo M. New P2Y12 blockers. *J Thromb Haemost.* 2009;7(Suppl 1):262-265.

49. Asai F, Jakubowski JA, Naganuma H, et al. Platelet inhibitory activity and pharmacokinetics of prasugrel (CS-747) a novel thienopyridine P2Y12 inhibitor: a single ascending dose study in healthy humans. *Platelets.* 2006;17(4):209-217.

50. Wiviott SD, Braunwald E, McCabe CH, et al. Prasugrel versus clopidogrel in patients with acute coronary syndromes. *N Engl J Med.* 2007;357(20):2001-2015.

51. Serebruany VL, Alberts MJ, Hanley DF. Prasugrel in the poststroke cohort of the TRITON trial: the clear and present danger. *Cerebrovasc Dis.* 2008;26(1):93-94.

52. Husted S, Emanuelsson H, Heptinstall S, Sandset PM, Wickens M, Peters G. Pharmacodynamics, pharmacokinetics, and safety of the oral reversible P2Y12 antagonist AZD6140 with aspirin in patients with atherosclerosis: a double-blind comparison to clopidogrel with aspirin. *Eur Heart J.* 2006;27(9): 1038-1047.

53. Best LC, McGuire MB, Jones PB, et al. Mode of action of dipyridamole on human platelets. *Thromb Res.* 1979;16(3-4):367-379.

54. Kim HH, Liao JK. Translational therapeutics of dipyridamole. *Arterioscler Thromb Vasc Biol.* 2008;28(3):s39-s42.

55. d'Esterre CD, Lee TY. Effect of dipyridamole during acute stroke: exploring antithrombosis and neuroprotective benefits. *Ann N Y Acad Sci.* 2010;1207:71-75.

56. Lenz T, Wilson A. Clinical pharmacokinetics of antiplatelet agents used in the secondary prevention of stroke. *Clin Pharmacokinet.* 2003;42(10):909-920.

57. Bousser MG, Eschwege E, Haguenau M, et al. "AICLA" controlled trial of aspirin and dipyridamole in the secondary prevention of athero-thrombotic cerebral ischemia. *Stroke.* 1983;14(1):5-14.

58. Persantine Aspirin Trial in cerebral ischemia. Part II: endpoint results. The American-Canadian Co-Operative Study group. *Stroke.* 1985;16(3):406-415.

59. The European Stroke Prevention Study (ESPS). Principal end-points. The ESPS Group. *Lancet.* 1987;2(8572):1351-1354.

60. Diener HC, Cunha L, Forbes C, Sivenius J, Smets P, Lowenthal A. European Stroke Prevention Study. 2. Dipyridamole and acetylsalicylic acid in the secondary prevention of stroke. *J Neurol Sci.* 1996; 143(1-2):1-13.

61. Halkes PH, van Gijn J, Kappelle LJ, Koudstaal PJ, Algra A. Aspirin plus dipyridamole versus aspirin alone after cerebral ischaemia of arterial origin (ESPRIT): randomised controlled trial. *Lancet.* 2006;367(9523):1665-1673.

62. Chamorro A. TP receptor antagonism: a new concept in atherothrombosis and stroke prevention. *Cerebrovasc Dis.* 2009;27(Suppl 3):20-27.

63. Bal Dit Sollier C, Crassard I, Simoneau G, Bergmann JF, Bousser MG, Drouet L. Effect of the thromboxane prostaglandin receptor antagonist terutroban on arterial thrombogenesis after repeated administration in patients treated for the prevention of ischemic stroke. *Cerebrovasc Dis.* 2009;28(5):505-513.

64. Osende JI, Shimbo D, Fuster V, Dubar M, Badimon JJ. Antithrombotic effects of S 18886, a novel orally active thromboxane A2 receptor antagonist. *J Thromb Haemost.* 2004;2(3):492-498.

65. Belhassen L, Pelle G, Dubois-Rande JL, Adnot S. Improved endothelial function by the thromboxane A2 receptor antagonist S 18886 in patients with coronary artery disease treated with aspirin. *J Am Coll Cardiol.* 2003;41(7):1198-1204.

66. Egan KM, Wang M, Fries S, et al. Cyclooxygenases, thromboxane, and atherosclerosis: plaque destabilization by cyclooxygenase-2 inhibition combined with thromboxane receptor antagonism. *Circulation.* 2005;111(3):334-342.

67. Hennerici MG, Bots ML, Ford I, Laurent S, Touboul PJ. Rationale, design and population baseline characteristics of the PERFORM vascular project: an ancillary study of the Prevention of cerebrovascular and cardiovascular Events of ischemic origin with teRutroban in patients with a history oF ischemic strOke or tRansient ischeMic attack (PERFORM) trial. *Cardiovasc Drugs Ther.* 2010;24(2):175-180.

68. Gaussem P, Reny JL, Thalamas C, et al. The specific thromboxane receptor antagonist S18886: pharmacokinetic and pharmacodynamic studies. *J Thromb Haemost.* 2005;3(7):1437-1445.

69. Bousser MG, Amarenco P, Chamorro A, et al. The Prevention of cerebrovascular and cardiovascular Events of ischemic origin with teRutroban in patients with a history oF ischemic strOke or tRansient ischeMic attack (PERFORM) study: baseline characteristics of the population. *Cerebrovasc Dis.* 2009; 27(6):608-613.

70. Bousser MG, Amarenco P, Chamorro A, et al. Rationale and design of a randomized, double-blind, parallel-group study of terutroban 30 mg/day versus aspirin 100 mg/day in stroke patients: the prevention of cerebrovascular and cardiovascular events of ischemic origin with terutroban in patients with a history of ischemic stroke or transient ischemic attack (PERFORM) study. *Cerebrovasc Dis.* 2009;27(5): 509-518.

71. Hong KW, Lee JH, Kima KY, Park SY, Lee WS. Cilostazol: therapeutic potential against focal cerebral ischemic damage. *Curr Pharm Des.* 2006;12(5):565-573.

72. Minami N, Suzuki Y, Yamamoto M, et al. Inhibition of shear stress-induced platelet aggregation by cilostazol, a specific inhibitor of cGMP-inhibited phosphodiesterase, in vitro and ex vivo. *Life Sci.* 1997;61(25):PL 383-389.

73. Tamai Y, Takami H, Nakahata R, Ono F, Munakata A. Comparison of the effects of acetylsalicylic acid, ticlopidine and cilostazol on primary hemostasis using a quantitative bleeding time test apparatus. *Haemostasis.* 1999;29(5):269-276.

74. Schror K. The pharmacology of cilostazol. *Diabetes Obes Metab.* 2002;4(Suppl 2):S14-S19.

75. Yasunaga K, Mase K. Antiaggregatory effect of oral cilostazol and recovery of platelet aggregability in patients with cerebrovascular disease. *Arzneimittelforschung.* 1985;35(7A):1189-1192.

76. Gotoh F, Tohgi H, Hirai S, et al. Cilostazol stroke prevention study: a placebo-controlled double-blind trial for secondary prevention of cerebral infarction. *J Stroke Cerebrovasc Dis.* 2000;9:147-157.

77. Matsumoto M. Cilostazol in secondary prevention of stroke: impact of the Cilostazol Stroke Prevention Study. *Atheroscler Suppl.* 2005;6(4):33-40.

78. Shinohara Y, Gotoh F, Tohgi H, et al. Antiplatelet cilostazol is beneficial in diabetic and/or hypertensive ischemic stroke patients. Subgroup analysis of the cilostazol stroke prevention study. *Cerebrovasc Dis.* 2008;26(1):63-70.

79. Huang Y, Cheng Y, Wu J, et al. Cilostazol as an alternative to aspirin after ischaemic stroke: a randomised, double-blind, pilot study. *Lancet Neurol.* 2008;7(6):494-499.

80. Shinohara Y, Katayama Y, Uchiyama S, et al. Cilostazol for prevention of secondary stroke (CSPS 2): an aspirin-controlled, double-blind, randomised non-inferiority trial. *Lancet Neurol.* 2010;9(10):959-968.

81. Kwon SU, Cho YJ, Koo JS, et al. Cilostazol prevents the progression of the symptomatic intracranial arterial stenosis: the multicenter double-blind placebo-controlled trial of cilostazol in symptomatic intracranial arterial stenosis. *Stroke.* 2005;36(4):782-786.

82. McNeely W, Goa KL. Triflusal. *Drugs.* 1998;55(6):823-833.

83. Anninos H, Andrikopoulos G, Pastromas S, Sakellariou D, Theodorakis G, Vardas P. Triflusal: an old drug in modern antiplatelet therapy. Review of its action, use, safety and effectiveness. *Hellenic J Cardiol.* 2009;50(3):199-207.

84. de la Cruz JP, Mata JM, Sanchez de la Cuesta F. Triflusal vs. aspirin on the inhibition of human platelet and vascular cyclooxygenase. *Gen Pharmacol.* 1992;23(2):297-300.

85. Matias-Guiu J, Alvarez-Sabin J, Codina A. Comparative study of the effect of low-dosage acetylsalicylic acid and triflusal in the prevention of cardiovascular events among young adults with ischemic cerebrovascular disease. *Rev Neurol.* 1997;25(147):1669-1672.

86. Matias-Guiu J, Ferro JM, Alvarez-Sabin J, et al. Comparison of triflusal and aspirin for prevention of vascular events in patients after cerebral infarction: the TACIP study: a randomized, double-blind, multicenter trial. *Stroke.* 2003;34(4):840-848.

87. Culebras A, Rotta-Escalante R, Vila J, et al. Triflusal vs. aspirin for prevention of cerebral infarction: a randomized stroke study. *Neurology.* 2004;62(7):1073-1080.

88. Hara H, Osakabe M, Kitajima A, Tamao Y, Kikumoto R. MCI-9042, a new antiplatelet agent is a selective S2-serotonergic receptor antagonist. *Thromb Haemost.* 1991;65(4):415-420.

89. Wiernsperger N. Serotonin 5-HT2 receptors and brain circulation. *J Cardiovasc Pharmacol.* 1990;16(Suppl 3):S20-S24.

90. Nishihira K, Yamashita A, Tanaka N, et al. Inhibition of 5-hydroxytryptamine receptor prevents occlusive thrombus formation on neointima of the rabbit femoral artery. *J Thromb Haemost.* 2006;4(1):247-255.

91. Uchiyama S, Ozaki Y, Satoh K, Kondo K, Nishimaru K. Effect of sarpogrelate, a 5-HT(2A) antagonist, on platelet aggregation in patients with ischemic stroke: clinical-pharmacological dose-response study. *Cerebrovasc Dis.* 2007;24(2-3):264-270.

92. Shinohara Y, Nishimaru K, Sawada T, et al. Sarpogrelate-Aspirin Comparative Clinical Study for Efficacy and Safety in Secondary Prevention of Cerebral Infarction (S-ACCESS): a randomized, double-blind, aspirin-controlled trial. *Stroke.* 2008;39(6):1827-1833.

93. Diener HC, Bogousslavs.ky J, Brass LM, et al. Aspirin and clopidogrel compared with clopidogrel alone after recent ischaemic stroke or transient ischaemic attack in high-risk patients (MATCH): randomised, double-blind, placebo-controlled trial. *Lancet.* 2004;364(9431):331-337.

94. Bhatt DL, Fox KA, Hacke W, et al. Clopidogrel and aspirin versus aspirin alone for the prevention of atherothrombotic events. *N Engl J Med.* 2006;354(16):1706-1717.

95. Kennedy J, Hill MD, Ryckborst KJ, Eliasziw M, Demchuk AM, Buchan AM. Fast assessment of stroke and transient ischaemic attack to prevent early recurrence (FASTER): a randomised controlled pilot trial. *Lancet Neurol.* 2007;6(11):961-969.

96. Markus HS, Droste DW, Kaps M, et al. Dual antiplatelet therapy with clopidogrel and aspirin in symptomatic carotid stenosis evaluated using doppler embolic signal detection: the Clopidogrel and Aspirin for Reduction of Emboli in Symptomatic Carotid Stenosis (CARESS) trial. *Circulation.* 2005;111(17):2233-2240.

97. Wong KS, Chen C, Fu J, et al. Clopidogrel plus aspirin versus aspirin alone for reducing embolisation in patients with acute symptomatic cerebral or carotid artery stenosis (CLAIR study): a randomised, open-label, blinded-endpoint trial. *Lancet Neurol.* 2010;9(5):489-497.

98. Furie KL, Kasner SE, Adams RJ, et al. Guidelines for the prevention of stroke in patients with stroke or transient ischemic attack: a guideline for healthcare professionals from the American Heart Association/ American Stroke Association. *Stroke.* 2011;42(1):227-276.

99. Guidelines for management of ischaemic stroke and transient ischaemic attack 2008. *Cerebrovasc Dis.* 2008;25(5):457-507.

Anticoagulation

8

Hen Hallevi
Eitan Auriel
Natan M. Bornstein

TOPICS

Anticoagulants are frequently prescribed for stroke prevention (both primary and secondary prevention). The most common indications are atrial fibrillation (AF) and prosthetic heart valves (see Table 8–1). Most of the evidence we have for the efficacy of anticoagulants in stroke prevention comes from the large atrial fibrillation trials. Six randomized controlled clinical trials have compared warfarin with either control or placebo for the prevention of stroke in patients with nonvalvular AF.[1-6] With the exception of the EAFT (European Atrial Fibrillation Trial), which was a secondary prevention trial,[3] all these trials studied primary stroke prevention. Warfarin was the oral vitamin K antagonist of choice in the primary prevention studies, whereas the EAFT study[3] used phenprocoumon or acenocoumarol. Despite significant variations in trial design and different intensities of anticoagulation and outcomes, the results were quite consistent. Meta-analyses of adjusted-dose warfarin in patients with AF showed a 60% reduction in the relative risk of stroke or systemic embolism and a 30% reduced all-cause mortality compared to placebo.[7] Warfarin was also superior to the combination of aspirin and clopidogrel.[8] Indeed there are few interventions in preventive medicine showing comparable efficacy. The mainstays of anticoagulant therapy are the coumarins (warfarin and acenocoumarol) that antagonize vitamin K activity in the liver and reduce the production of several clotting factors of the intrinsic coagulation pathway, including factors II, VII, IX, and X, as well as protein C and S. The result is prolongation of the prothrombin time and international normalized ratio (INR), and the partial thromboplastin time is relatively unaffected. Newer anticoagulants include the direct thrombin inhibitors and antagonists of factor Xa (see later). Anticoagulation for stroke prevention in patients with AF should be prescribed according to the CHADS$_2$ score (Table 8–2).[9] According to this simple clinical

Table 8–1. Causes of Cardioembolic Stroke

Location	Cause
Atrial	Atrial fibrillation Left atrial myxoma Sustained atrial flutter Patent foramen ovale Atrial septal aneurysm
Valvular	Rheumatic heart disease of the left heart Prosthetic mitral or aortic valve Infective endocarditis Marantic endocarditis Libman-Sacks endocarditis Fibroelastoma of the mitral or aortic valve
Ventricular	Left ventricular thrombus Recent anterior wall myocardial infarction Dilated cardiomyopathy Akinetic wall segment Apical aneurysm Severe congestive heart failure

tool the risk of stroke increases with age and additional risk factors such as hypertension, heart failure, diabetes, and previous embolization. Valvular disease of the left heart (although not part of the $CHADS_2$ score) also dramatically increases the risk for stroke[10] and must be taken into account when considering this treatment. Recently, a new score based on the $CHADS_2$ and the 2006 American College of Cardiology guidelines risk scheme was introduced, called CA_2DS_2-VASC.[11] This new scheme includes additional risk factors such as female sex and the presence of vascular risk factors. It has been validated on a large European cohort and was shown to be superior to the $CHADS_2$ score in identifying AF patients who are at high risk of stroke despite anticoagulation.[12] Its added usefulness over the $CHADS_2$ score in clinical practice remains to be determined. Anticoagulation therapy carries

Table 8–2. The $CHADS_2$ Score

Risk Factor	Points
Congestive heart failure	1
Hypertension	1
Age ≥75	1
Diabetes	1
Prior **S**troke/TIA/systemic embolus	2

a real risk for systemic and intracerebral hemorrhage. Although this risk can be minimized with careful attention to INR control within the therapeutic window,[13] it is the most common reason for failure to prescribe anticoagulation in a patient with a clear indication. The other common reason is patient preference not to take the drug because of the need for frequent blood draws and dietary limitations. The recent introduction of simple-to-use home self-monitoring tools should enhance patient comfort and compliance with the drug. It does seem, however, that self-monitoring does not reduce the rate of stroke and bleeding complication as compared to high-quality clinic visits.[14]

UTILIZATION OF VKA ANTAGONISTS IN ELDERLY PATIENTS

Elderly patients who stand to benefit most from anticoagulation are often denied this therapy. Recurrent falls, difficulty in drug management, and uncertain compliance are the most frequently quoted reasons. Primary care physicians, neurologists, and cardiologists all share this tendency, which results in significant underuse of warfarin in the elderly.[15] In a cross-sectional study of 11,082 patients with nonvalvular AF who could walk, only 59% with at least one risk factor for stroke and no specific contraindications received anticoagulation therapy.[15] Of these, 60.7% of those aged 65 to 74 years and 35.4% of those aged 85 years or older used warfarin.

High risk of falls is a significant barrier to treatment of elderly patients. Indeed, the risk of intracranial hemorrhage is increased in the elderly. When compared with patients 50 years of age, the unadjusted relative risk of patients 80 years of age or older having a life-threatening or fatal bleed on warfarin was 4.5 (95% confidence interval [CI], 1.3-15.6).[16] Careful monitoring of INR can minimize this risk. It appears that an INR of 2.0 to 3.0 provides the best balance between bleeding risk and stroke prevention benefit. One study showed that an INR of 3.5 to 3.9 was associated with an increased risk of intracranial hemorrhage (ICH) when compared to an INR of less than 2.0 (adjusted odds ratio [OR] 4.6; 95% CI, 2.3-9.4), but an INR of 2.0 to 3.0 was not (adjusted OR 1.3; 95% CI, 0.8-2.2).[13] In analyses from the SPORTIF III and SPORTIF V trials, higher rates of bleeding were seen among patients who had poor INR control compared with those with good control.[17]

With regard to the risk of hemorrhage in patients with "high risk" of falling, a meta-analysis of antithrombotic therapy in elderly patients at risk for falls concluded that the propensity for falling in elderly patients should not be an important factor when deciding whether or not to treat with anticoagulation in an elderly patient.[18] In this work, the quality-adjusted life expectancy was greatest for warfarin, followed by aspirin, followed by no therapy. This remained true unless the annual stroke risk was less than 2%. They found that an elderly patient taking warfarin would have to fall almost daily (300 times per year) for the risk of bleeding complications from falling to outweigh the benefits of warfarin therapy. Although this work may underestimate the risk-benefit ratio, it does appear that elderly patients with CHADS$_2$ score 2 or greater who are not at exceptionally high risk of fall and head trauma are more likely to benefit from anticoagulation in the setting of AF than not, provided that standard INR monitoring is done.

PHARMACOGENETIC DOSING OF WARFARIN

There is a great interindividual variability in the weekly dose of warfarin required for INR maintenance. This is related to clinical and demographic parameters such as height, weight, age, and race, as well as variations in two genes—cytochrome P450, family 2, subfamily C, polypeptide 9 (CYP2C9); and vitamin K epoxide reductase complex, subunit 1 (VKORC1).[19-22] Keeping in mind the importance of strict INR control, accounting for these variables becomes an important health care issue. A recent large, retrospective study of patients starting warfarin therapy compared three models for their success in predicting the stable weekly maintenance dose: a fixed-dose model (5 mg per day), a clinical model based on clinical variables such as weight and ethnicity, and a "pharmacogenetic" model using both clinical and genetic variables. The pharmacogenetic model was superior to both other models, and the clinical model was superior to the fixed-dose model, in the 46% of patients requiring warfarin doses outside the "midrange" (21-49 mg/wk). Interestingly, for the 54% of patients requiring the midrange, the pharmacogenetic model performed slightly better than the clinical model but was comparable to the fixed-dose model.[23] Another study comparing a pharmacogenetic versus a clinical model found that hospitalizations for hemorrhage were 28% less common in the group of patients for whom genetic information on CYP2C9 and VKORC1 had been supplied to prescribing physicians than in the control group.[24] Following this and other studies, the Food and Drug Administration (FDA) has recently revised the product label of warfarin suggesting the use of the pharmacogenetic model if genetic information is available.[25,26] We recommend that an effort is made to check the gene status of every patient considered for warfarin therapy and apply the pharmacogenetic model according to the FDA guidelines. If not feasible, one should resort to the clinical model. Web-based "warfarin calculators" that use both clinical and genetic data are freely available and simple to use. They should be used when starting or correcting warfarin dosing.[27]

Warfarin works by competitively inhibiting the enzymatic complex vitamin K epoxide reductase and is eliminated via the cytochrome P450 system in the liver. In addition, the drug is highly bound to plasma proteins (mainly albumin). These three points make warfarin quite sensitive to drug and dietary interactions that influence its therapeutic effect. Drugs may interact with warfarin through pharmacodynamic or pharmacokinetic mechanisms. Pharmacodynamic mechanisms for drug interactions with warfarin are synergism (impaired hemostasis, reduced clotting factor synthesis), competitive antagonism (vitamin K), and altered physiologic control loop for vitamin K metabolism (hereditary resistance). Pharmacokinetic mechanisms for drug interactions with warfarin are mainly enzyme induction, enzyme inhibition, and reduced plasma protein binding. There are many classes of drugs that can potentially influence the INR when coadministered with warfarin. Table 8–3 lists the common and important ones but many others exist that are not listed. It must be borne in mind that in every patient on warfarin, starting a new drug (including herbal remedies) or a change in his or her medical condition (hospitalization, heart failure, diarrhea, etc) mandates close INR monitoring until a new steady state has been achieved.

Table 8–3. Drug Classes and Foods That May Interact With Warfarin and Change (Increase or Decrease) the INR

Drugs	Foods Rich in Vitamin K
Analgesics	Cauliflower
Anesthetics, inhalation	Scallions (green onions)
Antiarrhythmics	Peas
Antibiotics[a]	Garbanzo beans (chick peas)
Aminoglycosides (oral)	Asparagus
Cephalosporins	Green/herbal teas, coffee
Macrolides	Liverwurst, beef liver
Penicillins	Soybean and canola oil
Quinolones	Spinach
Tetracyclines	Kale
Anticonvulsants (mostly "enzyme inducers")	Turnip greens, collard greens, mustard
Antidepressants	greens
Antineoplastics	Broccoli
Hypnotics	Cabbage
Hypolipidemics	Lettuce, parsley, watercress, endive
Bile acid-binding resins	Brussels sprouts
Fibric acid derivatives	
HMG-CoA reductase inhibitors	
Monoamine oxidase inhibitors	
Narcotics	
NSAIDs	
Proton pump inhibitors	
Psychostimulants	
SSRIs	
Steroids	
Thrombolytics	
Thyroid drugs	
Vitamins	

[a]Some interactions with antibiotics are due to a change in intestinal flora, rather than a pharmacokinetic drug-drug interaction.

HMG-CoA, -hydroxy- -methylglutaryl-coenzyme A; INR, international normalized ratio; NSAIDs, nonsteroidal anti-inflammatory drugs; SSRIs, selective serotonin reuptake inhibitors.

Vitamin K–rich foods such as spinach may reduce the effectiveness of warfarin (see Table 8–3). Although it is often recommended that patients reduce the dietary amounts of those foods and maintain a relatively stable diet, the diet that is best for stroke prevention is high in fruits and vegetables (see Chapter 3). An alternative approach to stabilizing INR is to add small amounts of vitamin K (100-500 μg per day); this may result in higher doses of warfarin, but can help to keep the INR within the therapeutic range.[28-31]

STARTING ANTICOAGULATION AFTER STROKE

Acute stroke patients present a special challenge when warfarin needs to be initiated. The most common scenario is a patient with cardioembolic stroke due to AF not previously treated with warfarin. In the immediate period following a stroke the risk for hemorrhagic transformation (HT) is elevated due to tissue and vessel damage within the ischemic area. Two patterns are observed: (1) Early HT that presents within three days of the stroke. It is mostly asymptomatic and requires no treatment. (2) Late HT occurring 9 to 12 days poststroke. Late HT is usually symptomatic (ie, worsens the patient's neurological status) and is related to treatment with low-molecular-weight heparin in combination with warfarin (so-called "bridging").[32] The decision to institute chronic anticoagulation (AC) with warfarin is often done while the patient is in the hospital. Typically, in patients with extensive and disabling infarct the decision may be deferred fearing ICH. But many physicians still anticoagulate patients with milder stroke in an attempt to prevent early stroke recurrence. This risk is actually small and the odds of a hemorrhagic complication outweigh the benefit.[33] In addition, many physicians are reluctant to start warfarin without bridging with either heparin or enoxaparin, aiming at prevention of warfarin-related hypercoagulable state and skin necrosis. This is in fact uncommon in routine clinical practice with most cases associated with protein C deficiency.[34] Patients with cardioembolic stroke without a large infarct and HT on follow-up computed tomography (CT) scan may be started on warfarin according to their expected maintenance dose several days after stroke onset. Aspirin 80 to 100 mg should be coadministered until the INR reaches therapeutic level. Heparin for deep vein thrombosis prophylaxis may also be given. Patients with transient ischemic attack (TIA) or minor stroke and no evidence of acute infarction may start warfarin upon admission. In cases of large infarcts or symptomatic HT we recommend waiting a month and reassessing the patient's condition before instituting anticoagulation.[32,35] Many experts, however, would begin anticoagulation after a week. Immediate anticoagulation with heparin or low-molecular-weight heparin should be reserved for situations where another indication exists such as deep vein thrombosis, pulmonary embolus, or mechanical mitral valve.

STOPPING WARFARIN BEFORE A PROCEDURE

It is common to encounter patients who are taking warfarin for primary or secondary stroke prevention and need to undergo an invasive procedure. They can (and often do) suffer a stroke in the periprocedural period due to several causes. The cessation and reinitiation of warfarin is associated with a prothrombogenic state. That, along with the stress of the procedure, puts the patient at increased risk for a stroke.[36-38] We recommend that any patient on warfarin who needs an invasive procedure be put on low-molecular-weight heparin at a therapeutic dose and stop warfarin a week before the procedure. The heparin may be stopped 12 hours before the procedure and restarted at the earliest possible time point. Warfarin then may be restarted at the usual maintenance dose.

NEW ORAL ANTICOAGULANTS

As mentioned, until recently the only available licensed oral anticoagulants were the vitamin K antagonists, such as warfarin.[39,40] Although effective, the treatment is associated with numerous limitations, including influence of daily food intake, different metabolism in the liver, and interaction with other medications leading to the need for routine monitoring, which is inconvenient and expensive.[39,40] A narrow therapeutic range and the need for regular monitoring impair the effectiveness and safety of warfarin. The INR level in many (or most) patients does not stay within the therapeutic range, even with frequent monitoring. Furthermore, oral anticoagulation using warfarin is associated with a significant risk of major bleeding. Limitations associated with warfarin hamper its use and have encouraged pharmaceutical companies to find a replacement for warfarin for long-term therapy. The latter have led to the development of new anticoagulants targeting different sites in the coagulation cascade (Figure 8–1).[41] These new agents target either thrombin or activated factor X (Xa).

Thrombin, also known as coagulation factor II (F2), is produced by the enzymatic cleavage of two sites on prothrombin by factor Xa. Thrombin converts fibrinogen to its active form fibrin. Thrombin also activates factor XI and factor XIII, and promotes platelet activation and aggregation. This positive feedback accelerates the production of thrombin.[39,40,42] Because thrombin is one of the final effectors in the coagulation cascade, it serves as a logical target for novel anticoagulants.

Ximelagatran, an oral direct thrombin inhibitor, and its active form, melagatran, have been compared against conventional anticoagulant therapy in many clinical settings, including venous thromboembolism and stroke prevention in patients with nonvalvular atrial fibrillation (NVAF). The agent was licensed in Europe but was withdrawn from the market and further development by the manufacturer shortly thereafter because of potential hepatotoxicity.[43]

Recently, based on the results of the RCT RE-LY (see below), the FDA approved the novel oral thrombin inhibitor dabigatran etexilate (dabigatran) in the fixed dose of 150 mg twice a day for the prevention of stroke in patients with NVAF, and licensed it as the only oral alternative to warfarin. In other countries (such as Canada), the 110-mg twice-daily dose has been approved; it would be more appropriate for patients with impaired renal function. We might see the use of warfarin supplanted in the near future if the manufacturer of dabigatran can price the drug appropriately.[44]

In contrast to ximelagstran, dabigatran is 80% renal excreted and therefore is not hepatotoxic and has no interaction with cytochrome P450 enzymes. However, some drugs that inhibit P-glycoprotein including verapamil, amiodarone, or quinidine, all used by patients with NVAF, may lead to an increased plasma concentration of dabigatran and consequently increased bleeding risk.

The Randomized Evaluation of Long-term anticoagulation therapy (RE-LY) was a global trial that evaluated two doses of dabigatran, 110 mg bid and 150 mg bid, against usual therapy with warfarin titrated to a target INR of 2.0 to 3.0 in 18,113 patients with NVAF in an open-label fashion.[45] The primary study outcome, at a median follow-up of two years, was stroke or systemic embolism. The primary safety outcome was major hemorrhage. Other outcomes included myocardial infarction, pulmonary embolism, transient ischemic attack, and death. Each primary and secondary outcome was adjudicated by two independent blinded investigators.

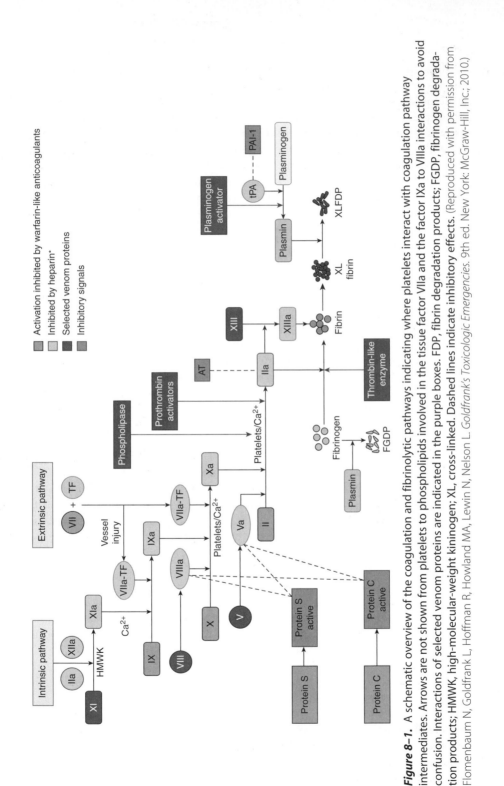

Figure 8-1. A schematic overview of the coagulation and fibrinolytic pathways indicating where platelets interact with coagulation pathway intermediates. Arrows are not shown from platelets to phospholipids involved in the tissue factor VIIa and the factor IXa to VIIIa interactions to avoid confusion. Interactions of selected venom proteins are indicated in the purple boxes. FDP, fibrin degradation products; FGDP, fibrinogen degradation products; HMWK, high-molecular-weight kininogen; XL, cross-linked. Dashed lines indicate inhibitory effects. (Reproduced with permission from Flomenbaum N, Goldfrank L, Hoffman R, Howland MA, Lewin N, Nelson L. *Goldfrank's Toxicologic Emergencies.* 9th ed. New York: McGraw-Hill, Inc.; 2010.)

In the primary analysis the lower dose was not inferior and the higher dose was superior to warfarin for prevention of stroke and systemic embolism (relative risk [RR] 0.90; 95% CI, 0.74-71.1; and RR 0.65; 95% CI, 0.52-50.81, respectively), whereas major bleeding rates were lower for the lower dose and similar for the higher dose compared with warfarin (RR 0.80; 95% CI, 0.70-70.93; and RR 0.93; 95% CI, 0.81-81.87, respectively). Intracranial bleeding rates were lower for both doses. For unknown reasons an increased rate of myocardial infarction was seen with dabigatran compared with warfarin, reaching statistical significance only for the high dose. More trial dropouts occurred with dabigatran than with warfarin, probably because treatment with the former was associated with a higher rate of dyspepsia.

The results of the RE-LY trial demonstrated that dabigatran has the potential to be more effective and safer than the traditional vitamin K antagonists. A recent RE-LY subanalysis showed that dabigatran is at least noninferior to warfarin in all subgroups of NVAF patients at low, moderate, or high risk of stroke.[46]

The RE-LY trial was the first trial to prospectively evaluate a new anticoagulant in warfarin-naïve and experienced populations. A prespecified analysis of the RE-LY trial compared these two subpopulations.[47] The rationale behind this substudy was the belief that patients who are experienced with the taking of vitamin K antagonists have demonstrated the ability to comply with the administration regimen and have a personalized dose of warfarin that achieves the therapeutic values. However, the results of this substudy demonstrated that previous warfarin exposure does not influence the benefit of dabigatran at either dose compared with warfarin.

As opposed to warfarin, dabigatran acts almost immediately; after oral administration patients are therapeutically anticoagulated within two hours, so no bridging therapy with a parenteral drug is required.[39,40] It has a predictable anticoagulant effect, so routine monitoring of its anticoagulant effect and dietary precautions are not necessary. Although it does not require regular dose monitoring, anticoagulant status can be assessed by measuring thrombin clotting time, which may be crucial in the setting of hemorrhage.[46]

Despite the obvious advantages of dabigatran in patients with NVAF compared to warfarin, including better efficacy and safety, and more convenient administration, the agent also has several disadvantages.[39,40,46] Dabigatran should be taken twice daily, in contrast with the traditional vitamin K antagonists, which are administrated only once a day. The need for multiple administrations during the day has been known to reduce adherence and may eventually lead to withdrawal of the medication in some noncompliant patients. The use of dabigatran is also problematic in patients with impaired creatinine clearance because it is 80% renally excreted.[48] The high rate of dyspepsia (~20% of patients) may also complicate intake and result in reduced compliance. The lack of regular monitoring prevents the ability to test patient adherence as it can with warfarin, and the issue of anticoagulation complicates decisions about administration of tissue plasminogen activator (tPA) in the setting of acute stroke. Finally, in contrast with the vitamin K antagonists, an antidote has not yet been developed to be given in cases of severe or life-threatening hemorrhage. Approaches to this problem were reviewed in 2010 by van Ryn et al.[49]

Factor X is activated into factor Xa (Xa), which acts by cleaving prothrombin in two places, consequently forming active thrombin, which serves as the first member of the final common pathway.[50] Therefore, fXa also serves as a good target for new agents. Direct as well as indirect inhibitors of fXa are in various stages of development for their antithrombotic effect. A new parenterally applicable fXa inhibitor is fondaparinux; it has been shown to be effective for several indications, including the prophylaxis and treatment of venous thromboembolism and coronary ischemia.[39,40]

Several other oral fXa inhibitors including the agents rivaroxaban, apixaban, and edoxaban have been studied for stroke prevention in patients with NVAF.[39,40]

The AVERROES trial was a double-blind, double-dummy superiority trial of apixaban 5 mg twice daily compared with ASA 81 to 324 mg once daily in patients with NVAF and at least one risk factor for stroke who had failed or were thought to be unsuitable for warfarin therapy.[51] Apixaban reduced the rate of stroke and systemic embolism by approximately half (hazard ratio [HR] 0.45; 95% CI, 0.32-0.62), with no increase in major or intracranial bleeding (HR 1.13; 95% CI, 0.74-1.75).[39,40]

ROCKET AF was a randomized, double-blind, double-dummy, event-driven trial that aimed to establish the noninferiority of rivaroxaban compared with warfarin in patients with NVAF who had a history of stroke or at least two additional independent risk factors for future stroke.[52] Rivaroxaban 20 mg once daily was noninferior to dose-adjusted warfarin (target INR of 2-3) for the prevention of stroke or systemic embolism (HR 0.79; 95% CI, 0.65-0.95) with no increase in major bleeding (HR 1.04; 95% CI, 0.90-1.20).[39,40]

These novel anticoagulant drugs were developed with the aim of an orally available agent that does not require monitoring and could be applied at a fixed dose. Currently, data from a phase 3 trial for stroke prevention in NVAF are available only for dabigatran and apixaban.[53]; however, the availability of new oral anticoagulants will help to optimize care in patients with NVAF and reduce the devastating complication of stroke.

REFERENCES

1. The effect of low-dose warfarin on the risk of stroke in patients with nonrheumatic atrial fibrillation. The Boston Area Anticoagulation Trial for Atrial Fibrillation Investigators. *N Engl J Med.* 1990;323(22): 1505-1511.

2. Stroke Prevention in Atrial Fibrillation Study. Final results. *Circulation.* 1991;84(2):527-539.

3. Secondary prevention in non-rheumatic atrial fibrillation after transient ischaemic attack or minor stroke. EAFT (European Atrial Fibrillation Trial) Study Group. *Lancet.* 1993;342(8882):1255-1262.

4. Connolly SJ, Laupacis A, Gent M, Roberts RS, Cairns JA, Joyner C. Canadian Atrial Fibrillation Anticoagulation (CAFA) Study. *J Am Coll Cardiol.* 1991;18(2):349-355.

5. Ezekowitz MD, Bridgers SL, James KE, et al. Warfarin in the prevention of stroke associated with nonrheumatic atrial fibrillation. Veterans Affairs Stroke Prevention in Nonrheumatic Atrial Fibrillation Investigators. *N Engl J Med.* 1992;327(20):1406-1412.

6. Petersen P, Boysen G, Godtfredsen J, Andersen ED, Andersen B. Placebo-controlled, randomised trial of warfarin and aspirin for prevention of thromboembolic complications in chronic atrial fibrillation. The Copenhagen AFASAK study. *Lancet.* 1989;1(8631):175-179.

7. Hart RG, Pearce LA, Aguilar MI. Meta-analysis: antithrombotic therapy to prevent stroke in patients who have nonvalvular atrial fibrillation. *Ann Intern Med.* 2007;146(12):857-867.

8. Connolly S, Pogue J, Hart R, et al. Clopidogrel plus aspirin versus oral anticoagulation for atrial fibrillation in the Atrial Fibrillation Clopidogrel Trial with Irbesartan for prevention of Vascular Events (ACTIVE W): a randomised controlled trial. *Lancet.* 2006;367(9526):1903-1912.

9. Gage BF, Waterman AD, Shannon W, Boechler M, Rich MW, Radford MJ. Validation of clinical classification schemes for predicting stroke: results from the National Registry of Atrial Fibrillation. *JAMA.* 2001;285(22):2864-2870.

10. Wolf PA, Abbott RD, Kannel WB. Atrial fibrillation as an independent risk factor for stroke: the Framingham Study. *Stroke.* 1991;22(8):983-988.

11. Lip GY, Nieuwlaat R, Pisters R, Lane DA, Crijns HJ. Refining clinical risk stratification for predicting stroke and thromboembolism in atrial fibrillation using a novel risk factor-based approach: the Euro Heart Survey on Atrial Fibrillation. *Chest.* 2010;137(2):263-272.

12. Lip GY, Frison L, Halperin JL, Lane DA. Identifying patients at high risk for stroke despite anticoagulation: a comparison of contemporary stroke risk stratification schemes in an anticoagulated atrial fibrillation cohort. *Stroke.* 2010;41(12):2731-2738.

13. Fang MC, Chang Y, Hylek EM, et al. Advanced age, anticoagulation intensity, and risk for intracranial hemorrhage among patients taking warfarin for atrial fibrillation. *Ann Intern Med.* 2004;141(10): 745-752.

14. Matchar DB, Jacobson A, Dolor R, et al. Effect of home testing of international normalized ratio on clinical events. *N Engl J Med.* 2010;363(17):1608-1620.

15. Flaker GC, McGowan DJ, Boechler M, Fortune G, Gage B. Underutilization of antithrombotic therapy in elderly rural patients with atrial fibrillation. *Am Heart J.* 1999;137(2):307-312.

16. Fihn SD, Callahan CM, Martin DC, McDonell MB, Henikoff JG, White RH. The risk for and severity of bleeding complications in elderly patients treated with warfarin. The National Consortium of Anticoagulation Clinics. *Ann Intern Med.* 1996;124(11):970-979.

17. White HD, Gruber M, Feyzi J, et al. Comparison of outcomes among patients randomized to warfarin therapy according to anticoagulant control: results from SPORTIF III and V. *Arch Intern Med.* 2007;167(3):239-245.

18. Man-Son-Hing M, Nichol G, Lau A, Laupacis A. Choosing antithrombotic therapy for elderly patients with atrial fibrillation who are at risk for falls. *Arch Intern Med.* 1999;159(7):677-685.

19. Anderson JL, Horne BD, Stevens SM, et al. Randomized trial of genotype-guided versus standard warfarin dosing in patients initiating oral anticoagulation. *Circulation.* 2007;116(22):2563-2570.

20. Aquilante CL, Langaee TY, Lopez LM, et al. Influence of coagulation factor, vitamin K epoxide reductase complex subunit 1, and cytochrome P450 2C9 gene polymorphisms on warfarin dose requirements. *Clin Pharmacol Ther.* 2006;79(4):291-302.

21. Caldwell MD, Awad T, Johnson JA, et al. CYP4F2 genetic variant alters required warfarin dose. *Blood.* 2008;111(8):4106-4112.

22. Schwarz UI, Ritchie MD, Bradford Y, et al. Genetic determinants of response to warfarin during initial anticoagulation. *N Engl J Med.* 2008;358(10):999-1008.

23. Klein TE, Altman RB, Eriksson N, et al. Estimation of the warfarin dose with clinical and pharmacogenetic data. *N Engl J Med.* 2009;360(8):753-764.

24. Epstein RS, Moyer TP, Aubert RE, et al. Warfarin genotyping reduces hospitalization rates results from the MM-WES (Medco-Mayo Warfarin Effectiveness study). *J Am Coll Cardiol.* 2010;55(25): 2804-2812.

25. Warfarin FDA product label. 2011. http://www.accessdata.fda.gov/drugsatfda_docs/label/2010/009218s108lbl.pdf (accessed March 20. 2011).

26. Wang L, McLeod HL, Weinshilboum RM. Genomics and drug response. *N Engl J Med.* 2011;364(12): 1144-1153.

27. Warfarin Dosing. http://www.warfarindosing.org/Source/Home.aspx (accessed March 20, 2011).

28. Ford SK, Misita CP, Shilliday BB, Malone RM, Moore CG, Moll S. Prospective study of supplemental vitamin K therapy in patients on oral anticoagulants with unstable international normalized ratios. *J Thromb Thrombolysis.* 2007;24(1):23-27.

29. Reese AM, Farnett LE, Lyons RM, Patel B, Morgan L, Bussey HI. Low-dose vitamin K to augment anticoagulation control. *Pharmacotherapy.* 2005;25(12):1746-1751.

30. Rombouts EK, Rosendaal FR, Van Der Meer FJ. Daily vitamin K supplementation improves anticoagulant stability. *J Thromb Haemost.* 2007;5(10):2043-2048.

31. Sconce E, Avery P, Wynne H, Kamali F. Vitamin K supplementation can improve stability of anticoagulation for patients with unexplained variability in response to warfarin. *Blood.* 2007;109(6): 2419-2423.

32. Hallevi H, Albright KC, Martin-Schild S, et al. Anticoagulation after cardioembolic stroke: to bridge or not to bridge? *Arch Neurol.* 2008;65(9):1169-1173.

33. Paciaroni M, Agnelli G, Micheli S, Caso V. Efficacy and safety of anticoagulant treatment in acute cardioembolic stroke: a meta-analysis of randomized controlled trials. *Stroke.* 2007;38(2):423-430.

34. Zeuthen EL, Lassen JF, Husted SE. Is there a hypercoagulable phase during initiation of antithrombotic therapy with oral anticoagulants in patients with atrial fibrillation? *Thromb Res.* Mar 15 2003;109(5-6): 241-246.

35. Adams HP, Jr., del Zoppo G, Alberts MJ, et al. Guidelines for the early management of adults with ischemic stroke: a guideline from the American Heart Association/American Stroke Association Stroke Council, Clinical Cardiology Council, Cardiovascular Radiology and Intervention Council, and the Atherosclerotic Peripheral Vascular Disease and Quality of Care Outcomes in Research Interdisciplinary Working Groups: the American Academy of Neurology affirms the value of this guideline as an educational tool for neurologists. *Stroke.* 2007;38(5):1655-1711.

36. Constans M, Santamaria A, Mateo J, Pujol N, Souto JC, Fontcuberta J. Low-molecular-weight heparin as bridging therapy during interruption of oral anticoagulation in patients undergoing colonoscopy or gastroscopy. *Int J Clin Pract.* 2007;61(2):212-217.

37. Spyropoulos AC, Bauersachs RM, Omran H, Cohen M. Periprocedural bridging therapy in patients receiving chronic oral anticoagulation therapy. *Curr Med Res Opin.* 2006;22(6):1109-1122.

38. Spyropoulos AC. Bridging of oral anticoagulation therapy for invasive procedures. *Curr Hematol Rep.* 2005;4(5):405-413.

39. Eikelboom J, Weitz JI. New oral anticoagulants for stroke prevention in atrial fibrilation. *Clinical Invest.* 2011;1(1):3-7.

40. Eikelboom JW, Weitz JI. New anticoagulants. *Circulation.* 2010;121(13):1523-1532.

41. Chaudhari D, Bhuriya R, Arora R. Newer anticoagulants as an alternate to warfarin in atrial fibrillation: a changing paradigm. *Am J Ther.* 2010. [Epub ahead of print]

42. Howard N, Abell C, Blakemore W, et al. Application of fragment screening and fragment linking to the discovery of novel thrombin inhibitors. *J Med Chem.* 2006;49(4):1346-1355.

43. Testa L, Bhindi R, Agostoni P, Abbate A, Zoccai GG, van Gaal WJ. The direct thrombin inhibitor ximelagatran/melagatran: a systematic review on clinical applications and an evidence based assessment of risk benefit profile. *Expert Opin Drug Saf.* 2007;6(4):397-406.

44. Spence JD. Secondary stroke prevention. *Nat Rev Neurol.* 2010;6(9):477-486.

45. Connolly SJ, Ezekowitz MD, Yusuf S, et al. Dabigatran versus warfarin in patients with atrial fibrillation. *N Engl J Med.* 2009;361(12):1139-1151.

46. Schirmer SH, Baumhakel M, Neuberger HR, et al. Novel anticoagulants for stroke prevention in atrial fibrillation: current clinical evidence and future developments. *J Am Coll Cardiol.* 2010;56(25): 2067-2076.

47. Ezekowitz MD, Wallentin L, Connolly SJ, et al. Dabigatran and warfarin in vitamin K antagonist-naive and -experienced cohorts with atrial fibrillation. *Circulation.* 2010;122(22):2246-2253.

48. Stangier J, Stahle H, Rathgen K, Fuhr R. Pharmacokinetics and pharmacodynamics of the direct oral thrombin inhibitor dabigatran in healthy elderly subjects. *Clin Pharmacokinet.* 2008;47(1):47-59.

49. van Ryn J, Stangier J, Haertter S, et al. Dabigatran etexilate—a novel, reversible, oral direct thrombin inhibitor: interpretation of coagulation assays and reversal of anticoagulant activity. *Thromb Haemost.* 2010;103(6):1116-1127.

50. Turpie AG. Oral, direct factor Xa inhibitors in development for the prevention and treatment of thromboembolic diseases. *Arterioscler Thromb Vasc Biol.* 2007;27(6):1238-1247.

51. Eikelboom JW, O'Donnell M, Yusuf S, et al. Rationale and design of AVERROES: apixaban versus acetylsalicylic acid to prevent stroke in atrial fibrillation patients who have failed or are unsuitable for vitamin K antagonist treatment. *Am Heart J.* 2010;159(3):348-353, e341.

52. Rivaroxaban-once daily, oral, direct factor Xa inhibition compared with vitamin K antagonism for prevention of stroke and Embolism Trial in Atrial Fibrillation: rationale and design of the ROCKET AF study. *Am Heart J.* 2010;159(3):340-347, e341.

53. Granger CB, Alexander JH, McMurray JJ, Lopes RD, Hylek EM, Hanna M et al. Apixaban versus warfarin in patients with atrial fibrillation. *N Engl J Med.* 2011;365:981-92.

Lipid-Lowering Therapy

J. David Spence

INTRODUCTION

The notion that an elevated serum cholesterol is not a risk factor for stroke is an old canard, a relic of the days when hypertension dominated stroke risk. When almost half of strokes were intracerebral hemorrhages or lacunar infarctions from hypertension, the effect of serum cholesterol, which is clearly a risk factor for strokes due to large artery disease, was harder to appreciate. In a community in which blood pressure had been controlled[1] and strokes due to hypertensive small vessel disease had much diminished,[2] we found that serum cholesterol was a significant predictor of stroke.[3]

REDUCTION OF STROKE RISK BY LIPID-LOWERING THERAPY

Most of the evidence on stroke reduction by lipid-lowering therapy comes from studies done in patients with coronary artery disease. Amarenco and Labreuche[4] reviewed the relation between lowering of low-density lipoprotein (LDL) cholesterol and reduction of stroke; the relationship is linear. Meta-analysis of randomized trials of statins in combination with other preventive strategies, including 165,792 individuals, shows that each 1 mmol/L (39 mg/dL) decrease in LDL cholesterol equates to a reduction in relative risk for stroke of 21.1% (95% confidence interval [CI], 6.3-33.5; $P = .009$). A large meta-analysis (of 170,000 participants in trials of intensive lipid-lowering therapy) showed that more intensive lipid-lowering regimens with statins reduced stroke by 16%, compared with less intensive regimens.[5] Another meta-analysis[6] showed an 18% reduction in the risk of stroke with more intensive statin therapy. The Stroke Prevention by Aggressive Reduction in Cholesterol Levels (SPARCL) trial similarly showed a 16% reduction of stroke by high-dose atorvastatin versus placebo.[7] However, the reduction of stroke risk was probably underestimated by the intention-to-treat analysis, because a high proportion (25.4%) of the participants randomized to placebo actually received statin therapy.

It seems likely that this rather modest benefit (compared to reduction of myocardial infarction) relates to stroke subtypes: strokes due to hypertensive small vessel disease, vasculitis, or dissection would be expected to benefit less than those from atherosclerosis. Indeed, among patients in the SPARCL trial who had carotid stenosis, high-dose statins reduced recurrent stroke by 33% and reduced major coronary events by 43%.[8] Probably even greater reductions are possible with intensive combination therapy. We found[9] that intensive medical therapy based on plaque measurement markedly reduced the two-year risk of myocardial infarction and stroke among patients with asymptomatic carotid stenosis, compared to usual care: the two-year risk of myocardial infarction declined from 7.6% to 1%, and the risk of stroke declined from 8.8% to 1%. These major reductions in risk were not achieved by more intensive statin therapy alone; the intensive therapy, guided by plaque measurements, included lifestyle modification, high-dose statins, and combination with ezetimibe and in some cases fibrates or niacin. Our evidence suggests[10] that treating arteries, as opposed to treating blood tests, was a major factor in these results.

COMBINATION THERAPY WITH STATINS

There are several groups of high-risk patients for whom statin therapy alone is not sufficient. This includes patients with atherosclerotic stroke, carotid stenosis, or a history of coronary artery disease or peripheral vascular disease who have not responded adequately to statins alone. Nonresponders would include those who have not achieved target levels of LDL cholesterol, those with progression of carotid plaque despite having achieved target levels of LDL, those with low levels of high-density lipoprotein (HDL), and those with high levels of triglycerides.

Ezetimibe is a logical addition to statins because it lowers cholesterol by a different mechanism. Statins work by inhibiting synthesis of cholesterol (mainly in the liver), whereas ezetimibe blocks intestinal absorption of cholesterol. The combination has a synergistic effect: 10 mg of atorvastatin plus 10 mg of ezetimibe lowers LDL cholesterol by as much as does 80 mg of cholesterol,[11] and nearly as much as does 40 mg of rosuvastatin.

The notion that ezetimibe may have harmful effects on the arteries is pure mythology, based on two clinical trials that measured the wrong endpoint[12]: carotid intima-media thickness is not truly atherosclerosis.[13] We suspect that ezetimibe was responsible for much of the risk reduction in the studies discussed above, and have evidence (as yet unpublished) that ezetimibe regresses carotid plaque. This is consistent with the reduction of cardiovascular events in the aortic stenosis trial[14] and in a trial in patients with chronic kidney disease[15] (results presented at the American Society of Nephrology in 2010).

For patients with high triglyceride levels, reduction of carbohydrate intake is crucial; the most effective drug therapy is niacin. Niacin not only has beneficial effects on lipoprotein profiles, including Lp(a), it also has antiatherosclerotic effects via inhibition of vascular inflammation.[16] Flushing is due to release of prostaglandin

D2 from skin mast cells; it usually wears off after five days[17] and is tolerable to most patients with adequate education. Maneuvers to increase the tolerability of niacin include pretreatment with nonsteroidal anti-inflammatory agents (because they inhibit synthesis of prostaglandins), gradual titration of niacin dose, slow-release preparations of niacin, and laropiprant,[18] a PGD-2 antagonist. Caution may be needed with the form of slow-release niacin, as too slow a pattern of absorption may favor the formation of toxic metabolites.[19] Apart from flushing, the main adverse effects of niacin are aggravation of gout and impairment of glucose tolerance. For patients who cannot take niacin, fibrates such as fenofibrate are an option.

DRUG INTERACTIONS WITH STATINS

Several of the most commonly used statins are metabolized by cytochrome P450 3A4 (CYP3A4). This is a problem not only because of interaction with drugs that inhibit CYP3A4, but also because grapefruit or grapefruit juice inhibits CYP3A4[20] to the same extent. Although the area under the curve of blood levels over time (AUC) of atorvastatin is "only" doubled by inhibitors of CYP3A4, simvastatin and lovastatin have the potential for 15-fold increases in AUC with inhibitors of CYP3A4. The reason is that simvastatin and lovastatin are only 5% bioavailable, because 95% of an oral dose is metabolized in the gut wall during absorption, to inactive metabolites. Thus if gut wall CYP3A4 is completely knocked out, there is a theoretical potential for 20-fold rises in blood levels. Inhibitors of CYP3A4 include grapefruit,[21,22] erythromycin, itraconazole, ketoconazole, clarithromycin, cyclosporine, and other drugs.

It is a myth, perpetuated soon after the discovery of this effect by our group,[23] that it is safe to take such drugs later in the day if grapefruit is taken in the morning, or that a large dose of grapefruit is required for this effect. Grapefruit is a "suicide inhibitor" of CYP3A4; a single glass of grapefruit juice has effects that persist for 36 hours, and consuming half of a whole grapefruit is sufficient. Rhabdomyolysis has been reported from a single exposure to grapefruit juice with simvastatin.[24] Because grocers seldom take a drug history when dispensing grapefruit,[25] these drugs therefore fall into the category of drugs with "complicated pharmacokinetics" and should be avoided now that other safer alternatives are available. Neither rosuvastatin nor pravastatin is affected by such drugs, although they are affected by inhibitors of the drug transport factor organic acid transporting polypeptide (OATP), such as gemfibrozil.[26]

In some patients, elevated levels of statins are due to underlying genetic abnormalities of statin absorption or metabolism; this has been reviewed by Vladutiu.[27]

ADVERSE EFFECTS OF STATINS AND HOW TO AVOID THEM

As discussed in Chapter 15, the long lists of adverse effects* provided by pharmacists are worse than useless because they list virtually all symptoms known to mankind, regardless of causality. Although it is widely believed that statins cause liver

---

* The term "side effects" is best replaced by "adverse effects." Many drugs have more than one action, not all harmful.

damage, this may be a myth.[28] Elevation of enzymes attributed to liver damage may be from muscle. Statins probably do not cause headache, dizziness, fatigue, nausea, diarrhea, constipation, and so on.

The notion that they may cause intracerebral hemorrhage is probably also a myth. If the increase in cerebral hemorrhage observed in the SPARCL trial had been causally related to atorvastatin, there should have been an association of lower LDL to intracerebral hemorrhage. That this was not observed suggests that a more likely reason for the association was that patients who stopped their statin because of adverse effects may have also stopped their antihypertensive medication. Day et al[29] found no association between statin therapy and microhemorrhage on magnetic resonance imaging (MRI), among patients with acute ischemic stroke.

There is, however, a causal relationship to muscle problems, including myalgia, myopathy, and rhabdomyolysis. Patients with statin-induced myalgia/myopathy will complain of aching and cramps, and sometimes weakness. This may be related to hypothyroidism,[30] an easily treated condition that raises plasma cholesterol and causes rheumatic complaints even in patients not on statins.[31] An elevation of plasma creatine phosphokinase (CK) may be due to exercise or minor injury, so borderline or temporary elevations of CK are not a strong reason to stop a drug that reduces stroke risk by approximately 30%. CK levels up to several times the upper limit of normal will usually be tolerated, although in patients with weakness a myopathy should be considered even if the CK level is normal,[32] so muscle biopsy may be warranted.[27] It is important to distinguish between myalgia/myopathy and pain from other causes such as arthritis: statins cause muscle pain, not joint pain, sciatica, or bursitis. This effect is not idiosyncratic; an equivalent strength of statin effect will produce the same problem regardless of the statin, so changing from one brand to another will not be effective, unless the new statin is weaker than the one that provoked the problem. (A theoretical issue that may bear out is that rosuvastatin and pravastatin may penetrate less into muscle cells, relating to lipophilicity.) Figure 9–1 shows the probable cause of statin myopathy, which is depletion of ubiquinone (coenzyme Q10 [CoQ10]), in susceptible individuals. CoQ10 is required for mitochondrial function, and depletion of CoQ10 causes muscle problems in patients with disorders of mitochondrial function. It is possible that the slight increase in diabetes with statins reported from a meta-analysis[33] might also be related to mitochondrial dysfunction. There is evidence that statins cause depletion of carnitine, with associated myositis,[34] and carnitine supplementation improves glycemia as well as improving the effects of statins on plasma lipids and lipoproteins, including Lp(a), in diabetics.[35,36] There are limited data supporting the use of CoQ10 supplements for treatment of myalgia[37]; likely reasons for negative results include low bioavailability of oral CoQ10. There is also limited evidence that supplementation with L-carnitine improves mitochondrial function and myopathy in patients on statins.[35,38]

Susceptibility Due to Mitochondrial Disorders

Patients who exhibit muscle problems with low doses of statins probably are susceptible to depletion of CoQ10[39] because of an inherited problem of mitochondrial

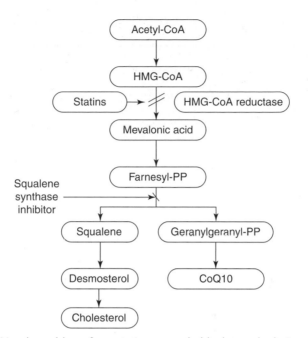

Figure 9–1. Muscle problems from statins are probably due to depletion of CoQ10. Statins probably cause myalgias because they deplete CoQ10 in patients who are susceptible to CoQ10 depletion because of an underlying deficiency of mitochondrial function. Because squalene synthase inhibitors block conversion of farnesyl-PP to squalene, they will not reduce levels of CoQ10 as do statins; indeed they may increase levels of CoQ10 as a result of shunting toward geranylgeranyl PP. (Reproduced by permission of the *International Journal of Stroke* from Spence JD. Pollypill: for Pollyanna. *Intl J Stroke.* 2008;3:92-97.)

function or energy metabolism. In a study published in 2006, Vladutiu et al looked at only three candidate genes among 100 patients with statin myopathy, but found marked increases in the prevalence of mutations for palmitoyl transferase deficiency II (13-fold), McCardle disease (20-fold), and myoadenylate deaminase deficiency (3.25-fold).[40] In muscle biopsies, significant abnormalities of mitochondrial function or fatty acid metabolism were found in 51%, with multiple abnormalities in 31%.[40] An important review of genetic predisposition to statin myopathy was published by Vladutiu in 2008.[27]

Avoiding Adverse Effects of Statins

Patients with stroke, particularly those with carotid stenosis, have a high risk of other cardiovascular events such as myocardial infarction. In stroke patients, statins not only reduce the risk of stroke by up to 30%, they also markedly reduce the risk of myocardial infarction. It is therefore not good practice to permit (even less, encourage) patients to stop statin therapy for invalid reasons. In patients with complaints

Table 9–1. Approaches to Avoiding Myalgia/Myopathy From Statins

Reduce the dose of statin
Avoid simvastatin and lovastatin because of potential for huge interactions
Add ezetimibe
Supplement with high doses of CoQ10 (eg, 150 mg twice daily)
? Supplement with carnitine (eg, 300 mg twice daily)
? Switch to rosuvastatin (? less penetration into muscle cells)
Switch to a squalene synthase inhibitor (when it becomes available; see Figure 9–1)

that are mistakenly attributed to statins (for example, vertigo, sciatica, low back pain, hypothyroidism), it may be sufficient to discuss causation of symptoms and educate the patient, and, for example, detect and treat the hypothyroidism. In extreme cases it may be necessary to conduct an N of 1 randomized trial, as discussed in Chapter 15.

However, in some cases, problems of myalgia/myopathy are indeed causally related, for the reasons discussed above. Table 9–1 outlines approaches to reducing muscle problems in patients taking statins: reducing the dose of statin, adding ezetimibe, supplementation with CoQ10, and possibly switching to a more hydrophilic statin such as rosuvastatin, and supplementation with carnitine.

In the future, switching to squalene synthase inhibitors, when they become available, may be an important option. Squalene synthase inhibitors will reduce the synthesis of cholesterol while increasing the synthesis of CoQ10 by shunting (Figure 9–1).

CONCLUSION

Cholesterol is an important risk factor for stroke, particularly atherosclerotic stroke. Lipid-lowering therapy reduces the risk of stroke by up to 30% in arteriopaths, and reduces the risk of major coronary events by 43%. It is therefore important to prescribe statins to stroke patients who are arteriopaths, and to find ways to help patients persist with statin therapy. Combination therapy with niacin or fibrates, and more intensive therapy based on carotid plaque measurement including lifestyle modification, may help reduce stroke and coronary events even further.

REFERENCES

1. Birkett NJ, Donner AP, Maynard M. Prevalence and control of hypertension in an Ontario county. *Can Med Assoc J.* 1985;132:1019-1024.

2. Spence JD. Antihypertensive drugs and prevention of atherosclerotic stroke. *Stroke.* 1986;17:808-810.

3. Hachinski V, Graffagnino C, Beaudry M, et al. Lipids and stroke: a paradox resolved. *Arch Neurol.* 1996;53:303-308.

4. Amarenco P, Labreuche J. Lipid management in the prevention of stroke: review and updated meta-analysis of statins for stroke prevention. *Lancet Neurol.* 2009;8:453-463.

5. Baigent C, Blackwell L, Emberson J, et al. Efficacy and safety of more intensive lowering of LDL cholesterol: a meta-analysis of data from 170,000 participants in 26 randomised trials. *Lancet.* 2010;376:1670-1681.

6. Josan K, Majumdar SR, McAlister FA. The efficacy and safety of intensive statin therapy: a meta-analysis of randomized trials. *CMAJ.* 2008;178:576-584.

7. The Stroke Prevention by Aggressive Reduction in Cholesterol Levels (SPARCL) Investigators. High-Dose Atorvastatin after Stroke or Transient Ischemic Attack. *N Engl J Med.* 2006;355:549-559.

8. Sillisen H, Amarenco P, Hennerici MG, et al. Atorvastatin reduces the risk of cardiovascular events in patients with carotid atherosclerosis: a secondary analysis of the Stroke Prevention by Aggressive Reduction in Cholesterol Levels (SPARCL) Trial. *Stroke.* 2008;39:3297-3302.

9. Spence JD, Coates V, Li H, et al. Effects of intensive medical therapy on microemboli and cardiovascular risk in asymptomatic carotid stenosis. *Arch Neurol.* 2010;67:180-186.

10. Spence JD, Hackam DG. Treating arteries instead of risk factors. A paradigm change in management of atherosclerosis. *Stroke.* 2010;41:1193-1199.

11. Stein E, Stender S, Mata P, et al. Achieving lipoprotein goals in patients at high risk with severe hypercholesterolemia: efficacy and safety of ezetimibe co-administered with atorvastatin. *Am Heart J.* 2004;148:447-455.

12. Spence JD. Is carotid intima-media thickness a reliable clinical predictor? *Mayo Clin Proc.* 2008;83:1299-1300.

13. Finn AV, Kolodgie FD, Virmani R. Correlation between carotid intimal/medial thickness and atherosclerosis. A point of view from pathology. *Arterioscler Thromb Vasc Biol.* 2010;30:177-181.

14. Rossebo AB, Pedersen TR, Boman K, et al. Intensive lipid lowering with simvastatin and ezetimibe in aortic stenosis. *N Engl J Med.* 2008;359:1343-1356.

15. Sharp Collaborative Group. Study of Heart and Renal Protection (SHARP): randomized trial to assess the effects of lowering low-density lipoprotein cholesterol among 9,438 patients with chronic kidney disease. *Am Heart J.* 2010;160:785-794.

16. Wu BJ, Yan L, Charlton F, Witting P, Barter PJ, Rye KA. Evidence that niacin inhibits acute vascular inflammation and improves endothelial dysfunction independent of changes in plasma lipids. *Arterioscler Thromb Vasc Biol.* 2010;30:968-975.

17. Stern RH, Spence JD, Freeman DJ, Parbtani A. Tolerance to nicotinic acid flushing. *Clin Pharmacol Ther.* 1991;50:66-70.

18. Maccubbin D, Koren MJ, Davidson M, et al. Flushing profile of extended-release niacin/laropiprant versus gradually titrated niacin extended-release in patients with dyslipidemia with and without ischemic cardiovascular disease. *Am J Cardiol.* 2009;104:74-81.

19. Stern RH, Freeman DJ, Spence JD. Differences in metabolism of time-release and unmodified nicotinic acid: explanation of the differences in hypolipidemic action? *Metabolism.* 1992;41:879-881.

20. Bailey DG, Malcolm J, Arnold O, Spence JD. Grapefruit juice-drug interactions. *Br J Clin Pharmacol.* 1998;46:101-110.

21. Kantola T, Kivisto KT, Neuvonen PJ. Grapefruit juice greatly increases serum concentrations of lovastatin and lovastatin acid. *Clin Pharmacol Ther.* 1998;63:397-402.

22. Lilja JJ, Kivisto KT, Neuvonen PJ. Grapefruit juice-simvastatin interaction: effect on serum concentrations of simvastatin, simvastatin acid, and HMG-CoA reductase inhibitors. *Clin Pharmacol Ther.* 1998;64:477-483.

23. Bailey DG, Spence JD, Munoz C, Arnold JM. Interaction of citrus juices with felodipine and nifedipine. *Lancet.* 1991;337:268-269.

24. Dreier JP, Endres M. Statin-associated rhabdomyolysis triggered by grapefruit consumption. *Neurology.* 2004;62:670.

25. Spence JD. Drug interactions with grapefruit: whose responsibility is it to warn the public? *Clin Pharmacol Ther.* 1997;61:395-400.

26. Schneck DW, Birmingham BK, Zalikowski JA, et al. The effect of gemfibrozil on the pharmacokinetics of rosuvastatin. *Clin Pharmacol Ther.* 2004;75:455-463.

27. Vladutiu GD. Genetic predisposition to statin myopathy. *Curr Opin Rheumatol.* 2008;20:648-655.

28. Bader T. The myth of statin-induced hepatotoxicity. *Am J Gastroenterol.* 2010;105:978-980.

29. Day JS, Policeni BA, Smoker WR, et al. Previous statin use is not associated with an increased prevalence or degree of gradient-echo lesions in patients with acute ischemic stroke or transient ischemic attack. *Stroke.* 2011;42:354-358.

30. Krieger EV, Knopp RH. Hypothyroidism misdiagnosed as statin intolerance. *Ann Intern Med.* 2009;151:72.

31. Bland JH, Frymoyer JW. Rheumatic syndromes of myxedema. *N Engl J Med.* 1970;282:1171-1174.

32. Mohaupt MG, Karas RH, Babiychuk EB, et al. Association between statin-associated myopathy and skeletal muscle damage. *CMAJ.* 2009;181:E11-E18.

33. Sattar N, Preiss D, Murray HM, et al. Statins and risk of incident diabetes: a collaborative meta-analysis of randomised statin trials. *Lancet.* 2010;375:735-742.

34. Bhuiyan J, Seccombe DW. The effects of 3-hydroxy-3-methylglutaryl-CoA reductase inhibition on tissue levels of carnitine and carnitine acyltransferase activity in the rabbit. *Lipids.* 1996;31:867-870.

35. Zammit VA, Ramsay RR, Bonomini M, Arduini A. Carnitine, mitochondrial function and therapy. *Adv Drug Deliv Rev.* 2009;61:1353-1362.

36. Malaguarnera M, Vacante M, Motta M, Malaguarnera M, Li VG, Galvano F. Effect of L-carnitine on the size of low-density lipoprotein particles in type 2 diabetes mellitus patients treated with simvastatin. *Metabolism.* 2009;58:1618-1623.

37. Caso G, Kelly P, McNurlan MA, Lawson WE. Effect of coenzyme q10 on myopathic symptoms in patients treated with statins. *Am J Cardiol.* 2007;99:1409-1412.

38. Arduini A, Peschechera A, Giannessi F, et al. Improvement of statin-associated myotoxicity by L-carnitine. Effects of simvastatin and carnitine versus simvastatin on lipoprotein(a) and apoprotein(a) in type 2 diabetes mellitus. *J Thromb Haemost.* 2004;2:2270-2271.

39. Baker SK, Tarnopolsky MA. Statin myopathies: pathophysiologic and clinical perspectives. *Clin Invest Med.* 2001;24:258-272.

40. Vladutiu GD, Simmons Z, Isackson PJ, et al. Genetic risk factors associated with lipid-lowering drug-induced myopathies. *Muscle Nerve.* 2006;5734:153-162.

Management and Prevention of Intracranial Atherosclerotic Disease

10

Yongchai Nilanont
Niphon Poungvarin

INTRODUCTION

Intracranial atherosclerotic disease (ICAD) is an important etiology of ischemic stroke worldwide, especially in Asian, Hispanic, and black populations.[1-3] ICAD may account for 8% to 10% of all ischemic strokes in whites,[3-5] 13% in Hispanics, and 17% in African Americans.[6] However, it accounts for the highest proportion of stroke in the Chinese population (33%-37%).[1,7]

Independent risk factors for ICAD include age, high blood pressure, high cholesterol level, and diabetes mellitus (DM).[8,9] Risk factors for recurrent ischemic stroke from ICAD are hypertension (systolic blood pressure [SBP] >140 mm Hg), hyperlipidemia (total cholesterol >200 mg/dL), no alcohol consumption, and DM.[10,11] Men are more likely to develop ICAD, whereas women appear to have a higher rate of recurrence.[12-14]

Patients with symptomatic ICAD are at high risk of subsequent stroke. Despite risk factor modification and the use of antithrombotic medication, the overall rates of recurrent stroke in the territory of a stenotic intracranial artery were 11% at one year and 14% at two years.[15] Moreover, 23% of patients with high-grade stenosis (>70%) went on to experience another ipsilateral ischemic stroke over the next year.[14] The purpose of this chapter is to review the existing clinical trial evidence concerning stroke prevention in patients with intracranial atherosclerotic disease.

CLINICAL PATTERNS OF INTRACRANIAL STENOSIS

The neurologic syndromes associated with ICAD are not unique. Other stroke mechanisms such as extracranial carotid stenosis or cardioembolism that cause cerebral infarction in the same vascular territory can produce similar neurological manifestations. However, a review of the history on temporal course of the neurological symptoms, patients' risk factor profile, and previous history of transient ischemic attack, as well as a meticulous physical examination may assist physicians to identify the most likely stroke etiology. (See Chapter 12 for a discussion of the crucial role of diagnosis in prevention of recurrent stroke.) For example, large vessel atherosclerotic disease may be more likely to occur in patients with atherosclerotic risk factors such as hypertension, diabetes, smoking, or hyperlipidemia. A prior history of recurrent stereotypical transient ischemic attacks (TIAs) should suggest intrinsic large artery disease (extracranial or intracranial large artery disease) or focal seizures, rather than embolism from the heart or aorta. Transient ischemic attacks tend to be more common in patients with extracranial carotid disease than in those with intracranial large vessel atherosclerotic disease. In one study of patients with stroke in the territory of the middle cerebral artery, the rate of TIA preceding stroke in patients with middle cerebral artery stenosis was 20%, compared to 64% in patients with extracranial carotid stenosis.[16] In addition, TIAs in patients with middle cerebral artery stenosis also occur in a shorter period than those associated with extracranial carotid occlusive disease.[16]

The cavernous portion of the internal carotid artery is the typical location of ICAD. Patients usually present with cerebral infarction in the middle cerebral artery (MCA) territory, with hemiparesis, aphasia (dominant hemisphere), anosognosia and neglect (nondominant hemisphere), hemisensory loss, and hemianopsia. Partial syndromes are frequently diagnosed depending on which branch (superior or inferior division of the MCA) is primarily involved. Cerebral infarction in the anterior cerebral artery (ACA) territory may also result from occlusion of the carotid siphon. Patients with an infarction in this territory typically present with leg weakness, or leg and face weakness, with relative sparing of the arm.

ICAD that involves the MCA typically affects the proximal portion (stem, M1 segment, as shown in Figure 10–1), but occasionally affects the superior division alone.[17] Patients with infarction of the entire MCA territory usually present with hemiplegia, hemisensory loss, forced gaze deviation to the affected hemisphere, hemianopsia, and aphasia (dominant hemisphere) or neglect (nondominant hemisphere). If infarction occurs in the superior division of the MCA, patients typically present with hemiplegia, hemisensory deficit, conjugate deviation of the eyes, contralateral neglect (nondominant hemisphere), and Broca aphasia (dominant hemisphere). Infarctions in the inferior division of the MCA territory in the dominant hemisphere cause Wernicke aphasia, hemianopsia, agitation, and confusion whereas confusion, agitation, hemianopsia, and poor drawing and copying are found in the mirror image infarct of the nondominant hemisphere.[18]

Patients with atherosclerotic disease of the proximal part of the MCA territory, which involves the origins of the lenticulostriate arteries, occasionally present with pure motor hemiparesis, resembling small vessel disease. Neuroimaging findings

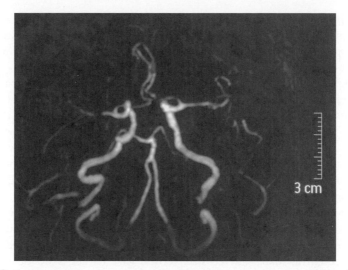

Figure 10-1. Magnetic resonance angiography (MRA) showed severe stenosis at proximal segment of the right middle cerebral artery.

include a moderate-sized (2-5 cm) infarction involving the internal capsule and basal ganglia (striatocapsular infarction) with sparing of the cortical areas supplied by the MCA. The relatively large size of subcortical infarction provides a hint that the stroke etiology involves the MCA (and not a single small penetrating artery).[19]

Anterior cerebral artery stenosis is uncommon in ICAD. Most infarctions in this territory are caused by artery-to-artery emboli from extracranial carotid stenosis, the heart, or the carotid siphon.[20] When atherosclerosis is present, it is usually distal to the stem of the anterior cerebral artery (A1 segment) and involves the territories supplied by the pericallosal or callosomarginal branches.[21] Lesions in these areas cause weakness in the leg, thigh, and foot, occasionally involving the shoulder, and producing cortical sensory disturbances. Language deficits, particularly mutism, can be found in the acute stage in patients with left anterior cerebral artery infarction; this is sometimes followed by mixed transcortical aphasia.[20]

The clinical syndromes of ICAD of the basilar artery depend on the vascular territory of the anatomical lesion, whether the lesion has involved the brainstem unilaterally or bilaterally, and whether distal embolism has occurred. Patients typically present with diplopia, vertigo or dysequilibrium, perioral numbness, dysarthria, paraplegia, or alternating hemiplegia.[22-24] In those with proximal basilar occlusion whose distal basilar artery and superior cerebellar artery are still patent (by retrograde flow from the posterior communicating arteries), the lesions are usually confined to the midline and paramedian structures in the pons. The pontine tegmentum and cerebellum are usually preserved because these structures receive blood supply from circumferential branches of the patent distal basilar artery and from the posterior inferior cerebellar artery. Therefore, patients with proximal basilar occlusion usually present with combinations of any of the following signs: hemiparesis (if brainstem involvement is unilateral), quadriparesis (if bilateral), pseudobulbar palsy, extraocular movement abnormalities, internuclear ophthalmoplegia, skew deviation, or one and a half syndrome.

In proximal basilar occlusion resulting in bilateral infarction of the basis pontis, patients typically present with severe weakness of the limbs and limitation of eye movements in which only eye blinking or vertical gaze are preserved, that is, the "locked-in" syndrome. Bilateral infarctions of the basis pontis may occasionally be due to nonstenotic atherosclerotic disease of the basilar artery, by occlusion (probably atheroembolic) of the orifices of paramedian penetrating branches of the basilar artery.[25] These patients may experience neurological deficits similar to those with proximal basilar artery occlusion.

Occlusion of the distal basilar artery produces signs of ischemia in the midbrain, thalamus, mesial temporal, and occipital lobes bilaterally. Midbrain ischemia causes pupillary and eye movement abnormalities including decreased pupillary reactivity, eccentric shape, altered size, vertical gaze palsies, skew deviation, and third nerve palsy. Peduncular hallucinosis is also described.[26] Thalamic infarction produces an impaired level of consciousness, memory disturbances, and sensory symptoms depending on the location and size of the lesion. Temporal and occipital infarctions are frequently accompanied by hemianopsia or cortical blindness (if both occipital lobes are involved), amnesia, and agitated behavior. In some cases, involvement of the visual association cortex may cause patients to become lost in familiar surroundings or fail to recognize faces (prosopagnosia). The "top of the basilar" syndrome is most often due to an embolus.[26,27]

Atherosclerosis of the posterior cerebral artery often involves the proximal part near the origin of the thalamogeniculate branches.[28] The ventroposterolateral thalamus and the medial temporal and the occipital lobes are typical infarct locations. Patients usually present with hemianopsia or hemisensory TIAs.[28] Common neurological signs and symptoms in those with cerebral infarction in the territory supplied by the posterior cerebral artery include contralateral hemisensory loss (ventroposterolateral thalamus), amnesia (medial temporal), contralateral hemianopsia, hemichromatopsia, alexia without agraphia, and visual agnosia (occipital).[29]

The posterior inferior cerebellar artery is usually involved in ICAD of the intracranial vertebral artery. The clinical syndromes depend on the location of the occlusion, whether the vertebral arteries are involved on one side or both, and whether the vertebral artery itself is the source of distal embolism. If occlusion occurs at the origin of the posterior inferior cerebellar artery, patients typically presents with a constellation of neurologic symptoms due to injury to the lateral part of the medulla (Wallenberg syndrome) including sensory deficits affecting the trunk and extremities on the opposite side of the infarction and sensory deficits affecting the face and cranial nerves on the same side as the infarction. Specifically, there is loss of pain and temperature sensation on the contralateral side of the body and ipsilateral side of the face. This crossed sensory loss is diagnostic for the syndrome. Other clinical signs and symptoms include dysphagia, dysarthria, ataxia, vertigo, nystagmus, ipsilateral Horner syndrome, and hiccups. If the lesion extends from one vertebral artery to the proximal basilar artery, or if both vertebral arteries are occluded, the clinical syndrome may be similar to that of intrinsic basilar artery occlusion. If the vertebral artery produces distal embolism, the emboli most commonly lodge at the top of the basilar artery or in the posterior cerebral arteries.[27]

MECHANISMS, AND LESION AND ANGIOGRAPHIC PATTERNS OF ICAD

Possible mechanisms for cerebral infarction in ICAD include plaque rupture with thrombosis leading to complete occlusion, artery-to-artery embolism, hemodynamic compromise, local branch occlusion, or a combination of these events. In a study exploring the mechanism by which MCA stenosis produces acute cerebral infarction using diffusion-weighted magnetic resonance imaging (DW-MRI) with microembolic signals (MES) detected by transcranial Doppler ultrasound (TCD), MES were found in 33.3% during 30 minutes of TCD monitoring in the acute stage.[30] This finding indicates that artery-to-artery embolism is an important stroke mechanism in patients with ICAD. In addition, MES were found to occur more frequently in patients with multiple infarctions than in those with single infarctions. Two previous studies also support that MCA stenosis is responsible for multiple MCA territory infarctions on DWI.[31,32]

The patterns of acute infarction within the MCA territory were categorized as cortical infarction, border zone infarction, and perforating artery infarction, on the basis of the location of the lesion according to map templates by Damasio.[33] Border zone infarctions include anterior border zone infarctions where the lesion is located between the ACA and MCA territories; posterior border zone infarctions occur when the infarction is between the MCA and the posterior cerebral artery (PCA) territories as in Figure 10–2, and internal border zone infarctions are between the deep and the superficial perforators of the MCA as shown in Figure 10–3.[34] Figure 10–4 demonstrates anterior and posterior, as well as internal border zone infarcts in the same patient. Perforating artery infarctions include striatocapsular infarctions or perforating vessel infarctions.

Three different angiographic patterns of the MCA cortical branches beyond the proximal MCA segment were identified as follows: (1) a normal pattern with both normal size and normal flow of the MCA branches; (2) a shift pattern of the angiographic ACA-MCA border zone toward the MCA side as compared to the normal side and decreased MCA vessel size, with relatively normal maintenance of the MCA flow; (3) a dilatation pattern of the MCA vessels with minimal shift of the border zone and slow MCA flow, as shown in Figure 10–5.[35] One study assessed an association between angiographic patterns in patients with symptomatic severe proximal middle cerebral artery infarction and presenting symptoms (stroke vs TIA), infarction patterns (border zone vs non–border zone), and perfusion status (mild vs moderate vs severe). Women were found to have the shift pattern more commonly than men. In addition, patients with the dilatation pattern are more likely to have strokes, border zone infarction, and decreased perfusion than those with the shift pattern.[35]

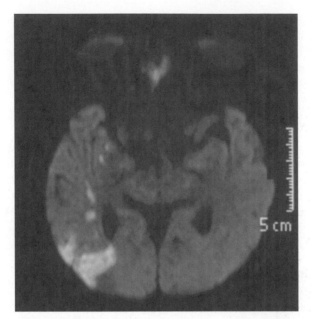

Figure 10–2. Diffusion-weighted magnetic resonance imaging (MRI) demonstrated acute cerebral infarction in the posterior border zone located between the MCA and the PCA territories.

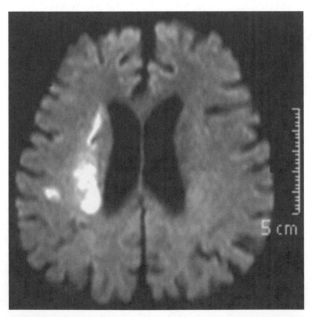

Figure 10–3. Diffusion-weighted magnetic resonance imaging (MRI) demonstrated an internal border zone infarction between deep and superficial perforators of the MCA territory.

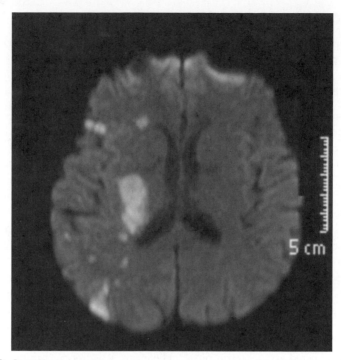

Figure 10–4. Diffusion-weighted magnetic resonance imaging (MRI) showed acute cerebral infarctions involving anterior, posterior, and internal border zone regions in the same patient.

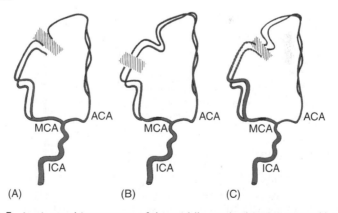

Figure 10–5. Angiographic patterns of the middle cerebral (MCA) cortical branches beyond the proximal segment: (A) normal flow and size of the MCA branches; (B) shift pattern as the ACA-MCA border zone (shaded area) is shifted toward the MCA side and the MCA cortical branches size get smaller, with relatively normal maintenance of the MCA flow; (C) dilatation pattern in which the MCA branches are dilated with slow flow. A minimal shift of the border zone is also demonstrated. (After Choi JW, Kim JK, Choi BS, et al. Angiographic pattern of symptomatic severe M1 stenosis: comparison with presenting symptoms, infarct patterns, perfusion status, and outcome after recanalization. *Cerebrovasc Dis.* 2010;29:297-303.)

RISK FACTOR MANAGEMENT

Few secondary stroke prevention trials have provided data on the effectiveness of risk factor management in symptomatic intracranial stenosis patients.

Blood Pressure Management

Hypertension is the most important modifiable stroke risk factor. A recent global health model demonstrated that approximately 54% of strokes worldwide are attributable to high blood pressure.[36] Secondary stroke prevention studies have shown that the risk of recurrent stroke can be reduced by optimal control of blood pressure in patients with various underlying causes of stroke.[37-39] (See Chapter 6 for a discussion of the management of hypertension in stroke prevention.) The Seventh Report of the Joint National Committee on Prevention, Detection, Evaluation, and Treatment of High Blood Pressure (JNC 7) recommended an optimal blood pressure of less than 140/90 mm Hg for stroke and cardiovascular prevention.[40] However, there has been an ongoing debate concerning an optimal target blood pressure in patients with atherosclerotic disease of the large cerebral arteries (internal carotid artery, middle cerebral artery, anterior cerebral artery, vertebral and basilar arteries). Moreover, previous studies and some expert opinions suggest that an increase in stroke risk might be related to lowering blood pressure in patients with severe carotid stenosis (particularly if the stenosis is bilateral) by creating a low flow state in the affected arterial territory.[41,42] Therefore, it is not uncommon in clinical practice to allow blood pressure to remain above 140/90 mm Hg in patients with intracranial stenosis. The Warfarin-Aspirin Symptomatic Intracranial Disease (WASID) study provided evidence that elevated systolic blood pressure (SBP) and diastolic blood pressure (DBP) were significantly associated with increased risk of stroke in the territory of the stenosed artery, and the overall risk of ischemic stroke.[15] In addition, subsequent subgroup analysis did not show any evidence of an increased risk of stroke with lower SBP in patients with severe ($\geq 70\%$) stenosis and those with stenosis of the posterior circulation arteries.[43] Therefore, it is advisable for clinicians to follow the JNC 7 recommendations in stroke prevention in patients with intracranial stenosis.

Hypercholesterolemia

Lipid-lowering therapy is discussed in Chapter 9. With regard to intracranial stenosis, elevated low-density lipoprotein (LDL) level was shown to be strongly associated with higher risk of subsequent stroke, myocardial infarction (MI), or vascular death in patients in a substudy of the WASID study.[11] (The main study is discussed below.)

Anticoagulation

The WASID study was a randomized, double-blind, multicenter clinical trial[15] comparing the safety and efficacy of aspirin 1300 mg daily with warfarin (target international normalized ratio [INR] 2.0-3.0) in patients with symptomatic intracranial stenosis. Between 1999 and 2003, patients aged 40 years or older were enrolled if they had TIA or nondisabling stroke (modified Rankin Score ≤3) within 90 days that was attributable to angiographically verified 50% to 99% stenosis of a major intracranial vessel (carotid, middle cerebral, vertebral, or basilar). Exclusion criteria included tandem 50% to 99% stenosis of the extracranial carotid artery, nonatherosclerotic stenosis of an intracranial artery, a cardiac source of embolism, a contraindication to aspirin or warfarin use, an indication for heparin use after being randomized, and a coexisting condition that limited survival to less than 5 years. The study was originally designed to enroll a total of 806 patients with a mean follow-up of 3 years. However, because of higher rates of death and hemorrhage in the warfarin group, the study was stopped early after 569 subjects had been randomly assigned with a mean follow-up period of 1.8 years. The primary endpoint, including ischemic stroke, brain hemorrhage, or death from vascular causes other than stroke, occurred in 22.1% and 21.8% among those assigned to aspirin and warfarin, respectively. The rate of death was significantly higher among patients taking warfarin (9.7% in the warfarin group vs 4.3% in the aspirin group). Myocardial infarction and major hemorrhages also occurred more often in patients assigned to warfarin. The results of WASID demonstrated that aspirin was safer and as effective as warfarin for stroke prevention in symptomatic intracranial atherosclerotic disease.

Antiplatelet Agents

After the publication of the WASID study, aspirin became the antithrombotic drug of choice for stroke prevention in symptomatic intracranial atherosclerosis patients. Although recent evidence demonstrated some benefits of clopidogrel plus aspirin over aspirin alone in reducing microembolic signals caused by symptomatic intracranial or carotid artery stenosis, a benefit of this combination with regard to a reduction of recurrent stroke risk remains to be confirmed. Apart from aspirin, cilostazol, a phosphodiesterase inhibitor, is the only antiplatelet agent tested in intracranial stenosis patients. The Trial of cilostazol in Symptomatic intracranial arterial Stenosis (TOSS) study aimed to test the efficacy and safety of cilostazol on prevention of progression against acute symptomatic intracranial artery stenosis in a multicenter, double-blind, placebo-controlled trial design.[44] During a six-month follow-up, there was no stroke or TIA in either the cilostazol plus aspirin or the placebo plus aspirin arm. However, the progression rate of symptomatic intracranial atherosclerosis was significantly lower in the cilostazol arm (6.7% vs 28.8%; $P = .008$). In addition, regression was also found more frequently in the cilostazol group (24.4% vs 15.4%). These findings led to a multicenter trial of Cilostazol in Symptomatic Intracranial Arterial Stenosis-II (TOSS-II) for which the results have not yet been published. The efficacy of cilostazol was also tested against aspirin in the second Cilostazol Stroke Prevention Study (CSPS 2).[45] The study aimed to compare the efficacy and safety of cilostazol versus aspirin in patients with non-cardioembolic ischemic stroke, with a mean follow-up of 29 months. The primary endpoint was the first occurrence of stroke including cerebral infarction, cerebral hemorrhage, or subarachnoid hemorrhage. At the end of the study, the primary endpoint occurred at yearly rates of 2.76% in the cilostazol group and 3.71% in the aspirin group (hazard ratio 0.743; 95% confidence interval [CI] 0.564-0.981; $P = .0357$). However, hemorrhagic stroke accounted for the majority of the difference in the primary endpoint; there was no significant difference in recurrent ischemic stroke.

Antiplatelet therapy is discussed in detail in Chapter 7.

Revascularization Strategies

SURGICAL TREATMENT

An international randomized trial of extracranial–intracranial arterial bypass to reduce the risk of ischemic stroke (EC/IC Bypass Study) included 1377 patients with recent stroke or TIA who had atherosclerotic narrowing or occlusion of the ipsilateral internal carotid or middle cerebral artery.[46] Of those, 714 were randomly assigned to the best medical care, and 663 to the same regimen with the addition of bypass surgery joining the superficial temporal artery and the middle cerebral artery. During the mean follow-up of 55.8 months, strokes were found to occur more frequently and earlier in the patients randomized to surgery. Of note, those with severe middle cerebral artery stenosis ($\geq$70%) had a significantly better outcome if treated medically (5.1% strokes per year of follow-up) as compared to those treated surgically (9.5% per year of follow-up). Based on this study, EC/IC bypass surgery is not recommended.

ENDOVASCULAR INTERVENTION

With prior development, success, and general acceptance of angioplasty and stenting for the treatment of peripheral and coronary artery disease, endovascular therapy has emerged as an important alternative treatment for symptomatic intracranial stenosis. The Stenting of Symptomatic Atherosclerotic Lesions in the Vertebral or Intracranial Arteries (SSYLVIA) study enrolled 61 patients with symptomatic intracranial and extracranial vertebral artery stenosis 50% or above for stenting.[47] Intracranial stenosis accounted for 70.5% of the lesions. A stent was successfully placed in 95% of patients. There were no deaths, and patients had relatively low rates (6.6%) of stroke at 30 days. Fourteen percent of the patients (6 of 43) with an intracranial stenosis experienced recurrent stroke within one year. Restenosis of more than 50% at six months occurred in 12 of 37 (32.4%) intracranial stent patients. The Cochrane Database review in 2006 did not find any randomized controlled trials of angioplasty and stenting.[48] However, a systematic review on outcome after stenting for intracranial atherosclerosis included 31 studies dealing with 1177 procedures that had mainly been performed in symptomatic (98%) intracranial high-grade stenosis (mean 78 ± 7%). A high success rate was reported (median 96%). The periprocedural stroke and death ranged from 0% to 50% with a median of 7.7%. Complications were significantly higher in the posterior versus the anterior circulation (12.1% vs 6.6%, $P < .01$). Restenosis greater than 50% occurred more frequently after the use of a self-expanding stent than a balloon-mounted stent (17.4% vs 13.8%) during a mean follow-up of 5.4 and 8.7 months, respectively. Long-term outcomes are not yet available and the studies do not include a randomized intensive medical therapy arm.[49]

In 2008, a large multicenter, randomized controlled trial (the Stenting vs Aggressive Medical Management for Preventing Recurrent Stroke in Intracranial Stenosis [SAMMPRIS]) was initiated to evaluate the safety and efficacy of intracranial angioplasty with stenting combined with intensive medical therapy, compared with intensive medical therapy alone. Participants were those who experienced a TIA or stroke within 30 days, with severe (70%-90%) symptomatic major intracranial artery stenosis. The primary endpoint was recurrent stroke in the distribution of the stenosed artery. Mean follow-up was planned at up to two years, with a target enrollment of 764 subjects. Recruitment was expected to be completed in five years. The angioplasty and stenting system used in the trial was the Gateway-Wingspan system.

The study was stopped early in April 2011, after 451 (59%) of the planned 764 patients had been enrolled from 50 participating sites in the United States. At the time of the most recent data safety monitoring board review, 14% of patients treated with angioplasty and stenting combined with intensive medical therapy experienced a stroke or died within the first 30 days after enrollment compared with 5.8% of patients treated with intensive medical therapy alone, a highly significant difference. Within 30 days after enrollment, there were five stroke-related deaths, all in the stenting arm, and one non–stroke-related death was found in the medical arm. Beyond 30 days, the rates of stroke in the territory of the stenotic artery were similar in the two groups, but fewer than half the patients had been followed for one year. Therefore, follow-up of currently enrolled patients and comprehensive analysis of the total trial data set are important in the final interpretation of this study. As a result, the trial data currently available indicate that intensive medical management alone is superior to angioplasty combined with stenting in patients with symptomatic high-grade intracranial arterial stenosis.

CONCLUSION

Symptomatic ICAD is associated with a high risk of subsequent stroke. WASID demonstrated that aspirin is as effective as warfarin and resulted in fewer hemorrhagic complications. Aggressive blood pressure management according to the JNC 7 guidelines and reducing LDL level can lower the risk of recurrent stroke. Patients with severe (70%-99%) stenosis of ICAD with recent symptoms represent the highest-risk subgroup. Although intracranial stenting appears to be a promising interventional therapy, a currently available clinical study showed that aggressive medication management and risk factor control was associated with a lower risk of recurrent stroke and death at 30 days. However, long-term follow-up results have yet to be determined.

REFERENCES

1. Wong KS, Hung YN, Gao S, Lam WW, Chan YL, Kay R. Intracranial stenosis in Chinese patients with acute stroke. *Neurology.* 1998;50(3):812-813.

2. Kim JT, Yoo SH, Kwon JH, Kwon SU, Kim JS. Subtyping of ischemic stroke based on vascular imaging: analysis of 1,167 acute, consecutive patients. *J Clin Neurol.* 2006;2(4):225-230.

3. Sacco RL, Kargman DE, Gu Q, Zamanillo MC. Race-ethnicity and determinants of intracranial atherosclerotic cerebral infarction. The Northern Manhattan Stroke Study. *Stroke.* 1995;26(1):14-20.

4. Arenillas JF, Molina CA, Chacon P, et al. High lipoprotein (a), diabetes, and the extent of symptomatic intracranial atherosclerosis. *Neurology.* 2004;63(1):27-32.

5. Qureshi AI, Ziai WC, Yahia AM, et al. Stroke-free survival and its determinants in patients with symptomatic vertebrobasilar stenosis: a multicenter study. *Neurosurgery.* 2003;52(5):1033-1039; discussion 9-40.

6. White H, Boden-Albala B, Wang C, et al. Ischemic stroke subtype incidence among whites, blacks, and Hispanics: the Northern Manhattan Study. *Circulation.* 2005;111(10):1327-1331.

7. Huang YN, Gao S, Li SW, et al. Vascular lesions in Chinese patients with transient ischemic attacks. *Neurology.* 1997;48(2):524-525.

8. Bae HJ, Lee J, Park JM, et al. Risk factors of intracranial cerebral atherosclerosis among asymptomatics. *Cerebrovasc Dis.* 2007;24(4):355-360.

9. Kostner GM, Marth E, Pfeiffer KP, Wege H. Apolipoproteins AI, AII and HDL phospholipids but not APO-B are risk indicators for occlusive cerebrovascular disease. *Eur Neurol.* 1986;25(5):346-354.

10. Wong KS, Li H. Long-term mortality and recurrent stroke risk among Chinese stroke patients with predominant intracranial atherosclerosis. *Stroke.* 2003;34(10):2361-2366.

11. Chaturvedi S, Turan TN, Lynn MJ, et al. Risk factor status and vascular events in patients with symptomatic intracranial stenosis. *Neurology.* 2007;69(22):2063-2068.

12. Passero S, Rossi G, Nardini M, et al. Italian multicenter study of reversible cerebral ischemic attacks. Part 5. Risk factors and cerebral atherosclerosis. *Atherosclerosis.* 1987;63(2-3):211-224.

13. Moossy J. Pathology of cerebral atherosclerosis. Influence of age, race, and gender. *Stroke.* 1993; 24(12 Suppl):I22-I23; I31-I32.

14. Kasner SE, Chimowitz MI, Lynn MJ, et al. Predictors of ischemic stroke in the territory of a symptomatic intracranial arterial stenosis. *Circulation.* 2006;113(4):555-563.

15. Chimowitz MI, Lynn MJ, Howlett-Smith H, et al. Comparison of warfarin and aspirin for symptomatic intracranial arterial stenosis. *N Engl J Med.* 2005;352(13):1305-1316.

16. Caplan L, Babikian V, Helgason C, et al. Occlusive disease of the middle cerebral artery. *Neurology.* 1985;35(7):975-982.

17. Hinton RC, Mohr JP, Ackerman RH, Adair LB, Fisher CM. Symptomatic middle cerebral artery stenosis. *Ann Neurol.* 1979;5(2):152-157.

18. Caplan LR, Kelly M, Kase CS, et al. Infarcts of the inferior division of the right middle cerebral artery: mirror image of Wernicke's aphasia. *Neurology.* 1986;36(8):1015-1020.

19. Chimowitz MI, Furlan AJ, Sila CA, Paranandi L, Beck GJ. Etiology of motor or sensory stroke: a prospective study of the predictive value of clinical and radiological features. *Ann Neurol.* 1991;30(4):519-525.

20. Bogousslavsky J, Regli F. Anterior cerebral artery territory infarction in the Lausanne Stroke Registry. Clinical and etiologic patterns. *Arch Neurol.* 1990;47(2):144-150.

21. Kazui S, Sawada T, Naritomi H, Kuriyama Y, Yamaguchi T. Angiographic evaluation of brain infarction limited to the anterior cerebral artery territory. *Stroke.* 1993;24(4):549-553.

22. Archer CR, Horenstein S. Basilar artery occlusion: clinical and radiological correlation. *Stroke.* 1977;8(3):383-390.

23. Thompson JR, Simmons CR, Hasso AN, Hinshaw DB Jr. Occlusion of the intradural vertebrobasilar artery. *Neuroradiology.* 1978;14(5):219-229.

24. Pessin MS, Gorelick PB, Kwan ES, Caplan LR. Basilar artery stenosis: middle and distal segments. *Neurology.* 1987;37(11):1742-1746.

25. Fisher CM, Caplan LR. Basilar artery branch occlusion: a cause of pontine infarction. *Neurology.* 1971;21(9):900-905.

26. Caplan LR. "Top of the basilar" syndrome. *Neurology.* 1980;30(1):72-79.

27. Castaigne P, Lhermitte F, Gautier JC, et al. Arterial occlusions in the vertebro-basilar system. A study of 44 patients with post-mortem data. *Brain.* 1973;96(1):133-154.

28. Pessin MS, Kwan ES, DeWitt LD, Hedges TR 3rd, Gale D, Caplan LR. Posterior cerebral artery stenosis. *Ann Neurol.* 1987;21(1):85-89.

29. Pessin MS, Lathi ES, Cohen MB, Kwan ES, Hedges TR 3rd, Caplan LR. Clinical features and mechanism of occipital infarction. *Ann Neurol.* 1987;21(3):290-299.

30. Wong KS, Gao S, Chan YL, et al. Mechanisms of acute cerebral infarctions in patients with middle cerebral artery stenosis: a diffusion-weighted imaging and microemboli monitoring study. *Ann Neurol.* 2002;52(1):74-81.

31. Roh JK, Kang DW, Lee SH, Yoon BW, Chang KH. Significance of acute multiple brain infarction on diffusion-weighted imaging. *Stroke.* 2000;31(3):688-694.

32. Min WK, Park KK, Kim YS, et al. Atherothrombotic middle cerebral artery territory infarction: topographic diversity with common occurrence of concomitant small cortical and subcortical infarcts. *Stroke.* 2000;31(9):2055-2061.

33. Damasio H. A computed tomographic guide to the identification of cerebral vascular territories. *Arch Neurol.* 1983;40(3):138-142.

34. Bladin CF, Chambers BR. Clinical features, pathogenesis, and computed tomographic characteristics of internal watershed infarction. *Stroke.* 1993;24(12):1925-1932.

35. Choi JW, Kim JK, Choi BS, et al. Angiographic pattern of symptomatic severe M1 stenosis: comparison with presenting symptoms, infarct patterns, perfusion status, and outcome after recanalization. *Cerebrovasc Dis.* 2010;29(3):297-303.

36. Lawes CM, Vander Hoorn S, Rodgers A. Global burden of blood-pressure-related disease, 2001. *Lancet.* 2008;371(9623):1513-1518.

37. Randomised trial of a perindopril-based blood-pressure-lowering regimen among 6,105 individuals with previous stroke or transient ischaemic attack. *Lancet.* 2001;358(9287):1033-1041.

38. Rashid P, Leonardi-Bee J, Bath P. Blood pressure reduction and secondary prevention of stroke and other vascular events: a systematic review. *Stroke.* 2003;34(11):2741-2748.

39. Gueyffier F, Boissel JP, Boutitie F, et al. Effect of antihypertensive treatment in patients having already suffered from stroke. Gathering the evidence. The INDANA (Individual Data Analysis of Antihypertensive intervention trials) Project Collaborators. *Stroke.* 1997;28(12):2557-2562.

40. Chobanian AV, Bakris GL, Black HR, et al. The Seventh Report of the Joint National Committee on Prevention, Detection, Evaluation, and Treatment of High Blood Pressure: the JNC 7 report. *JAMA.* 2003;289(19):2560-2572.

41. Flemming KD, Brown RD Jr. Secondary prevention strategies in ischemic stroke: identification and optimal management of modifiable risk factors. *Mayo Clin Proc.* 2004;79(10):1330-1340.

42. Rothwell PM, Howard SC, Spence JD. Relationship between blood pressure and stroke risk in patients with symptomatic carotid occlusive disease. *Stroke.* 2003;34(11):2583-2590.

43. Turan TN, Cotsonis G, Lynn MJ, Chaturvedi S, Chimowitz M. Relationship between blood pressure and stroke recurrence in patients with intracranial arterial stenosis. *Circulation.* 2007;115(23): 2969-2975.

44. Kwon SU, Cho YJ, Koo JS, et al. Cilostazol prevents the progression of the symptomatic intracranial arterial stenosis: the multicenter double-blind placebo-controlled trial of cilostazol in symptomatic intracranial arterial stenosis. *Stroke.* 2005;36(4):782-786.

45. Shinohara Y, Katayama Y, Uchiyama S, et al. Cilostazol for prevention of secondary stroke (CSPS 2): an aspirin-controlled, double-blind, randomised non-inferiority trial. *Lancet Neurol.* 2010;9(10):959-968.

46. Failure of extracranial-intracranial arterial bypass to reduce the risk of ischemic stroke. Results of an international randomized trial. The EC/IC Bypass Study Group. *N Engl J Med.* 1985;313(19): 1191-1200.

47. Stenting of Symptomatic Atherosclerotic Lesions in the Vertebral or Intracranial Arteries (SSYLVIA): study results. *Stroke.* 2004;35(6):1388-1392.

48. Cruz-Flores S, Diamond AL. Angioplasty for intracranial artery stenosis. *Cochrane Database Syst Rev.* 2006;3:CD004133.

49. Groschel K, Schnaudigel S, Pilgram SM, Wasser K, Kastrup A. A systematic review on outcome after stenting for intracranial atherosclerosis. *Stroke.* 2009;40(5):e340-e347.

Appropriate Endarterectomy and Stenting for Carotid Stenosis

11

J. David Spence
Alastair M. Buchan
Henry J. M. Barnett
Joyce S. Balami

TOPICS

INTRODUCTION

Patients with carotid stenosis are severe arteriopaths, with a higher risk of coronary events than that of patients with known coronary artery disease (CAD): in the Scandinavian Simvastatin Survival Study,[1] the six-year risk of a myocardial infarction in the patients randomized to placebo was 26%; in the approximately contemporaneous Veterans Administration study of surgery for asymptomatic carotid stenosis (ACS), the four-year risk of a coronary event among patients with ACS but no previous history of CAD was 33%.[2] Thus patients with carotid stenosis have a very high risk that warrants intensive medical therapy. Although carotid endarterectomy is clearly beneficial for symptomatic stenosis,[3] and stenting is a viable option for selected patients, it is increasingly clear that with more intensive medical therapy, only a minority of patients with asymptomatic carotid stenosis can benefit from these procedures.

SYMPTOMATIC CAROTID STENOSIS

Patients with symptomatic severe carotid stenosis (≥70%) are the ones who will clearly benefit from endarterectomy. In the North American Symptomatic Carotid Endarterectomy Trial (NASCET) they had a 26% two-year risk of stroke or death that was reduced by endarterectomy to 9%.[4] The number needed to treat (NNT) to prevent one stroke was only six for patients age below 75, and only three for those aged 75 or older; for patients with moderate stenosis (50%-69%), the NNT was 15.[5] The importance of timely endarterectomy for symptomatic stenosis is discussed in Chapter 1.

NASCET, in 2700 randomized patients with symptoms appropriate to carotid stenosis, showed that the highest risk and greatest benefit increased with the degree of stenosis[3]; elderly men with no evidence of other organ failure get the most benefit[6]; unless other risk factors exist, women with moderate stenosis do not benefit[7]; in patients with contralateral occlusion the immediate risk is higher, but there is long-term benefit from carotid endarterectomy (CEA).[8] Symptomatic patients with intracranial stenosis of moderate degree do not have increased risk of CEA.[9] When leukoaraiosis (white matter disease) is widespread (and in all four horizontal quadrants, in the magnetic resonance [MR] image), CEA is risky and should be avoided. If the sole symptom is vascular *amaurosis fugax* with only moderate stenosis, unless other risk factors exist, CEA is not beneficial.[10]

Similar results were shown in the European Carotid Surgery Trial (ECST), with a clear benefit from endarterectomy in patients with severe carotid stenosis (≥80%).[11] The difference in defining severe stenosis was due to the different measurement methods used by the two trials. Moreover, there were differences in the definitions of outcome events. However, a reanalysis of the final results of ECST with a measurement of the prerandomization degree of stenosis measured by the NASCET method showed that the two studies yielded comparable findings. Patients with moderate stenosis (50%-69%) had some benefit but not in all the measured outcomes, whereas patients with severe stenosis (70%-99%) without near occlusion had major benefits from surgery[12,13] (Table 11–1 summarizes the findings from NASCET, ECST, and the pooled analysis). A recent Cochrane meta-analysis displayed similar results.[14]

Candidates for CEA should all receive thorough cardiac investigation and appropriate management strategies before proceeding to CEA. This may include the need for a coronary artery bypass graft (CABG). Surgeons with little CEA experience and who are unable to affirm a less than 6% risk of stroke and death should not be permitted by their institution to perform CEA unless accompanied by an expert who can match or fall below the allowable complication rate. When the carotid narrowing reaches more than 95%, abundant anastomoses of intracranial and extracranial type internal carotid beyond the stenosis will be much narrowed and of lesser diameter than the companion external carotid in the neck. This phenomenon has been dubbed near-occlusion.[15] Fox et al have reviewed the course and treatment for this lesion.[16] It can be corrected by CEA without undue risk, but without CEA it carries only moderate risk and often will go on to complete occlusion, usually without new symptoms. No CEA should be done, other than by experienced surgeons capable of CEA with minimal complications.

Stenting carries a higher risk than endarterectomy,[17] and this difference increases with advancing age.[18] Stenting should therefore be reserved for selected patients: younger patients at high risk from surgery because of concomitant medical conditions.[19,20] Paraskevas et al reviewed in 2011 reasons why endarterectomy is the treatment of choice for most patients with carotid stenosis.[20] Additional reasons for preferring stenting over endarterectomy would include previous endarterectomy or

Table 11–1. NNT and Relative Risk in the Surgery Group in NASCET, ECST, and Pooled Analysis

	NASCET	ECST	Pooled Analysis
Patients With Symptomatic Severe Stenosis (70%-99%)			
Any stroke			
NNT	8	5	6
RR (95% CI)	0.62 (0.45-0.82)	0.36 (0.22-0.51)	0.52 (0.40-0.64)
Ipsilateral ischemic stroke			
NNT	6	5	6
RR (95% CI)	0.41 (0.25-0.58)	0.31 (0.16-0.45)	0.39 (0.28-0.51)
Disabling or ipsilateral ischemic stroke			
NNT	11	14	14
RR (95% CI)	0.31 (0.10-0.52)	0.39 (0.12-0.67)	0.39 (0.21-0.58)
Patients With Symptomatic Moderate Stenosis (50%-69%)			
Any stroke			
NNT	13	18	13
RR (95% CI)	0.76 (0.57-0.95)	0.74 (0.49-0.99)	0.72 (0.58-0.86)
Ipsilateral stroke			
NNT	15	34	22
RR (95% CI)	0.70 (0.47-0.93)	0.81 (0.49-1.13)	0.75 (0.56-0.94)
Disabling or ipsilateral stroke			
NNT	29	83	43
RR (95% CI)	0.46 (0.12-0.79)	0.85 (0.35-1.35)	0.68 (0.36-1.07)

CI, confidence interval; NNT, number needed to treat; RR, relative risk.

stenosis due to radiation for cancer (because the scarring after surgery makes second operations more difficult and risky), and high stenosis not readily accessible to the surgeon. (Tables 11–2 and 11–3 summarize the advantages and disadvantages as well as the complications associated with CEA and carotid stenting [CAS].)

ASYMPTOMATIC CAROTID STENOSIS

Stenting or endarterectomy is not justifiable, however, in the great majority of patients with ACS. Even when there was a 30% relative risk reduction with surgery, the reduction in absolute risk was small. Moreover, any benefit may be nullified by higher perioperative complication rates and only centers with complication rates less than 3% should perform surgery in asymptomatic individuals.[21] However, with more intensive medical therapy, the risk of asymptomatic carotid stenosis with medical therapy is now below the risk of surgery or stenting. The annual risk of stroke is now below 1% per year; this has been shown in a vascular prevention clinic setting,[22] a meta-analysis,[23] and a prospective population-based study.[24]

Table 11–2. Advantages and Disadvantages of Carotid Endarterectomy and Stenting

Procedure	Advantages	Disadvantages
Endarterectomy	Gold standard for symptomatic severe carotid stenosis ↓ microembolic events ↓ restenosis	General anesthesia and ↑ systemic complications ↑ cranial nerve injury ↑ wound-derived complications
Stenting	Suitable in stenosis not accessible to surgery Suitable in patients with previous CEA, radiation arteritis Local anesthesia ↓ hospitalization and convalescence	Requires angiography (↑ complications) ↑ microembolic events ↑ restenosis ↑ local complications

No significant difference between CEA and CAS in the risk of stroke or death in the long term, but higher risk of stroke with stenting.

For that reason, current practice in the United States, where 90% or more of carotid endarterectomy and stenting is for asymptomatic stenosis,[25] is deplorable. Spence has reviewed some of the reasons for this practice[26]; they do not stand up to scrutiny. Malpractice is not too strong a word for this situation. These procedures are being justified by historical data that have been superseded, and there are concerns that procedures are being done more for the benefit of the operator than for the patient.[27]

That the risk of stroke or death was reduced marginally (although to a statistically significant degree) in the Asymptomatic Carotid Artery Surgery (ACAS)

Table 11–3. Complications Associated With Carotid Endarterectomy (CEA) and Carotid Stenting (CAS)

Endarterectomy	Stenting
Peri- and postoperative stroke	Peri- and postoperative stroke
Hyperperfusion syndrome	Hyperperfusion syndrome
Cranial nerve injury	Myocardial infarction
Wound bleeding	Renal dysfunction
Wound pain	Access-related complications
Parotitis	Distal embolization
Infection	Stent fracture
Labile blood pressure	Bradycardia and hypotension

trial[28] and the Asymptomatic Carotid Surgery Trial (ACST)[29] is no longer justification for these procedures in the face of recent evidence that with medical therapy, the risk of ACS has markedly declined.[22-24] A future prospective trial could be based on stratification of cerebrovascular risk using clinical, biochemical, and ultrasonographic characteristics in asymptomatic patients with carotid stenosis to select those who may benefit from surgical treatment.[30]

The CREST and ICSS Trials

The recent publication of the **Carotid Revascularization Endarterectomy versus Stenting Trial (CREST)** promises to exacerbate the already inappropriate use of endarterectomy and stenting for ACS in the United States and elsewhere. The CREST trial was funded to study symptomatic patients. Because of poor accrual rates, a major protocol change determined that asymptomatic subjects, with their low risk of stroke, were henceforth to be added to the database, and the analyses implied that the two groups of patients could be added together.[18] Contrarians have published their reasons[31] for believing that CREST failed to add to our knowledge of indications for the use of stenting in symptomatic patients or asymptomatic patients. CREST was originally designed to enroll symptomatic patients, for whom the sample size may have been reasonable. However, when problems with recruitment of patients drove the investigators to change the design to include asymptomatic patients, the study became underpowered for either symptomatic or asymptomatic patients. Because the risks for these two groups of patients are so different, it is not appropriate to combine them in analyses of the results.

The periprocedural risk of stroke for ACS in CREST, at 2.5% for stenting and 1.4% for endarterectomy (with 4-year risks of 4.5% and 2.7%), does *not* warrant uncritical intervention in ACS.[32] Spence et al[33] reported in 2005 that intervention could not benefit 90% of patients with ACS, because their 1-year risk of stroke was only 1%. By 2010, the proportion of patients who could benefit from intervention had declined to less than 5% with more intensive medical therapy[34]: the 2-year risk of stroke or myocardial infarction is now 1%. In both these studies it was shown that the patients who might benefit could be identified by the presence of microemboli on transcranial Doppler (TCD) ultrasound (Figure 11–1), and that patients without microemboli had a risk lower than that of intervention. More recently, that finding was validated in an international multicenter study of TCD embolus detection.[35] Two recent reports have shown that the risk of ACS is lower with medical therapy than with intervention in CREST.[23,24] Derdeyn in 2007 called for a moratorium on carotid stenting outside of clinical trials with a medical arm.[36] Recent evidence has proven him right.

Among patients with ACS, there are some indications that high-risk patients who may benefit from intervention can be identified. Spence et al[37] reported in 2005 that TCD detection of microemboli identified a subgroup of 10% of patients with a two-year stroke risk of 15%, whereas those without microemboli had only a 1% risk of stroke. This was substantiated by the report of the Asymptomatic Carotid Emboli Study (ACES),[35] in which ACS patients with microemboli had a significantly higher risk of stroke. However, with more intensive medical therapy,

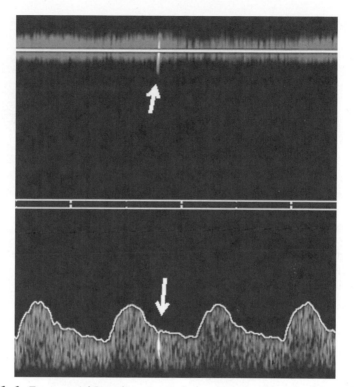

Figure 11–1. Transcranial Doppler microembolus detection identifies high-risk asymptomatic carotid stenosis. The microembolus can be seen in the upper channel (white arrow), which is an M-mode image of the middle cerebral artery. The lower channel shows the high-intensity transit (HIT) signal (white arrow) in the Doppler velocity spectrum. (Figure courtesy of Dr. Claudio Muñoz.)

both the prevalence of microemboli and the risk of stroke have declined markedly. Comparing their experience before and after 2003, when they implemented a regimen of more intensive medical therapy based on carotid plaque measurements,[38] Spence et al[22] found that the prevalence of microemboli in ACS patients declined from 12.6% to 3.7% of patients. More importantly, the two-year risk of stroke declined from 8.8% to 1%, and the two-year risk of myocardial infarction declined from 7.6% to 1%.

Madani et al[39] found that in patients with asymptomatic carotid stenosis, plaque ulceration detected by three-dimensional carotid ultrasound (Figure 11–2) also identified high-risk patients: those with three or more ulcers had a stroke risk equivalent to that of patients with microemboli; the combination of microemboli and ulcers increased to 10% the proportion of patients with ACS who now stand to benefit from endarterectomy or stenting. Besides microembolus detection and ulceration, new approaches to identifying high-risk patients based on imaging of vulnerable plaque are now being developed.[40] A small study suggests that intra-plaque hemorrhage on MRI is a promising approach to this problem.[41]

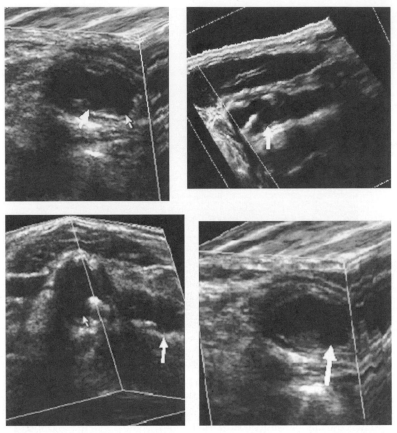

Figure 11–2. Carotid ulceration on three-dimensional ultrasound also identifies high-risk asymptomatic carotid stenosis. The white arrows show ulcers in carotid plaques in patients with asymptomatic stenosis. Patients with three or more ulcers (the total in both carotid arteries) have a risk equivalent to that of patients with microemboli. (Permission granted by Lippincott, Williams & Wilkins to reproduce from Madani A, Beletsky V, Tamayo A, Munoz C, Spence JD. High-risk asymptomatic carotid stenosis: ulceration on 3D ultrasound versus TCD microemboli. *Neurology.* 2011;77:744-750.)

The International Carotid Stenting Study (ICSS)[42] was designed to evaluate the safety of stenting versus endarterectomy. The short-term results from the interim analysis showed that stenting is less safe than endarterectomy, with a 3.3% higher risk of stroke, death, or procedural myocardial infarction within 120 days of randomization. In the per-protocol analysis the rate of adverse events in the stenting group was more than twice the rate in endarterectomy group. Even if there is no significant difference in disabling or fatal strokes between the two groups, there is an excess of nondisabling strokes in the stenting group, with a likely poor outcome because of the possible increased risk of dementia associated with stroke.[43] Although final data are still expected, there is no evidence so far to prefer stenting to endarterectomy in carotid stenosis patients with severe or moderate stenosis.

CONCLUSION

Carotid endarterectomy is beneficial for patients with severe symptomatic carotid stenosis. Stenting will only be warranted in such patients if they have had a previous endarterectomy, or in the presence of an occasional lesion that is difficult to access surgically. There is only moderate benefit for patients with only moderate stenosis or near occlusion. Below 50% stenosis, CEA will be more likely to be harmful. For approximately 90% of patients with asymptomatic carotid stenosis, the treatment of choice would be intensive medical therapy.

REFERENCES

1. Scandinavian Simvastatin Survival Study Group. Randomized trial of cholesterol lowering in 4,444 patients with coronary heart disease: the Scandinavian Simvastatin Survival Study (4S). *Lancet.* 1994;344:1383-1389.
2. Chimowitz MI, Weiss DG, Cohen SL, Starling MR, Hobson RW. Cardiac prognosis of patients with carotid stenosis and no history of coronary artery disease. Veterans Affairs Cooperative Study Group 167. *Stroke.* 1994;25:759-765.
3. Barnett HJM, Taylor DW, Eliasziw M, et al. Benefit of carotid endarterectomy in patients with symptomatic moderate or severe carotid stenosis. *N Engl J Med.* 1998;339:1415-1425.
4. North American Symptomatic Carotid Endarterectomy Trial Collaborators. Beneficial effect of carotid endarterectomy in symptomatic patients with high-grade carotid stenosis. *N Engl J Med.* 1991;325:445-507.
5. Barnett HJ. The inappropriate use of carotid endarterectomy. *CMAJ.* 2004;171:473-474.
6. Alamowitch S, Eliasziw M, Algra A, Meldrum H, Barnett HJ. Risk, causes, and prevention of ischaemic stroke in elderly patients with symptomatic internal-carotid-artery stenosis. *Lancet.* 2001;357:1154-1160.
7. Alamowitch S, Eliasziw M, Barnett HJ. The risk and benefit of endarterectomy in women with symptomatic internal carotid artery disease. *Stroke.* 2005;36:27-31.
8. Gasecki AP, Eliasziw M, Ferguson GG, Hachinski V, Barnett HJ. Long-term prognosis and effect of endarterectomy in patients with symptomatic severe carotid stenosis and contralateral carotid stenosis or occlusion: results from NASCET. North American Symptomatic Carotid Endarterectomy Trial (NASCET) Group. *J Neurosurg.* 1995;83:778-782.
9. Kappelle LJ, Eliasziw M, Fox AJ, Sharpe BL, Barnett HJ. Importance of intracranial atherosclerotic disease in patients with symptomatic stenosis of the internal carotid artery. The North American Symptomatic Carotid Endarterectomy Trail. *Stroke.* 1999;30:282-286.
10. Streifler JY, Eliasziw M, Benavente OR, et al. The risk of stroke in patients with first-ever retinal vs hemispheric transient ischemic attacks and high-grade carotid stenosis. North American Symptomatic Carotid Endarterectomy Trial. *Arch Neurol.* 1995;52:246-249.
11. European Carotid Surgery Trialists' Collaborative Group. Randomised trial of endarterectomy for recently symptomatic carotid stenosis: final results of the MRC European Carotid Surgery Trial (ECST). *Lancet.* 1998;351:1379-1387.
12. Rothwell PM, Eliasziw M, Gutnikov SA, et al. Analysis of pooled data from the randomised controlled trials of endarterectomy for symptomatic carotid stenosis. *Lancet.* 2003;361:107-116.
13. Rothwell PM, Gutnikov SA, Warlow CP. Reanalysis of the final results of the European Carotid Surgery Trial. *Stroke.* 2003;34:514-523.
14. Rerkasem K, Rothwell PM. Carotid endarterectomy for symptomatic carotid stenosis. *Cochrane Database Syst Rev.* 2011;4:CD001081.
15. Morgenstern LB, Fox AJ, Sharpe BL, Eliasziw M, Barnett HJ, Grotta JC. The risks and benefits of carotid endarterectomy in patients with near occlusion of the carotid artery. North American Symptomatic Carotid Endarterectomy Trial (NASCET) Group. *Neurology.* 1997;48:911-915.
16. Fox AJ, Eliasziw M, Rothwell PM, Schmidt MH, Warlow CP, Barnett HJ. Identification, prognosis, and management of patients with carotid artery near occlusion. *AJNR Am J Neuroradiol.* 2005;26:2086-2094.
17. Rothwell PM. Poor outcomes after endovascular treatment of symptomatic carotid stenosis: time for a moratorium. *Lancet Neurol.* 2009;8:871-873.

18. Brott TG, Hobson RW, II, Howard G, et al. Stenting versus endarterectomy for treatment of carotid-artery stenosis. *N Engl J Med.* 2010;363:11-23.

19. Yadav JS, Wholey MH, Kuntz RE, et al. Protected carotid-artery stenting versus endarterectomy in high-risk patients. *N Engl J Med.* 2004;351:1493-1501.

20. Paraskevas KI, Veith FJ, Riles TS, Moore WS. Is carotid artery stenting a fair alternative to carotid endarterectomy for symptomatic carotid artery stenosis? *Eur J Vasc Endovasc Surg.* 2011;41:717-719.

21. Chambers BR, Donnan GA. Carotid endarterectomy for asymptomatic carotid stenosis. *Cochrane Database Syst Rev.* 2005;CD001923.

22. Spence JD, Coates V, Li H, et al. Effects of intensive medical therapy on microemboli and cardiovascular risk in asymptomatic carotid stenosis. *Arch Neurol.* 2010;67:180-186.

23. Abbott AL. Medical (nonsurgical) intervention alone is now best for prevention of stroke associated with asymptomatic severe carotid stenosis: results of a systematic review and analysis. *Stroke.* 2009;40:e573-e583.

24. Marquardt L, Geraghty OC, Mehta Z, Rothwell PM. Low risk of ipsilateral stroke in patients with asymptomatic carotid stenosis on best medical treatment: a prospective, population-based study. *Stroke.* 2010;41:e11-e17.

25. Vogel TR, Dombrovskiy VY, Haser PB, Scheirer JC, Graham AM. Outcomes of carotid artery stenting and endarterectomy in the United States. *J Vasc Surg.* 2009;49:325-330.

26. Spence JD. Asymptomatic carotid stenosis: mainly a medical condition. *Vascular.* 2010;18:123-126.

27. Naylor AR, Gaines PA, Rothwell PM. Who benefits most from intervention for asymptomatic carotid stenosis: patients or professionals? *Eur J Vasc Endovasc Surg.* 2009;37:625-632.

28. Executive Committee for the Asymptomatic Carotid Atherosclerosis Study. Endarterectomy for asymptomatic carotid artery stenosis. *JAMA.* 1995;272:1421-1428.

29. Halliday A, Mansfield A, Marro J, et al. Prevention of disabling and fatal strokes by successful carotid endarterectomy in patients without recent neurological symptoms: randomised controlled trial. *Lancet.* 2004;363:1491-1502.

30. Nicolaides AN, Kakkos SK, Kyriacou E, et al. Asymptomatic internal carotid artery stenosis and cerebrovascular risk stratification. *J Vasc Surg.* 2010;52:1486-1496.

31. Barnett HJ, Pelz DM, Lownie SP. Reflections by contrarians on the post-CREST evaluation of carotid stenting for stroke prevention. *Int J Stroke.* 2010;5:455-456.

32. Naylor AR. Riding on the CREST of a Wave! *Eur J Vasc Endovasc Surg.* 2010;39:523-526.

33. Spence JD, Tamayo A, Lownie SP, Ng W, Ferguson GG. Absence of microemboli on transcranial Doppler identifies low-risk patients with asymptomatic carotid stenosis who do not warrant endarterectomy or stenting. *Stroke.* 2005;36:2373-2378.

34. Spence JD, Coates V, Li H, et al. Effects of Intensive medical therapy on microemboli and cardiovascular risk in asymptomatic carotid stenosis. *Arch Neurol.* 2010;67:180-186.

35. Markus HS, King A, Shipley M, et al. Asymptomatic embolisation for prediction of stroke in the Asymptomatic Carotid Emboli Study (ACES): a prospective observational study. *Lancet Neurol.* 2010;9:663-671.

36. Derdeyn CP. Carotid stenting for asymptomatic carotid stenosis: trial it. *Stroke.* 2007;38:715-720.

37. Spence JD, Tamayo A, Lownie SP, Ng WP, Ferguson GG. Absence of microemboli on transcranial Doppler identifies low-risk patients with asymptomatic carotid stenosis. *Stroke.* 2005;36:2373-2378.

38. Spence JD, Hackam DG. Treating arteries instead of risk factors. A paradigm change in management of atherosclerosis. *Stroke.* 2010;41:1193-1199.

39. Madani A, Beletsky V, Tamayo A, Munoz C, Spence JD. High-risk asymptomatic carotid stenosis: ulceration on 3D ultrasound versus TCD microemboli. *Neurology.* 2011;77:744-750.

40. Spence JD. Cerebrovascular disease: identifying high-risk patients from carotid plaque composition. *Nat Rev Cardiol.* 2010;7:426-428.

41. Altaf N, Daniels L, Morgan PS, et al. Detection of intraplaque hemorrhage by magnetic resonance imaging in symptomatic patients with mild to moderate carotid stenosis predicts recurrent neurological events. *J Vasc Surg.* 2008;47:337-342.

42. Ederle J, Dobson J, Featherstone RL, et al. Carotid artery stenting compared with endarterectomy in patients with symptomatic carotid stenosis (International Carotid Stenting Study): an interim analysis of a randomised controlled trial. *Lancet.* 2010;375:985-997.

43. Pendlebury ST, Rothwell PM. Prevalence, incidence, and factors associated with pre-stroke and post-stroke dementia: a systematic review and meta-analysis. *Lancet Neurol.* 2009;8:1006-1018.

Finding the Cause of the TIA or Stroke: The Key to Appropriate Therapy

12

J. David Spence
Henry J. M. Barnett

INTRODUCTION

Diagnosis is absolutely crucial to the successful management of patients presenting with a sudden central nervous system (CNS) deficit. We prefer the term "stroke" because it is deliberately agnostic about the cause, thereby minimizing the risk of leaping to conclusions and thereby missing treatable specific causes. The term CVA, for "cerebrovascular accident," is abhorrent to most stroke experts; we call it "cursory vascular analysis." The term "cerebral thrombosis" is particularly inappropriate, because about 20% of strokes are hemorrhagic, and because with the rapid blood flow there is no time for polymerization of fibrin, so thrombosis does not happen in arteries until the artery is occluded. Most cerebral infarctions are embolic. First it must be determined if the patient has had a vascular event—about 15% of patients presenting to an emergency department have stroke mimics,[1] and

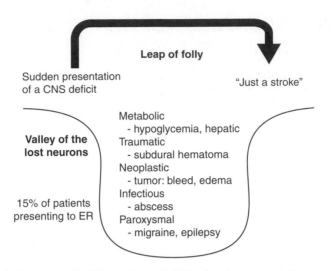

Figure 12–1. "Just a stroke." Approximately 15% of patients presenting to an emergency department with an apparent stroke have some other cause.

assuming that the event is vascular is a leap of folly (Figure 12–1). Once it has been determined that the problem is vascular, it is first necessary to determine whether it was hemorrhagic or ischemic. Then it is necessary to determine as specifically as possible the pathogenesis of the event (Table 12–1). The reason diagnosis is crucial is that the appropriate treatment to prevent another event depends on the cause.

The importance of a team approach, with collaboration of stroke neurologists and cardiologists, was shown in our NASCET report on this subject.[2]

Perhaps the most common mistake we see being made in emergency departments is doubling the dose of aspirin, or fussing about the choice of antiplatelet agent, in a patient presenting with a transient ischemic attack (TIA) or cerebral infarction while already taking aspirin. We showed in a randomized trial in patients undergoing carotid endarterectomy that low-dose aspirin is more effective than high-dose aspirin,[3] possibly because higher doses inhibit production of prostacyclin from the endothelium for longer. However, in that trial the patients were only followed for 90 days. There were not sufficient patients to analyze separately for each of the doses tried (81, 325, 925, and 1300 mg). There was a trend only suggesting that 325 mg was superior to 81 mg or 925 mg. The dose question is therefore unsettled; some feel the empirical use of 325 mg (enteric coated) may be best.

However, the key issue is not the dose of aspirin; the error is in focusing on the dose of aspirin, or the choice of antiplatelet agent, rather than the underlying cause of the event. Antiplatelet agents will only prevent a fraction of ischemic strokes: those due to embolization of platelet aggregates. If a patient has a cerebral ischemic event while taking aspirin, this means that the cause of the event was probably not an embolus of platelet aggregates, so we need to ask what did cause the event: was it from giant cell arteritis, for which the treatment is corticosteroids, or embolization

Table 12–1. Pathogenesis of Stroke

Ischemic (80%)
Occlusive:
Large vessel occlusion
Intraplaque hemorrhage, plaque rupture, dissection
Small vessel disease ("lacunar")
Fibrinoid necrosis, hyaline degeneration
Embolic:
Artery-to-artery:
Carotid stenosis, vertebral, intracranial, cardiogenic
Atrial fibrillation, recent MI, ventricular aneurysm/dyskinesia
SBE, marantic, verrucous, paradoxical, atrial myxoma
Unusual: air, fat, amniotic fluid (watershed)
Stasis:
Watershed ischemia
Ipsilateral carotid occlusion
Intracranial stenosis
Blood constituents
WBC, RBC, platelets, Sickle, immunoglobulins
Venous infarction
Vasculitis:
Giant cell arteritis, syphilis, SLE, etc
Hemorrhagic (20%)
Intracerebral hemorrhage (ICH)
Hypertensive (base of brain)
Amyloid angiopathy (lobar)
Arteriovenous malformation, cavernous angioma
Subarachnoid hemorrhage (SAH)
Berry aneurysm
Mycotic aneurysm
Cerebral vein thrombosis

Note that "cerebral thrombosis" does not occur in arteries until they have been occluded by another process.

RBC, red blood cells; SBE, subacute bacterial endocarditis; SLE, systemic lupus erythematosus; WBC, white blood cells.

of atheromatous debris from carotid stenosis, for which the treatment is endarterectomy, or embolization of red thrombus from a cardiac cause such as atrial fibrillation, for which the treatment is anticoagulants?

The history is of utmost importance; it is not good enough to say that the patient cannot give a history because of aphasia or coma—as much information as possible must be obtained from ambulance attendants, the family, the primary care physician, the contents of a purse, employee records, and previous hospital records. Case 1 illustrates this principle.

Case 1   In the spring of 1974, a comatose 26-year-old woman was brought into the Emergency Department of Victoria Hospital in London, Canada. JDS, then the senior resident in neurology, was called to see her. The ambulance attendants stated that they were called to the office where she did clerical work because she was found unconscious under her desk. On arrival she had no vital signs and resuscitation was initiated. A call to her workplace revealed that she was fine when she came in to work at 8:30 AM, but at 9:15 she was found unconscious by her coworkers, lying face down with her head under her desk. The Human Resources person with access to her personnel file (which might reveal some information about her medical history) was away for the day, and the files were locked. However, her purse remained in her desk and within it was a bottle of headache capsules, prescribed by her family physician. A call to the family physician revealed that she had presented a week before to another emergency department with a sudden severe headache, which was called migraine, and a spinal tap was not performed. Thus her sentinel leak had been missed. There was not yet a computed tomography (CT) scanner in the hospital, so a clinical diagnosis of catastrophic subarachnoid hemorrhage was made and resuscitation was called off. Autopsy revealed that rupture of a left middle cerebral artery aneurysm had destroyed her left hemisphere and ruptured into the ventricle. The diagnosis took approximately 10 minutes, requiring an interview with the ambulance attendant, a phone call to her place of employment, and a phone call to her family physician.

STROKE MIMICS ("JUST A STROKE")

In the past, when a patient came to the emergency department with the sudden presentation of a CNS deficit, there was a tendency for physicians to leap to the conclusion that the problem was "just a stroke." That term embodied a number of assumptions, including the feeling that there was nothing to be done. This has been less common since the advent of effective therapy for acute stroke, but still there are problems with early assessment of patients presenting with stroke. Perhaps the most common nonstroke referrals to a stroke team are syncope and vertigo from a vestibular problem. Syncope is loss of consciousness due to global reduction of cerebral blood flow, most commonly from postural hypotension, and often related to excessive vagal stimulation. Arrhythmias such as tachycardia/bradycardia syndrome, obstruction to the circulation of blood by a cardiac tumor or atrial myxoma, severe aortic stenosis (during exercise), or a large pulmonary embolus are other causes to be considered. Vertigo from any cause may be accompanied by nausea (amounting to motion sickness) and ataxia, but vertebrobasilar ischemia almost always has other associated focal symptoms. Diplopia, dysarthria, numbness, tingling, weakness, dysphagia, or visual symptoms such as flashing lights, blurring or loss of vision, hemianopsia or becoming lost in familiar surroundings, and transient global amnesia would be other clues to vertebrobasilar ischemia that should be inquired about in a patient presenting with vertigo as the chief complaint. A careful examination of the cranial nerves, including testing for nystagmus, loss of corneal sting sensation, and loss of nasal tickle (from a lesion in the spinal trigeminal nucleus) would all be negative in a patient whose vertigo is due to a peripheral vestibular problem.

Stroke mimics that need to be considered are shown in Figure 12–1, which symbolizes the missed opportunities when these causes are ignored. Perhaps most important among these is a treatable condition that is disastrous if missed (a "treatable disaster"). Such are subdural hematoma and hypoglycemia. Perhaps the most common stroke mimic is post-ictal paralysis[1] after an unwitnessed seizure, but all need to be considered before concluding that the problem is vascular.

All of these considerations must be entertained quickly because thrombolytic therapy, to be effective, must be given as soon as possible; indeed many patients are excluded by the brain imaging that is now routine prior to initiation of thrombolytic therapy. However, a blood glucose (or a finger-prick glucose done in the emergency room) must be included in the initial blood work drawn.

STROKE SUBTYPES

Of course hemorrhage must be differentiated from ischemic stroke, but that is not enough. It is important to define as precisely as possible the pathogenesis and etiology of the event (Table 12–1 and Table 12–2), because the appropriate treatment depends on the cause. Case 2 illustrates the problem for hemorrhagic stroke.[2]

Case 2   A 19-year-old woman presented to the emergency department of Victoria Hospital with severe headache that had persisted for approximately three hours. It came on abruptly, but on a background of two weeks of malaise, fever, and night sweats preceded by pain, swelling, and redness of the left ankle. On examination by JDS, she was a pale, slender young woman who looked ill. Her temperature was 38.6°C, with a blood pressure of 108/66 mm Hg and heart rate 110 and regular. There was a grade 2 systolic murmur loudest at the aortic area; she had splenomegaly and a splinter hemorrhage in the index finger of the right hand.

Table 12–2. Classification of Stroke

Powers	Passage	Passenger
Heart	**Vessels**	**Contents**
Recent MI	Atherosclerosis	Atheromatous debris
Old MI	Vasculitis	Fat embolism
Arrhythmia	- SLE, GCA, etc	Air embolism
- A Fib	Trauma	Blood: too much
Paradoxical	-dissection	RBCs
Endocarditis	Venous	- sickle
-marantic	Lacunar	WBCs
-bacterial		Protein
-Libbman-Sacks		-Waldenstrom's

This classification, adapted from classifications for causes of dystocia or bowel obstruction, occurred to JDS during an examination for qualification in neurology. It may be a helpful aide-memoir to a busy clinician in the emergency department.

GCA, giant cell arteritis; MI, myocardial infarction; RBCs/WBCs, red and white blood cells, in polycythemia and leukemia; SBE, subacute bacterial endocarditis.

She was drowsy but oriented, and able to respond lucidly to questioning. She had photophobia and slight meningismus. The left plantar response was extensor; the remainder of the neurological examination was normal. A diagnosis of subacute bacterial meningitis with subarachnoid hemorrhage from a mycotic aneurysm was made clinically, and was confirmed subsequently by investigations. The mycotic aneurysm was in a branch of the right pericallosal artery.

THE AORTA AS A SOURCE OF EMBOLIC ISCHEMIA CAUSING STROKE

Atheromatous lesions of the ascending aorta, seen on transesophageal echocardiography, were identified as a recognizable cause of stroke by Amarenco et al. in Paris.[4] This should be sought if there are no cardiac or large vessel (carotid) causes of a stroke to be found, particularly in patients whose presentation suggests a central source of emboli. If threatening emboli recur despite antithrombotic therapy, it is possible in skilled hands to replace the ascending aorta surgically.

INTRACRANIAL HEMORRHAGE

Whereas acute extradural or subdural hemorrhage is almost always from obvious trauma, subacute subdural hemorrhage may seemingly be spontaneous, from such causes as severe vomiting or a minor head injury weeks or months ago. Patients taking anticoagulants must be suspected of harboring a subdural hematoma if they develop progressive headache and/or drowsiness, with or without focal symptoms. Most patients presenting with hemorrhagic stroke will have spontaneous sudden hemorrhages, and the appropriate treatment depends on the cause. Rarely hemorrhages may be, as described in Case 2, from rupture of a mycotic aneurysm.

HYPERTENSIVE INTRACEREBRAL HEMORRHAGE

In jurisdictions where hypertension is poorly controlled, the most common cause of intracerebral hemorrhage will be hypertension. These lesions result from rupture of a small resistance vessel at the base of the brain, in the territory called by Hachinski the "vascular centrencephalon." The substrates involved are the internal capsule, basal ganglia, thalamus, brainstem, and cerebellum. In these vascular territories, short, straight arteries with few branches transmit pressure right through from large arteries to small resistance vessels over a short distance. High pressure in the resistance vessels damages the arterioles, causing hyaline degeneration and fibrinoid necrosis, and the formation of microaneurysms.[5] Rupture of these small damaged vessels, or the microaneurysms, leads to hemorrhage under high pressure. (When these same small vessels of the centrencephalon, brainstem, and cerebellum occlude, rather than burst, they will produce lacunar infarcts—see below.)

Although the hemorrhage may disrupt tracts and cause permanent damage, often recovery may be surprisingly good because the hemorrhage tends to push aside rather than disrupt brain tissue. Appropriate treatment of this condition is currently under investigation. Probably controlling hypertension is beneficial; early administration of clotting factors such as factor VIII may also be beneficial, and the appropriate role of surgical removal of clot, or lysis of clot with fibrinolytic agents so that the clot can be aspirated or clear spontaneously more rapidly, is being defined in clinical trials. Another promising possibility that should be investigated for large hemorrhages is hemicraniectomy, which has been extremely effective for malignant middle cerebral territory infarction (see Chapter 17).[6]

SUBARACHNOID HEMORRHAGE

Most subarachnoid hemorrhages are due to rupture of a berry aneurysm. The classic presentation of the sudden explosive onset of the headache (thunderclap headache), usually described as "the worst headache I ever had," with photophobia, neck stiffness, meningismus, vomiting, and sometimes focal neurological symptoms and signs, is easy to diagnose and often confirmed early with a CT scan that shows hemorrhage. Identifying the offending aneurysm and dealing with it, either by surgical clipping or by catheterization and coiling or related therapies, is necessary (when feasible) to prevent fatal rebleeding. In such cases it is best not to perform a spinal tap, as the sudden drop in cerebrospinal fluid (CSF) pressure may precipitate a new hemorrhage. (This is not just a theoretical concern; on Dr Charles Drake's busy aneurysm service in the mid-1970s we used to see a subarachnoid hemorrhage on the operating table about once a month, precipitated by placement of the Aitken drain.) The spinal tap should be done in the patient with suspected subarachnoid hemorrhage who has a normal CT scan and is about to be discharged home as "probably migraine," in order to avoid missing the sentinel bleed and the subsequent disastrous hemorrhage about a week later. Dissection aneurysms of the vertebral artery, from neck injury or chiropractic manipulation, are difficult to diagnose early, because the sharp neck pain from the initial dissection will not be associated with blood on the CT scan until the later rupture of the aneurysm. The spinal tap will be negative when the aneurysm has not yet ruptured, so only an angiogram will reveal it.

AMYLOID (CONGOPHILIC) ANGIOPATHY

In contrast to the vascular centrencephalon, the cortex is supplied by long arteries with many branches, rather like a step-down transformer. Blood pressure in cortical arteries is therefore low, and lobar hemorrhages from cortical arteries are more indolent than hypertensive hemorrhages. The principal cause is amyloid or congophilic angiopathy, a disease of the elderly, with some possible relation to Alzheimer disease. This condition accounts for a much higher proportion of intracerebral hemorrhage in jurisdictions where blood pressure is well controlled, and is increasing in frequency with the aging of the population. At present there is little to be offered; there is slight evidence that blood pressure control makes a difference. An increased incidence occurs in patients on long-term anticoagulant therapy, so withholding antiplatelet agents or anticoagulants may be prudent, but this is problematic in patients with atrial fibrillation. Because atrial fibrillation also increases dramatically with age,[7] the coincidence of atrial fibrillation and amyloid angiopathy is not rare. In such cases, one approach that may be worth consideration is surgical removal of the atrial appendage. (Clinical trials of devices to occlude the atrial appendage have so far not been very promising, and such surgery can now be done with minimally invasive approaches using thoracoscopy and robotic instruments.[8])

CORTICAL VEIN THROMBOSIS

Localized cortical hemorrhage and hemorrhagic infarction may be from cortical vein thrombosis, with infarction from stasis of blood flow, and hemorrhage into the infarcted tissue because outflow is obstructed. Thrombosis of the sagittal sinuses must be suspected, and despite the hemorrhage, treatment with anticoagulants or infusion of thrombolytics into the thrombosed sinus may be necessary.

Two of the most common situations resulting in cerebral vein thrombosis were the postpartum state and in patients in postoperative periods.[9] In considering other causes of the venous thrombosis, besides investigation for the usual clotting factors such as factor V Leiden, it must be remembered that hyperhomocysteinemia, the most common hypercoagulable state (~20% of the population), increases the risk of venous thrombosis, including thrombosis of cerebral veins and venous sinuses.[10] Deficiency of vitamin B_{12}, including that from inflammatory bowel disease, is a likely cause; this is discussed in Chapter 3.

VASCULAR MALFORMATIONS

Hemorrhage from arteriovenous malformations (AVMs), and particularly from cavernous angiomas, tends to be so indolent that focal seizures from the irritation due to hemosiderin are perhaps more likely than symptoms due to bleeding per se. Surgery can be very difficult; for large AVMs awake surgery with brain stimulation to map and avoid damage to functional cortex may be important. Preoperative embolization to occlude large feeding arteries may be helpful. Cavernous angiomas are often multiple, so surgical management, or approaches such as gamma knife irradiation, may in some cases be more appropriately reserved for lesions in strategic locations such as the brainstem, where a small bleed may cause a large deficit.

CEREBRAL ISCHEMIA

In a patient presenting with a TIA or nondisabling stroke, the appropriate treatment required to prevent a subsequent major stroke depends crucially on the underlying cause. A patient whose amaurosis fugax is due to giant cell arteritis (GCA) does not need to double the dose of his or her aspirin; he or she needs urgent initiation of high-dose corticosteroid, such as prednisone 50 mg daily. The initiation of corticosteroid should not wait until a biopsy confirms the diagnosis; preventable permanent blindness can develop within hours or days. Indeed, because the lesions of GCA are focal, they may be missed on a blind temporal artery biopsy, and absence of tissue confirmation should not prevent appropriate treatment. Because the ophthalmic branch of the superficial temporal artery may be useful for anastomotic purposes in subjects who go on to carotid artery occlusion, some prefer to make a diagnostic occipital artery biopsy. Patients with GCA

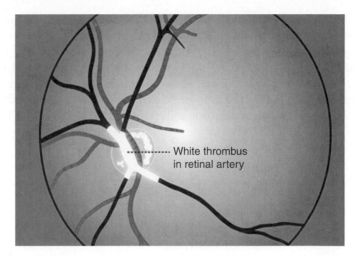

White thrombus
in retinal artery

Figure 12–2. White thrombus in the retinal arteries during amaurosis fugax. This
was first described by C. Miller Fisher in a patient whose amaurosis and retinal white
thrombus were observed by many participants in Grand Rounds. JDS has seen it twice.
(Reproduced by permission of Vanderbilt University Press from Spence JD. *How to Prevent
Your Stroke.* Vanderbilt University Press; 2006.)

are elderly, and apart from the common occurrence of polymyalgia rheumatica,
most feel fatigued and anorexic, some have low-grade fever, and they commonly
have tenderness over scalp arteries. The sedimentation rate is high. Hamrin et al
suggested direct temporal artery angiography to identify where biopsies should be
made; using this approach they confirmed GCA in half of patients with polymyalgia
rheumatica.[11] Table 12–1 lists most of the many causes of ischemic stroke; it is
obvious that the appropriate treatment will be different for many of these causes.
Perhaps the most common distinction that needs to be made is whether the event
was caused by large artery disease, small vessel disease (lacunar), or a cardioembolic source. Large artery disease with embolization of platelet aggregates is really
the only clear indication for antiplatelet agents; the treatment for embolization of
atheromatous debris is carotid endarterectomy. If the event was due to embolism
from the heart, the appropriate treatment is anticoagulation; antiplatelet agents are
only a third as effective.[7] A key distinction that is under-recognized is that between
"white thrombus" and "red thrombus."[12,13] White thrombus consists of platelet
aggregates; it can be seen in the retinal arteries of a patient who is having an episode
of amaurosis fugax (Figure 12–2). This is what antiplatelet agents are for; they will
not prevent the formation and embolization of red thrombus, which is essentially
a fibrin polymer with entrapped red cells; for this anticoagulation is needed.

ARTERIAL DISSECTION

Particularly since the perfection of magnetic resonance (MR) angiography, arterial dissections are increasingly being diagnosed. They are most common in the
extracranial portion of the internal carotid artery and more dramatically seen in

the vertebral arteries. Infrequently they may be found to solely involve intracranial major branches in either the anterior or posterior circulation. They generally occur in younger patients. JDS has reported that the most common cause of traumatic vertebrobasilar ischemia is motor vehicle crashes.[14] An interesting issue is that whereas strokes from chiropractic manipulation are seldom missed, it is usual for strokes from motor vehicle crashes to be missed. This may be due to the subjective nature of diagnosis: physicians don't like chiropractic, and they don't like the adversarial nature of medicolegal proceedings, so they backpedal when they hear the term "whiplash."

The average age of patients in a recent large series was 44 years—about half the age of patients with large-artery atherosclerotic stroke. Approximately half of these arterial lesions occur without apparent trauma, or with minor trauma such as sneezing or Valsalva maneuvers; the rest are related to more obvious trauma. Fibromuscular dysplasia is an arterial lesion that may predispose to dissection, and other genetically determined abnormalities of collagen, elastin, and other supporting elements in the vessel wall may predispose to dissection with even minor trauma.[15]

The list of the traumatic mechanisms that have been recognized as causes and triggers of dissection continues to grow. Saver et al[16] put together a classic chapter on arterial dissections with a series of remarkable images telling the story of the pathogenesis very lucidly. Barnett made reference to the subject in the Robert Wartenberg Lecture of the American Academy of Neurology.[17] Figure 12–3 gives a clear pathogenic illustration of the mechanism of arterial injury, illustrating the impingement upon the arterial lumen by a cervical transverse process (C2) when the neck is turned forcibly to one side in full hyperextension. The vertebral artery in the vertebral canal comes suddenly in contact with the tip of the transverse process. This trauma to the vessel wall allows blood under arterial pressure to dissect between the media and adventitia. The dissection proceeds cephalad, creating a false secondary lumen. At the C1-C2 level the artery may completely occlude, with or without formation of a false aneurysm. Rear-end automobile collisions and chiropractic neck manipulations are most commonly causal.[14] Frequently drivers or front-seat passengers are turning to talk to another passenger beside them or in the back seat at the moment of the collision.

Recognized as other causes for carotid or vertebral dissections may be prolonged operation of an overhead construction crane, violent sexual intercourse (presumably with hyperextension of the neck), repeated indulgence in prolonged military parade ground drill, vigorous yoga, and sky-diving. A former editor of *Stroke* had a vertebrobasilar stroke while reaching under his desk to retrieve a piece of paper. A younger person with a stroke and a contralateral Horner syndrome has almost certainly suffered a carotid artery dissection. The autonomic supply to the muscles of the pupil encircles the carotid artery. Older people with limited neck movement from cervical spondylosis and lack of suppleness are not as commonly victims of traumatic neck dissections, especially of the vertebral artery.

Treatment strategies for dissections must bear in mind that the condition commonly heals itself and also that no comparative randomized trials have been

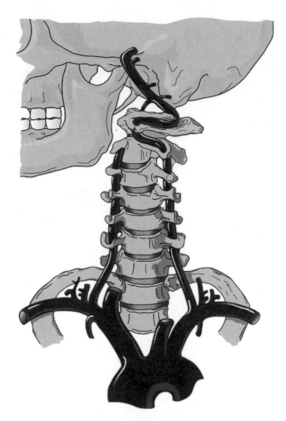

Figure 12–3. Susceptibility of the vertebral artery to trauma during motor vehicle collisions or chiropractic manipulation. (Reproduced by permission of the publisher from Spence JD. *How to Prevent Your Stroke.* Vanderbilt University Press; 2006.)

feasible. Despite its hemorrhagic nature, but because of its tendency to distal embolization from the top of the dissection, the use of heparin followed by warfarin may be rational. Residual aneurysmal dilatations have been handled with surgical or interventional treatment, judging cases on their merit but demanding expert operators. Again there are no proper randomized trials upon which to rely.

CARDIOEMBOLIC STROKE

It is particularly important to consider a cardiac source and anticoagulation in several groups of patients: the elderly, in whom atrial fibrillation is much more common; the young patient with cryptogenic stroke; and patients with multiple territory events (either simultaneously or sequentially). Because the risk of recurrent stroke is highest soon after an event, anticoagulation should be instituted when clinical suspicion is high, while investigations to identify a cardiac source are being put in process, and before the results are available. Atrial fibrillation may account for more than 25% of stroke in the elderly,[18] and this can be expected to increase as other causes of stroke are reduced by more intensive medical therapy.[19]

Prolonged monitoring of cardiac rhythm may be needed to detect intermittent atrial fibrillation.[18] There are serious problems with under-anticoagulation of patients with atrial fibrillation, particularly the elderly, in whom the relative benefit of anticoagulation over antiplatelet therapy is greatest.[7] This problem may be alleviated in the future with the advent of new anticoagulants that do not require dose adjustment and monitoring of blood tests. Dabigatran is approved for stroke prevention in atrial fibrillation,[20] and apixaban and rivaroxaban are soon likely to be approved; however, cost, difficulty of reversing anticoagulation, and drug interactions are issues with those newer drugs.

A cause of stroke that is commonly missed is paradoxical embolism, which now accounts for 5.5% of TIA or stroke,[21] and a higher proportion among young patients with normal arteries and normal blood pressure. Paradoxical embolism occurs when a patient with a pulmonary embolus has a right-to-left shunt; for this reason such patients should be anticoagulated, at least initially. (There is unwarranted controversy over this; who would not anticoagulate a patient with a pulmonary embolus who has not sustained a stroke?) In few cases, the right-to-left shunt will be through a pulmonary arteriovenous malformation, often associated with hereditary telangiectasia. Hart and Miller[22] found that 2% of strokes in patients below age 20 were from this condition. Some will be via an atrial septal defect or ventricular septal defect. Most, however, will be due to a patent foramen ovale (PFO). The difficulty is that because 25% of healthy people have a patent foramen ovale, and only 5.5% of TIA or stroke is due to this condition, about 80% of PFOs in patients with stroke are incidental. This is why randomized clinical trials of percutaneous closure of PFO are doomed to failure, unless clinical clues to paradoxical embolism[21] (Table 12–3) are appropriately taken into account. Transcranial Doppler bubble studies are more sensitive than echocardiography to detect right-to-left shunting.[23]

Table 12–3. Clinical Clues to Paradoxical Embolism

Young patient without other causes of stroke
Dyspnea,[a] tachycardia at onset of stroke
Low pO_2 and CO_2
Loud P2, pulmonic regurgitation murmur
Loss of consciousness at the onset of a carotid stroke
Long ride in a plane or car,[a] sitting in front of a computer
Swollen leg, previous DVT,[a] varicose veins[a]
Previous pulmonary embolism[a]
Valsalva maneuver at the onset of stroke[a]
Waking up with stroke[a]
Sleep apnea[a]

[a]Significantly more common ($P < .05$) in patients with confirmed patent foramen ovale (PFO) in the study by Ozdemir et al,[21] compared with patients with cryptogenic stroke and negative transcranial Doppler bubble studies and transesophageal echocardiogram.

Permission obtained from J. Wiley and Sons to reproduce from Spence JD. Clinical clues to paradoxical embolism. *Intl J Stroke.* 2010;5(6):514.

LACUNAR INFARCTION

When the small blood vessels in the centrencephalon, including the small penetrators to the brainstem and cerebellum, occlude rather than rupturing, they cause tiny ischemic infarcts known as lacunes. There will be one of several clinical syndromes produced (primary motor stroke, primary sensory stroke, ataxic hemiparesis, dysarthria–clumsy-hand syndrome). In company with a normal MRI or with one or several small (2 mm) infarctions, they can be clinically recognizable. A recent editorial and manuscript in *Neurology* repeats the known fact that they carry an immediate outlook for a quick initial recovery from clinical symptoms,[24] but at 12 years they carry a high risk for other vascular complications and risk of death from heart disease, and other serious vascular complications.[25] As most lacunar infarctions are from hypertension or diabetes, effective management of these conditions is crucial (see Chapters 3 and 10).

CONCLUSION

Appropriate management of the patient who presents with a TIA or stroke includes taking steps to minimize the risk of recurrent stroke. In order to know what therapy is needed, the diagnosis of the pathogenesis and etiology of the event is necessary. This diagnosis requires a thorough history and physical examination, judicious use of laboratory investigations, clinical acumen, and judgement.

REFERENCES

1. Norris JW, Hachinski VC. Misdiagnosis of stroke. *Lancet.* 1982;1:328-331.
2. Barnett HJ, Gunton RW, Eliasziw M, et al. Causes and severity of ischemic stroke in patients with internal carotid artery stenosis. *JAMA.* 2000;283:1429-1436.
3. Taylor DW, Barnett HJ, Haynes RB, et al. Low-dose and high-dose acetylsalicylic acid for patients undergoing carotid endarterectomy: a randomised controlled trial. ASA and Carotid Endarterectomy (ACE) Trial Collaborators. *Lancet.* 1999;353:2179-2184.
4. Amarenco P, Duyckaerts C, Tzourio C, Henin D, Bousser MG, Hauw JJ. The prevalence of ulcerated plaques in the aortic arch in patients with stroke. *N Engl J Med.* 1992;326:221-225.
5. Pickering G. *Hypertension: Causes, Consequences and Management.* 2nd ed. Edinburgh and London: Churchill Livingstone; 1974.
6. Vahedi K, Hofmeijer J, Juettler E, et al. Early decompressive surgery in malignant infarction of the middle cerebral artery: a pooled analysis of three randomised controlled trials. *Lancet Neurol.* 2007;6: 215-222.
7. Spence JD. Stroke: atrial fibrillation, stroke prevention therapy and aging. *Nat Rev Cardiol.* 2009;6: 448-450.
8. Kiaii B, McClure RS, Skanes AC, et al. Robotic-assisted left atrial ligation for stroke reduction in chronic atrial fibrillation: a case report. *Heart Surg Forum.* 2006;9:E533-E535.
9. Barnett HJ, Hyland HH. Noninfective intracranial venous thrombosis. *Brain.* 1953;76:36-49.
10. Martinelli I, Battaglioli T, Pedotti P, Cattaneo M, Mannucci PM. Hyperhomocysteinemia in cerebral vein thrombosis. *Blood.* 2003;102:1363-1366.
11. Hamrin B, Jonsson N, Landberg T. Arteritis in "polymyalgia rheumatica." *Lancet.* 1964;1:397-401.
12. Deykin D. Thrombogenesis. *N Engl J Med.* 1967;276:622-628.
13. Caplan LR, Fisher M. The endothelium, platelets, and brain ischemia. *Rev Neurol Dis.* 2007;4: 113-121.

14. Beaudry M, Spence JD. Motor vehicle accidents: the most common cause of traumatic vertebrobasilar ischemia. *Can J Neurol Sci.* 2003;30:320-325.

15. Mayer SA, Rubin BS, Starman BJ, Byers PH. Spontaneous multivessel cervical artery dissection in a patient with a substitution of alanine for glycine (G13A) in the alpha 1 (I) chain of type I collagen. *Neurology.* 1996;47:552-556.

16. Saver JL, Hart RG, Easton JD. Dissections and trauma of cervico-cerebral arteries. In: Barnett HJM, Stein BM, Mohr JP, Yatsu FM, eds. *Stroke: Pathophysiology, Diagnosis, and Management.* 2nd ed. New York: Churchill, Livingstone; 1992:671-688.

17. Barnett HJ. Progress towards stroke prevention: Robert Wartenberg lecture. *Neurology.* 1980;30: 1212-1225.

18. Tayal AH, Callans DJ. Occult atrial fibrillation in ischemic stroke: seek and you shall find. *Neurology.* 2010;74:1662-1663.

19. Spence JD, Coates V, Li H, et al. Effects of intensive medical therapy on microemboli and cardiovascular risk in asymptomatic carotid stenosis. *Arch Neurol.* 2010;67:180-186.

20. Connolly SJ, Ezekowitz MD, Yusuf S, et al. Dabigatran versus warfarin in patients with atrial fibrillation. *N Engl J Med.* 2009;361:1139-1151.

21. Ozdemir AO, Tamayo A, Munoz C, Dias B, Spence JD. Cryptogenic stroke and patent foramen ovale: clinical clues to paradoxical embolism. *J Neurol Sci.* 2008;275:121-127.

22. Hart RG, Miller VT. Cerebral infarction in young adults: a practical approach. *Stroke.* 1983;14: 110-114.

23. Anzola GP. Transcranial Doppler: Cinderella in the assessment of patent foramen ovale in stroke patients. *Stroke.* 2004;35:e137.

24. Potter GM, Roman G. Cerebral small-vessel disease: what lies beyond the early years? *Neurology.* 2011;76:684-685.

25. Melkas S, Putaala J, Oksala NK, et al. Small-vessel disease relates to poor poststroke survival in a 12-year follow-up. *Neurology.* 2011;76:734-739.

Thoughts on the Hazards of Relying on Publications: Cautions Needed Before Applying Published Results to Evidence-Based Medicine

13

Henry J. M. Barnett

Over the last few decades there has been an avalanche of advances in stroke diagnosis and therapy. In two recent communications, one relating to the 40th anniversary of the journal *Stroke*[1] and the other through the Karolinska Stroke Award Lecture,[2] I have sketched these revolutionary changes. Of these huge advances none has been more critical in opening the door to evidence-based medicine than the introduction and continuing refinement of the randomized (blinded) controlled clinical trial (RCT).

Enquiring readers can usually, but not always, accept the conclusions drawn from articles appearing in the most reputable clinical journals. They rely on the wisdom and integrity of the authors and of the careful peer reviews known to be practiced by the journal in question through its editorial staff. Even in the best circumstances, mistakes will slip through the cracks. Detection of these errors requires that the reader be aware of items that are essential to the assessment of a credible report. I summarize them here.

The blinded randomized trial with an acceptable control arm of identical patients has become the basis for modern-day data gathering and is standard for evaluating innovative therapy as well as additions to proven therapy as the solid basis for clinical decision making. Evidence-based medicine can be said to have been born when this strategy replaced reliance on experiential and authoritarian dogma. In therapeutic neurology it is a demand of all who engage in practice involving stroke prevention and treatment that they check carefully all manuscripts describing putative changes in patient management. Did mistakes or omissions from the method mistakenly mislead the reader?

A full description of the methods to be employed must be published in advance of the manuscript describing results and conclusions. The methods paper will outline all the specifics of the analyses to be performed. The nature of the trials' outcome events must be detailed. Patients to be included and excluded must be clearly defined.

The methods report must outline the secure and doubly blinded method of randomization. The plans for analyses are the province of the biostatistician with assistance from the epidemiologist and clinician principal investigator (PI). The expert clinician (the PI) must scrutinize the entire research plan, and then select and instruct the team of clinical investigators and be in a position to assure involved investigators that the trial is feasible and practical. The recruited team of investigators should be experts in the field under study, or at the very least be led by one. An estimate must be made of the number of patients needed to provide the totality of outcomes expected in each treatment group. The clinicians, including radiologists along with statisticians and epidemiologists, should be involved in this exercise.

The Fort Knox of the RCT is the outcomes data-bank. There should never be more than one key to this fortress and it should be in the possession of the biostatistician, never to be made available to industry, the investigators, or the patients until the analyses are complete and poised for publication. The principal biostatistician will be empowered to make scrupulously secret interim analyses at predetermined intervals with predescribed stopping rules to ensure that harm is not being done or unexpected substantial good occurring and denied to the trial patients. Unless the statistician is also a clinician skilled in the subject under inquiry, he or she should not lead a clinical trial. The key will be turned when stopping rules are due and again when the final analyses are to be conducted. These analyses should await the verification of all outcomes in both treatment groups. This will obviate the need for a preliminary and then a later report that may be contradictory. The new treatment may have been recommended or erroneously denied based on the publication of incomplete and at times misleading premature preliminary information.

Any subgroup(s) to be followed and eventually analyzed at the end of the trial must be identified in the protocol. Outcome events in these subgroups must be meticulously documented at follow-up visits. Observational revelations not anticipated in the methods paper may result from new entities recognized from the patients under study. It is wrong to ignore such careful observations, but equally wrong to regard their perceived treatment differences as final. Unanticipated observations may add to our understanding of disease. A good example of this is the unfolding in NASCET (the North American Symptomatic Carotid Endarterectomy Trial) of the previously overlooked distinct entity of near occlusion.[3,4]

Occasionally, only observational data can substitute for proof by randomized trials. Two examples will be given: First, asbestos has been proven to be a cause of lung cancer without a control group and without any RCT formally conducted.

The only control possible for asbestos hazards was a population in the same community who had never worked with asbestos. These subjects were to be found in the community. The scientific world, compensation boards, and insurance companies rightly accept the cause and effect relationship derived from thousands of observations in those who mined asbestos and those who did not. Second, in the search for the connection between lung cancer and tobacco the 25,000 British doctors studied by Sir Richard Doll provided him a control group. It turned out that nearly half of his registrants had never smoked, thereby producing a control group identical to his smoking group. An observational study converted itself into a comparative trial.[5] The overwhelming relationship of tobacco to deadly illness including stroke has been accepted by all except the tobacco barons, and one wonders if in the quiet of their own living rooms they do not recognize the obvious and secretly marvel at their duplicity. Surely they must by now know that they cause more premature deaths than do the drug barons. Tobacco barons are accepted in exclusive clubs; drug barons are accepted in prisons.

Melding the gold bricks of solid evidence stored in the data-bank requires that all the investigators be aware that a trial's outcome events are the gold dust from which the bricks of solid evidence will be formed. Before going into the bank, the details of every outcome event must be meticulously examined by the study principals blinded to the treatment arm. To make the study results believable these centers' investigators must be bona fide experts in this field of study. Outcomes should be certified by blinded collaborators in the participating centers and by the central office of the study, and not left for verification by paid employees of the manufacturer of the device or pharmaceutical. External auditors must be appointed and should consider the details of the handling of data, checking both on the adherence of the entrants' clinical picture to the protocol and for the accuracy of what is claimed to be an appropriate outcome. They will be kept blinded. In the author's experience, in multicenter trials, a weekly outcomes meeting with all central office staff and specialties that are part of the trial gives an opportunity for an interdisciplinary, blinded session of brainstorming about the outcome event. After this, the data will be sent to the auditors and then finally to the data-bank. We commonly found that some further investigation or clinical inquiry was required to verify that an acceptable outcome had occurred. The costs of this potential requirement must be built into the budget of every important RCT. Granting agencies must accept this budgetary item as an important part of a trial calculated to alter the practice of medicine.

Because regular communication between all investigators and the PI at the central office is the sine qua non of achieving a meticulous and complete database, the PI must be prepared for a serious time commitment to a funded trial. Follow-up data should be gathered by experts in the field under study. Telephone contact is a cheap but poor substitute for investigators to learn of the presence and details of an outcome event. Administrative databases are notoriously sparse of data. Excessively busy practitioners should not enter patients into an important trial if they do not have the will, the time, or the staff for personal ongoing contact. Patients will be lost or will skip follow-ups and become dropouts if they are not in regular contact with the investigator or his or her skilled staff. The ideal trial should have few dropouts. Patients known to be erratic and unpredictable or have drug or alcohol dependency should not be randomized in therapeutic trials. If a substantial number of the entrants drop out and their fate is unknown, the trial is fatally skewed and the center's data should not be accepted. If funding is not going to be available for visits and tests needed to clarify an outcome, the center ideally should not be in the trial or should be prepared to scramble to provide the extra funding needed to make a diagnosis that is as accurate and as scrupulous as possible.

The failure to record and pursue any of these methodological items constitutes a breach of scientific integrity. At its worst, the critical reader may worry that undisclosed plans could provoke the investigators to present unusual analyses that favor the innovative therapy. Sadly, it is no longer a rarity for investigators, even senior academics, to be influenced by financial arrangements with industry.[6]

Attempts have been made of late to add data together from a series of studies to increase the population studied and purportedly make the conclusions more rigorous and credible. I have never been convinced that in every one of these compilations of studies it was known with assurance that all in the series were studying the same disorder at the same phase in the disease, following the same protocol exactly, and that the compiler of the data was aware of how carefully decisions were made about the entry characteristics and how certain it was that the outcome events had been fully verified. Unless their completeness of data is known, outcome events should not be placed in the compiler's data-bank. Only then should the results of the analyses be ready and appropriate for meta-analysis. I remain a contrarian as far as accepting the value of many published meta-analyses. Burning therapeutic issues demand a trial with enough numbers to be acceptable for stand-alone definitive answers to the question for which all practitioners require an answer. Good trials are expensive. More costly is medical practice without verification of new treatment strategy by good trials.

Physicians should look with suspicion on any trial where the data are held in a data-bank exclusive to industry. There is a strong ethical requirement for all the data relative to published conclusions to be transparent and shared. Mistrust of the results and of the trial are surely justified if this disclosure is denied.

Several examples neglecting the rules of RCTs follow, given from the trials evaluating **surgery** and **stenting** in stroke prevention, and finally a few worrisome comments about some of **the antithrombotic trials**. The application of these treatments is covered in specific chapters that follow.

SURGICAL INTERVENTION IN SYMPTOMATIC PATIENTS WITH CAROTID STENOSIS

Soon after the introduction by Felix Easton of the concept of surgery on the carotid artery, the late William Fields published the results of a randomized trial involving patients with symptomatic stenosis. Benefit was claimed in stroke reduction.[7] There were several flaws in the design and execution. First, there were too few patients and outcome events to allow a convincing difference and confirmation of benefit. Second, there was too large a loss to follow-up. Third, the protocol allowed randomization of patients with only vertebral-basilar symptoms and asymptomatic carotid stenosis. I mention this historic but flawed document because I recall that some junior colleagues used Fields' "positive" conclusions in querying the need for another and larger trial. They had failed to examine critically the design and methods of this early attempt. The RCT was still a novelty, and its key but absolutely essential elements were still being defined and fully described.

Three other large trials of **symptomatic disease** followed: EC/IC, NASCET, and ECST, none of which were methodologically perfect, but all were in the next phase of RCTs approaching perfection.

The EC/IC Bypass trial[8] breached its protocol requirement that all follow-ups be conducted by an expert neurologist. This requirement was so seriously against Japanese custom that we had to allow them an exception to the protocol. They had not yet adopted the concept of interdisciplinary research. Akita was the exception with its interdisciplinary Neuroscience Institute. A handful of North American centers found neurologists too busy or insufficiently interested to perform follow-ups. These had to be done by the surgical operator. This is analogous to asking representatives of a drug manufacturer to verify outcome events. The Japanese surgeon evaluator was not necessarily blinded to the treatment arm. The data could conceivably be examined for complications by the person who performed the surgical procedure. Rothwell and Warlow studied the results of the European Carotid Surgery trial and detected a seven-fold increase in complications when reported by physicians compared to supposedly unbiased surgeons.[9]

The EC/IC Bypass trial was accused of getting and announcing a falsely negative result because one of the enthusiastic and disappointed surgeons telephoned some of the busiest American centers, which told them that from time to time (against their written pledges) they operated on eligible patients without putting them in the trial. This was a breach of methods difficult for the central office or the protocol to anticipate. They confessed to operating outside the trial on 11% of the total eligible patients. Total patient numbers within each subgroup remained adequate for our statisticians to perform significant but negative analyses. Leaving out all patients from the cheating centers also left adequate numbers of patients to confirm overall negative benefit for bypass. In time, the accusations and the rebuttal were published by the *New England Journal of Medicine*, and in due course Medicare, Blue Cross, etc, withdrew payment.[10–15] The principle has clearly been enunciated by David Sackett (and I paraphrase), "It is the patients who are in the trial and not those who are outside the trial who are pertinent to the analyses."

Problems are perceived in the ECST trial.[16] First, it had an inadequate budget to retrieve and check its outcome data as rapidly as and, just possibly, as thoroughly as it would have liked and as is desirable. The result was that for patients symptomatic with moderate stenosis (50%-69%), it reported an early negative postsurgical benefit,[16] and two years later a final contrary and positive report about benefit[17] (albeit minor). This final result published two years later was comparable to the initial finding of definite but minor benefit reported in NASCET in its patients with moderate stenosis. Second, the ECST (as in the ACST trial; see below) investigators were unable to perform the extra test(s) needed to identify "stroke by cause": assign stroke to large artery, lacunar (small artery) cardioembolic, or "other" causation. Third, in the absence of bilateral arteriograms and intracranial images they could not reliably describe the extent of collateral circulation and its impact on the risk and benefit of carotid endarterectomy (CEA). Finally, and most worrying, this trial allowed its surgeons to perform CEA outside the trial if they *believed* they could help the patient. This reverted the methodology to the selecting out of an unknown number of its eligible patients by the dubious pre-existing stratagem of "personal experience and authoritarianism." The purpose of the carotid trial was to liberate decisions about the indications for CEA from these "personal judgments" and to introduce "evidence-based decision making" to this surgical therapy. "Gut feelings" may lead to hypotheses but should not be part of an RCT. This strategy allowed for a decreased proportion of "severe stenosis" patients, compared to NASCET's data.

SURGICAL INTERVENTION IN ASYMPTOMATIC SUBJECTS WITH CAROTID STENOSIS

Three large RCTs have been conducted on **asymptomatic** patients: the VA trial,[18] the American trial (ACAS),[19] and the European trial (ACST).[20]

The VA trial must be discounted because it was flawed in the choice of outcome events, and furthermore the risk of surgery was too high. It did not establish that stroke was reduced by CEA, as was the aim of the trial, but only that transient ischemic attacks (TIAs) were diminished in the surgical arm. Few people would submit to the risk of immediate stroke to rid themselves of ongoing transient and nondisabling events lasting an average of a few minutes. This would be especially true if they were made aware of the surgical risk in their particular surgical environment. It is now generally recognized that a 30-day postoperative risk of stroke and death after CEA for asymptomatic subjects above 3% denies the subject benefit— indeed it is harmful. The 30-day post-CEA risk in the VA trial was 4.5%. No reports claiming success for the VA trial have made mention of its unacceptably high perioperative stroke risk.

The American ACAS and the European ACST both reported similar results (with approximately 1% absolute annual reduction in stroke risk with an equal number needed to treat [NNT] of approximately 65 to prevent one stroke in two years). Because of this purported apparent similarity the investigators of ACAS editorialized in the *BMJ* that the time had come to screen entire populations for asymptomatic carotid atheromatous narrowing,[21] directing many to the operating room hopefully to avert the stroke for which they have no more than 2% risk per year.[22] The question of any indication for surgery in asymptomatic patients is covered in extenso in Chapter 11. This chapter looks only at the design problems lurking in these reports.

What the *BMJ* article and the ACST report neglected to note was that the protocols of ACAS and ACST have two glaring differences: First, *ipsilateral* stroke was the primary outcome event in ACAS, and *stroke in any cerebral vascular territory* was the primary event in the European trial. This was a curious departure from the title of the manuscript that indicated the reader was to expect "the risk within the distribution of an asymptomatic artery." Moreover, the investigators could decide to operate outside the study if they *felt* they could reduce the risk for individual patients. This decision to operate was to be based on experience rather than scientifically sound facts. Both of these major trial differences negate any suggestion that the trials are similar (let alone "almost identical," as written in the *BMJ* editorial) and that the results may therefore be combined. This is not true, and is an example of failure of the review process.

Neither of these large trials on asymptomatic subjects gathered requisite data and failed to report on "stroke by cause." This was unfortunate because NASCET had already published data indicating that a strong minority (~40%) of strokes in association with asymptomatic carotid lesions are not of large-artery origin and thus not so likely to benefit from CEA.[23]

CAROTID ARTERY STENTING

Carotid artery stenting was developed by cardiologists who, after coronary artery stenting, explored the carotid artery and if they encountered stenosis, started to perform stenting at that site. The enthusiasm with which this was promoted was remarkable. It was driven by genuine belief that it might be a safer way than CEA to prevent threatening stroke, and probably also by financial gain. Knowledge of the brain, of the manifestations of cerebral ischemia, of the innocence of the low risk of stroke annually from patients with asymptomatic stenosis, and of the subtleties of vertebral-basilar versus carotid ischemia were regularly less apparent than one would have preferred to see and hear. Most of the many claims of benefit were based on single-operator case reports, and most were without controls. Such reports are notoriously unreliable and should rarely, if ever, be accepted for publication. Protective "umbrella" devices to entrap emboli from passing beyond the stent began to be introduced. The problem is that the insertion of the device carries a risk of embolic stroke. None have been convincingly of value in stroke prevention by properly controlled positive trials.

Controlled trials of carotid stenting have appeared in the literature from France, Germany, Australia, and the United Kingdom. Agreement and assurance about the use of stenting for carotid disease remains elusive and should be accepted only as experimental work-in-progress. This section concentrates on the flaws and misleading aspects of any positive claims yet published for stenting versus endarterectomy. The first North American randomized trial designed to test the efficacy of carotid stenting compared with CEA recruited a mere 100 symptomatic patients and only 234 asymptomatic subjects. The investigators made their analysis on the comparison of the two treatment strategies (SAPPHIRE TRIAL),[24] utilizing the combined groups. Furthermore, they added myocardial infarction (MI) to stroke and death to make their "compound endpoint." Again, as in the CREST report (see below), no mention was made of the extremely different stroke risk facing those with symptoms and those who were asymptomatic. In addition, they are quite mistaken in their assumption that the asymptomatic subjects with 80% or more stenosis are at a higher risk of stroke. The two large American (ACAS) and

European asymptomatic (ACST) trials both reported that there was no change in the risk or benefit associated with the higher degrees of stenosis. Data supporting the concept of higher risk of stroke for asymptomatic patients with the highest degrees of stenosis are simply lacking. This was opposite to the findings in the NASCET and ECST trials, both finding that the higher degrees of stenosis conferred extra risk and extra benefit of surgery in symptomatic stenosis. This misleading assumption was overlooked by the reviewers. By entering patients with disparate risks (low for asymptomatic, high for symptomatic) they breached the rule of **ceteris paribus** (all other things being equal).[25] In the writer's opinion this combination of seriously different levels of risk in the study population skews the SAPPHIRE trial and helps make it of little significance.

All entrants were described as being high risk for CEA. In Table I of the study, the investigators list the reasons for calling the entrants "high risk." Among the reasons given was the presence of serious heart disease. They neglected to tell us which of the entrants and in what numbers each of these putative high-risk situations were detected in each treatment arm. This is not acceptable because serious heart disease (MI) was called an outcome event of equal weight to stroke and death. This is bizarre because it could never be expected to be altered by improved cerebral revascularization, which was the goal of the trial. We need also to know if these outcomes were read with the investigator blinded to the treatment arm and whether or not the MI was clinically significant. We were told only that the MIs were "commonest in the postoperative CEA period." The timing of the MI post-treatment was not given. For sure MI was an indirect complication of the procedure, but we can state with certainty that the cardiac symptoms were not directly related to the catheterization. It has been reasoned that if the patients had all been given a complete cardiac workup prior to the invasive procedure they might have been subjected to coronary artery bypass graft (CABG) to remove the possibility of an irrelevant MI. My statistical colleague Eliasziw removed the irrelevant outcome of MI and repeated the analyses.[26] Stroke was not diminished in the stenting arm of the SAPPHIRE trial; thus it is not possible to argue that stenting in stroke-threatened patients has been shown to be equal to CEA.

Finally, they introduce no evidence that the protective device that they utilized has any proven merit. The proof of value of any such device remains unknown despite many claims from a variety of manufacturers. Sound evaluations are lacking. It sounds worthy, but like all therapeutic advances, it is only hypothetical until subjected to a rigorous randomized trial. The fact that they were acceptable to the Food and Drug Administration (FDA) is not proof of efficacy. Like good journals, they make mistakes.

The SAPPHIRE trial was terminated prematurely due to slowness of recruitment. They reported small numbers of events and had a mere 100 symptomatic patients. No significant answer to the differential value of the two treatment strategies applied to two very separate disorders can be attached to this trial. One wonders how and why this report passed the scrutiny of careful and critical reviewers.

A German trial (SPACE),[27] which eventually entered 1214 symptomatic patients, found noninferiority after 30 days. At two years of follow-up for stenting versus CEA, the stroke rate was the same but with a detected higher rate of restenosis (up to at least 70%) in the stenting group.[28] The French trial was cancelled after 500 patients due to excessive stroke and death outcomes in the stenting group.

There were flaws readily perceived in the attempt by Martin and his colleagues in the learning days of experience with endovascular technique compared with endarterectomy (the CAVATAS trial).[29] Three problems stand out: First, CEA and stenting both averaged unacceptably high post-treatment stroke and death (approaching 10% in both treatment arms). Second, there is no acceptable evidence to support the concept that vertebral-basilar symptoms will benefit from the removal of carotid artery stenosing lesions. Third, in this document they presented no evidence of the experience of the surgeons or interventionalists and indeed they lacked proof of excellent past experience. Finally, they did not introduce stents until late in the trial. They utilized balloon dilatation, the standard in the early days of therapy by interventional cerebral catheterization. They were ahead in their attempts to evaluate this developing technology. CAVATAS should be accepted only as a run-in to the later trial.

All of these perceived faults in trial design and proof of operator skills and trial execution were corrected before their final and quite definitive later report. An international team of well-trained interventionists reported that poststenting complication rates of stroke and death significantly exceeded those in the CEA group.[30]

The CREST study received an NINDS grant for 2500 patients with symptoms related to carotid stenosis randomly assigned to determine whether either stenting or CEA was superior or equivalent to the other in safety and long-term freedom from stroke.[31] Stroke neurologists and surgeons felt comfortable that this carefully designed protocol would put stenting of the carotid artery into the realm of evidence-based medicine. After four years, facing lagging recruitment, with only about a quarter of their target numbers recruited, the investigators felt that they had no choice but to make a midstream major protocol change. They had belatedly recruited Canadian sites, but had burned their bridges to German, French, UK, and Australian investigators. All of the rejected centers decided to start their own trials. CREST radically altered their trial design and dashed all hopes of success when it began to recruit asymptomatic patients, unfortunately a group well known to be at significantly lower risk than the original recruits. In doing this it breached the dictum laid down by Lilienfeld, the distinguished biostatistician/epidemiologist from Johns Hopkins who proposed that subjects submitted to treatment comparisons should comply with what he described in a famous lecture on the art and science of RCT as exhibiting ***ceteris paribus*** (all other things being equal).[25] All subjects in an RCT should be at equal risk of the primary outcome event, in this case ipsilateral stroke. This principle was violated. Even worse, its results paper made no mention of this devious distortion of its protocol to make sure that it had randomized the previously promised number of individuals. It gave no impressive statistical reason allowing it to study and analyze such a disparate mixture of patients as if they were one entity.

By this strategy only, CREST obtained close to its original total numbers set out in its grant application, but half of them were of the variety (symptomatic) in their original protocol. In their results paper, the investigators concluded that both potential revascularization treatments were of nearly equal value. There were fewer perioperative strokes in the CEA group, but there were more MIs in this CEA arm. Only by adding MI as part of a compound endpoint with stroke and death was there a difference detected between the two treatment strategies. This compound endpoint was not part of their original design. Surely, the plan of the trial was not to determine if stenting should be used in carotid stenosis to avoid MI! The goal at the start of this trial was to examine the usefulness of stenting instead of CEA in stroke prevention. Unhappily, cerebral events were more common after stenting.

Plainly, it is incumbent on those who would use either of these techniques to forestall stroke to make a thorough cardiac examination. These authors, at meetings that I have attended, reject the complications of cerebral ischemic events from stenting reported by Martin (which, incidentally, was now significantly different from and favoring CEA). They fail altogether to cite Martin and his colleagues' latest careful and improved international study in their references.[30]

The CREST investigators made light of and failed to comment on the known low risk of stroke anticipated in asymptomatic subjects. With their paucity of outcomes their 1250 subjects could never answer the burning question about the value of stenting in managing the asymptomatic subject. Unhappily, the media, including the neurological news magazine sponsored by the American Academy of Neurology (*Neurology Today*),[32] have written of this widely read paper as though there was good evidence that both treatments (stenting and CEA) confer equal benefit on individuals with carotid stenosis. CREST produced no good evidence that stenting has a role to play in either symptomatic or asymptomatic carotid lesions.

It is a great pity that the enthusiasts for carotid stenting did not get behind the original CREST trial and that European and Australian experts were not asked to join them and randomize the needed number of symptomatic patients to obtain a credible result. Unhappily, it may be predicted that as long as Medicare, Blue Cross, and others will pay for the procedure, the negative trials will not be attended to by the enthusiasts. The evidence favoring stenting as an alternative to CEA is far less than robust. It will be difficult to explain the use of stenting to an intelligent and alert patient with and especially without symptoms (more on this in Chapter 11). Modern patients are rightly asking for evidence-based arguments for new treatments. A contrarian's view about the use of stenting to control stenotic lessons has been published.[33]

PLATELET-INHIBITING DRUG TRIALS

These are covered rather more briefly than the surgical trials, and in full detail in Chapter 7. This section stresses the mistakes and serious omissions encountered in the reporting of the RCTs, starting with the serious breaches of modern methodology as applied to trials of aspirin, sulfinpyrazone, and then clopidogrel. RCTs of the newest antiplatelet agents are in progress.

Aspirin was the first antiplatelet drug proven to be of value in preventing disorders of thrombogenic origin. Overlooked by those of us who have written in the early days on the subject are two manuscripts from the *Mississippi Valley Medical*

Journal in 1953 and again in 1956.[34,35] They were merely serial observations, carefully recorded in an obscure journal, but should have been given earlier attention in view of what followed. The first report observed a reduction in coronary artery thrombosis in the aspirin-takers, and the second included a reported decrease in cerebral vascular problems. These observational trials, without controls, clearly pointed to the antithrombotic properties of aspirin.

Clumped platelets and cholesterol-containing debris had been observed passing through the retinal arterioles in patients with amaurosis fugax[36] (Figure 13–1) and in the cerebral arteries at postmortem by Gunning, Ross Russell, and colleagues.[37] They have been seen in the intramyocardial arteries in patients dying with unstable angina (Figure 13–2). Not long afterward, Fraser Mustard and Marian Packham identified two drugs (aspirin and sulfinpyrazone) that altered platelet function.[38] Mustard bespoke of the writer, an RCT, to evaluate a possible role for either or both of them to prevent stroke. A trial of factorial design was formulated; the hypothesis was that one or both or neither drug would prevent stroke. The trial was dubbed RRPCE (Recent Recurrent Presumed Cerebral Emboli of Arterial Origin). Errors crept into the design of this trial and its published analysis.[39] First there were too few patients (a mere 585). Perceived as more serious was the fact that without adding it to the methods paper, separate analyses were performed by sex. We found benefit from aspirin for all subjects, particularly significant in men, but did not detect benefit in women analyzed separately. It was never said that there "was no benefit," simply that "we did not detect it." This unannounced sex

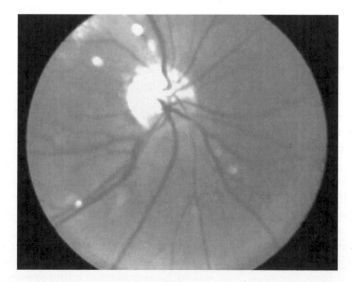

Figure 13–1. Retina in a patient with transient monocular blindness, showing atheromatous debris in retinal arterioles that has embolized from an ulcerative carotid lesion. The bright spots (Hollenhorst plaques) are thought to be cholesterol crystals. In some patients, as shown in Chapter 12, white thrombus (platelet aggregates) may be seen transiently in the retinal arteries during an episode of amaurosis fugax.

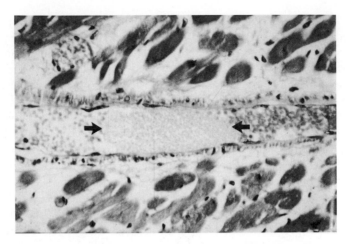

Figure 13–2. Intramyocardial branch of a coronary artery in which is visualized a platelet-fibrin embolic plug, in a postmortem examination of a patient suffering many clinical attacks diagnosed as "unstable angina." (Image courtesy of Dr. John Kaufmann.)

analysis and the small numbers of randomized patients were strongly criticized by Lilienfeld and Kurtzke, and later Dyken.[40] Nobody at that time recognized the differential prognosis, favoring women presenting with TIA or stroke. The four arms of the factorial-design trial were aspirin alone, sulfinpyrazone alone, both drugs together, or double placebo. The investigators of this initial RCT utilized 1300 mg daily of acetylsalicylic acid (ASA), a customary dose tolerated by arthritics. Critics including the Oxford Platelet Inhibiting Collaborators looked at all antiplatelet trials, but mistakenly overlooked the factorial design of this study and have failed to report on an analysis to examine the two aspirin-containing arms versus placebo.[41] There was negativity of the sulfinpyrazone arms. Serious doubt was expressed at the Princeton Conference about the possibility of synergism between the two drugs. There simply were too few patients in all arms to settle this with finality.

Within two years of our publication a total of approximately 6000 patients had entered into trials evaluating aspirin versus placebo as an antithrombotic.[42,43] The data were sufficiently robust that the FDA licensed aspirin as a drug to be prescribed in stroke-threatened patients. The later trials contained an adequate number of women to establish a lesser but significant benefit in women versus men. Our "mistake" opened up a previously unrecognized sex difference. Sex subgroups are now treated as part of all stroke RCTs.

In an attempt to test the value of sulfinpyrazone alone in monocular blindness a surgeon randomized to it or placebo a large number of patients said to have amaurosis fugax. The result was said to be positive for sulfinpyrazone and the Ciba-Geigy Company began an advertising campaign promoting sulfinpyrazone for "TIA patients." By questions asked probing the design and method of this trial, we learned that there was imperfect identification of vascular monocular visual loss in this trial. There was serious doubt about patient selection. The numbers randomized from this surgeon's general hospital patients exceeded the number of patients entered into NASCET from the aggregate of all our 10 participating stroke centers across Canada. Upon inquiry it transpired that none of his patients had been verified as having vascular/embolic monocular visual loss by experts in neurology or in ophthalmology. None had been examined for carotid disease, and none had been examined by even the bare minimum of ophthalmoscopy. In due course this spurious study was entered into the compiled meta-analysis being conducted in Oxford, erroneously making sulfinpyrazone an established and attractive platelet inhibitor. It behooves neurologists and trialists to look closely at the expertise applied in validating entrants into stroke trials. Neglecting to study the methods plan for any study is a substantial mistake. This report was a prime example of this serious blunder.

Long after the importance of identifying stroke by cause was recognized[44] a huge (18,000 patients) trial was launched to determine the relative benefits of anticoagulants versus aspirin. The fatal mistake is this: The AST trial[45] failed to insist on distinguishing between the causes of stroke. It was already firmly established that warfarin was the antithrombotic of choice preventing cardioembolism-causing stroke. By not identifying them, any conclusions from this trial were negated. Studying the "genus" stroke had become obsolete. The evidence was already sound and repeated in several trials that warfarin is superior to aspirin and is the treatment of choice in preventing cardioembolism. It is not the choice for large-artery stroke. With collection of proper data, cardiologists working with neurologists can identify cardioembolic stroke with reasonable certainty.

Clopidogrel (sold as Plavix) has been a marketing and financial success story. Failure to follow the rules for credible RCTs leaves their scientific basis less certain. Unhappily, the CAPRIE study cannot be held up as anything close to a model of an RCT.[46] The most condemning and glaring fault is the lack of a separate predisclosure of final results by a methods paper published in advance of the results paper. This is a necessity for a credible RCT. This is lacking in CAPRIE. This absence is particularly unfortunate because the analysis introduced the novelty in their results paper of a combined outcome event. Did these analyses occur in this manner because stroke patients failed to show a reduction in stroke recurrence? With the database guarded by the company, we will never be certain of this pivotal point. Patients with one of three different entities were eligible for randomization: recent MI, recent stroke, and symptomatic peripheral vascular disease. In separate analyses there was only an insignificant benefit for stroke, negative benefit for patients with MI as defined in this trial, and a strikingly significant benefit for peripheral vascular disease (PVD). The primary analysis compared the combined outcomes in all three areas with the combined outcomes in the control subjects. The data were all held in secret by the manufacturer, and despite several letters exchanged over a two-year period with the PI (incidentally a statistician), it was not possible to learn how the evaluation of the outcome endpoints was pursued, the cause of the strokes in the stroke group, or of the rigor with which they had evaluated each and every outcome in the three separate organ systems. With his sharp eyes focused on anything related to stroke prevention, Professor Saren

Jonas detected two FDA cautionary letters posted for all to see on the Internet, which warned the manufacturer against continuing to advertise the value of Plavix beyond what it had authorized. Many trials of Plavix alone or in combination have been conducted. A separate MI trial, using a restrictive and different definition of MI, was conducted and declared positive. All data are held by the company. What is needed and what is not likely to be conducted is a stroke and threatened stroke trial of Plavix versus aspirin. This will be expensive, but so too is Plavix compared with aspirin (by a huge factor of about 60). This author does not believe that there are adequate data to justify the use of Plavix in patients with stroke or with stroke-threatening symptoms, with the possible exception of those who also have symptomatic PVD. With only one nonsignificant trial standing alone and never repeated, this author is skeptical of Plavix's "lavish" promotion as a drug preventing stroke. The common practice of adding clopidogrel to the regimen when aspirin alone fails to stop all TIAs is deplored. Hankey et al remarked on the value of this combination after MI, but advised against it after cerebral ischemic events because of the risk of brain hemorrhage.[47] A Danish study condemned the use of clopidogrel added to aspirin.[48] It is regrettable that so many trees in the Boreal forests had to be turned into so many glossy pages of promotion for Plavix, when the absolute (rather than the relative) risk reduction is so marginal.

Chapter 7 is devoted to recommendations about the use of antiplatelet agents in stroke-threatened patients. The prolonged-release form of dipyridamole has not become widely embraced. Headache is a common reason for abandoning it; it is unduly expensive and the alleged long duration of action amounts to only about three hours.[49] The reader is advised to check the original studies that were accepted as giving prolonged action. Another daily dose of standard dipyridamole is no more than a minor inconvenience, if one can endure the headache. Dipyridamole cannot be used in the Aggrenox form for those sensitive to aspirin. Differences in absolute risk reduction between aspirin and any combinations with dipyridamole in Aggrenox are marginal and expensive. It is difficult to recommend the drug on the basis of what has been published by the company and its clinical adherents.

In conclusion, I have pointed out how peer review even in the best of medical journals can lead to erroneous conclusions. This is most glaring in RCTs evaluating the surgical management of asymptomatic carotid stenosis and in the several flaws identifiable in the reporting and interpretation of trials designed to evaluate the use of clopidogrel in stroke prevention. Aspirin remains the treatment of choice for patients after stroke or with stroke-threatening symptoms. In patients who have TIA or stroke despite the use of aspirin, it is more important to look for the cause of the event than to put emphasis on the choice of antiplatelet agent (see Chapter 12).

REFERENCES

1. Barnett HJM. Forty years of progress in stroke. *Stroke.* 2010;41:1068-1072.
2. Barnett HJM. Reflections on the carotid artery: 438 BC-2009 AD. The Karolinska Award Lecture in Stroke Research. *Stroke.* 2009;40:3143-3148.
3. Morgenstern L, Fox AJ, Sharp BL, Eliasziw M, Barnett HJM, Grotta JC. (NASCET) Carotid endarterectomy in patients with near-occlusion of the carotid artery. *Neurology.* 1997;48:911-915.

4. Fox AJ, Eliasziw M, Rothwell PM, Smith MH, Warlow CP, Barnett HJM. Prognosis and management of patients with carotid near-occlusion. *Am J Neuroradiol.* 2006;26:2086-2094.

5. Keating C. *Smoking Kills. The Revolutionary Life of Richard Doll.* Northampton, ME: Interlink Publishing; 2010.

6. Bernat JL. An exposé on the corrupting effects of money and power (book review of 'White Coat, Black Hat' by Carl Elliot). *Neurol Today.* 2010;10(24):17.

7. Fields W, Maslenikov V, Meyer JS, et al. Progress report of prognosis following surgery or non-surgical treatment for transient cerebral ischemic attacks and cervical carotid artery lesions. *JAMA.* 1970;211:1903-2003.

8. Steering Committee of NASCET: International Cooperative Study of Extracranial/Intracranial Arterial Anastomosis (EC/IC Bypass Study). Methodology and entry characteristics. *Stroke.* 1985;16:397-405.

9. Rothwell PM, Warlow CP. Interpretation of the operative risks of individual surgeons; on behalf of the European Carotid Surgery Trialists' Collaborative Group. *Lancet Neurol.* 1999;353(9161):1325.

10. The EC/IC Bypass Study Group: failure of extracranial-intracranial arterial bypass to reduce the risk of ischemic stroke. *N Eng J Med.* 1985;313:891-893.

11. Sundt TM. Was the international randomizer trial of extracranial-intracranial arterial bypass representative of the population at risk? *N Engl J Med.* 1987;316:814-816.

12. Sackett D, Taylor DW, Haynes B, et al. Are the results of the Extracranial-Intracranial Bypass Trial generalizable? *N Engl J Med.* 1987;316:820-824.

13. Relman AS. The Extracranial-Intracranial Arterial Bypass Study. What have we learned? *N Engl J Med.* 1987;316:809-810.

14. The EC/IC Bypass Study correspondence. *N Engl J Med.* 1987;317:1080-1081.

15. Barnett HJM, Fox A, Hachinski V, Haynes B, Peerless SJ, Sackett D, Taylor DW. Further conclusions from the Extracranial-Intracranial Bypass Trial. *Surg Neurol.* 1986;26:227-235.

16. European Carotid Surgery Trialists' Collaborative Group. Endarterectomys for moderate symptomatic stenosis; interim results from the MRC European Carotid Surgery Trial. *Lancet Neurol.* 1996;347: 1591-1593.

17. European Carotid Surgery Trialists' Collaborative Group. Randomised trial of endarterectomy for recently symptomatic carotid stenosis: final results of the MRC European Carotid Surgery Trial (ECST). *Lancet Neurol.* 1998;351:1379-1387.

18. Hobson RW, Weiss DG, Fields WS, et al. The Veterans Affairs Study Group. Efficacy of carotid endarterectomy for asymptomatic carotid stenosis. *N Engl J Med.* 1993;328:221-227.

19. Executive Committee for the asymptomatic Carotid Atherosclerosis Study. Endarterectomy for asymptomatic carotid stenosis (ACAS). *JAMA.* 1995;273:1421-1428.

20. The European Carotid Surgery Trialists' Collaborative Group (ACST). Risk of stroke in the distribution of an asymptomatic carotid artery. *Lancet.* 1995;345(8944):209-212.

21. Toole JF. Carotid artery stenosis, surgery for carotid artery stenosis. *BMJ.* 2004;329:635.

22. Barnett HJM, Meldrum HE, Thomas DJ, Eliasziw M. Treatment of asymptomatic arteriosclerotic carotid artery disease. *Adv Neurol.* 2003;92:319-328.

23. Inzitari D, Eliasziw M, Gates P, et al. The causes and risk of stroke in subjects with an asymptomatic internal carotid artery. *N Engl J Med.* 2000;283(11):1429-1436.

24. Yadav JS, Wholey MH, Kuntz RE, et al. Protected carotid-artery stenting versus endarterectomy in high-risk Patients. *N Engl J Med.* 2004;352(15):1493-1501.

25. Lilienfeld AM. Ceteris paribus. *Bull Hist Med.* 1982;56:1-18.

26. Eliasziw M, Barnett HJM. [Letter] (Stenting vs endarterectomy). *N Engl J Med.* 2005;352(6):625.

27. Ringleb P, Allenburg JR, Berger J, et al. 30-day results from the SPACE trial of stent-protected angioplasty versus carotid endarterectomy in symptomatic patients: a randomized non-inferiority trial. *Lancet Neurol.* 2006;368:1239-1247.

28. Eckstein HH, Ringleb P, Allenburg JR, et al. Results of the stent-protected angioplasty versus carotid endarterectomy (SPACE) study to treat symptomatic stenosis at 2 years: a multinational, prospective randomized trial. *Lancet Neurol.* 2008;7(10):893-902.

29. CAVATAS Investigators. Endovascular versus surgical treatment in patients with carotid stenosis in the carotid and vertebral artery. Transluminal angioplasty study (CAVATAS): a randomized trial. *Lancet Neurol.* 2001;357:1729-1737.

30. International Carotid Stenting Study Investigators, Ederle J, Dobson J, et al. Carotid artery stenting compared with endarterectomy in patients with symptomatic carotid stenosis (International Carotid Stenting Study): an interim analysis of a randomised controlled trial. *Lancet Neurol.* 2010;375(9719):985-997.

31. Brott G, Hobson RW II, Howard G, et al. Stenting versus endarterectomy for treatment of carotid-artery stenosis; for the CREST investigators. *N Engl J Med.* 2010;363:11-23.

32. Laino C. CREST puts stents, surgery on equal footing. *Neurol Today.* 2010;10:13-15.

33. Barnett HJM, Pelz DM, Lownie SP. Reflections by contrarians on the post-CREST evaluation of carotid stenting for stroke prevention. *Int J Stroke.* 2010;5:455-456.

34. Craven LL. Experiences with aspirin (acetylsalicylic acid) in the nonspecific prophylaxis of coronary thrombosis. *Mississippi Valley Medical Journal.* Third Prize, 1952, Mississippi Valley Medical Society Essay Contest:38-44.

35. Craven LL. Prevention of coronary and cerebral thrombosis. *Mississippi Valley Medical Journal (Quincy, IL).* 1956;78(5):213-215.

36. Fisher CM. Observations on the fundus oculi in transient monocular blindness. *Neurology.* 1959;9: 333-347.

37. Gunning AJ, Pickering, GW, Robb-Smith AHT, Russell RR. Mural thrombosis of the internal carotid artery and subsequent embolism. *Quart J Med.* New Series XXXIII. 1964;129:155-196.

38. Smythe HA, Ogryzle MA, Murphy EA, Mustard JF. The effect of sulfinpyrazone (sulfinpyrazone) on platelet economy and blood coagulation in man. *Can Med Assoc J.* 1965;92:818-821.

39. The Canadian Cooperative Stroke Study Group. A randomized trial of aspirin and sulfinpyrazone in threatened stroke. *N Engl J Med.* 1978;299:53-59.

40. Rice TR, Nelson E (eds.). *Eleventh Princeton Conference on Cerebrovascular Diseases, March 1978.* New York: Raven Press; 1978.

41. Antiplatelet Trialists' Collaboration. Collaborative overview of randomized trials of antiplatelet therapy, I: prevention of death, myocardial infarction, and stroke by prolonged antiplatelet therapy in various categories of patients. *BMJ.* 1994;308:81-106.

42. Bousser MG, Eschwege E, Haguenau M, et al. "AICLA" controlled trial of aspirin and dipyridamole in the secondary prevention of athero-thrombotic cerebral ischemia. *Stroke.* 1983;14:5-14.

43. UK-TIA Study Group. The United Kingdom transient ischaemic attack (UK-TIA) aspirin trial: final results. *J Neurol Neurosurg Psychiatry.* 1991;54:1044-1045.

44. International Stroke Trial Collaborative Group. The International Stroke Trial (IST): a randomized trial of aspirin, subcutaneous heparin, both, or neither among 19,435 patients with acute ischaemic stroke. *Lancet Neurol.* 1997;349:1569-1581.

45. Barnett HJM, Gunton RW, Eliasziw M, et al. Causes and severity of ischemic stroke in patients with internal carotid artery stenosis. *JAMA.* 2000;283(11):1429-1436.

46. CAPRIE Steering Committee. A randomized blinded trial of clopidogrel versus aspirin in patients at risk in ischemic events. *Lancet Neurol.* 1996;348:1329-1339.

47. Hankey GJ, Sudlow CLM, Dunbabin DW. Thienopyridines or aspirin to prevent stroke and other serious vascular events in patients at high risk of vascular disease?: a systematic review of the evidence from randomized trials. *Stroke.* 2000;31:1779-1784.

48. Sorensen R, Hunsen NL, Abildstrom SZ, et al. Risk of bleeding in patients with acute myocardial infarction treated with different combinations of aspirin, clopidogrel, and vitamin K antagonists in Denmark: a retrospective analysis of nationwide registry data. *Lancet Neurol.* 2009;374:1967-1974.

49. Dresse A, Chevolet C, Delapierre D, et al. Pharmacokinetics of oral dipyridamole (Persantine) and its effect on platelet adenosine uptake in man. *Eur J Clin Pharmacol.* 1982;23:229-234.

Prospects for Prevention of Dementia by Prevention of Stroke

14

Philip B. Gorelick

INTRODUCTION

Alzheimer disease (AD) and vascular dementia (VaD) traditionally have been thought of as distinct pathophysiologic entities. AD has been construed as a neurodegenerative disease with brain neurofibrillary tangles and amyloid plaques, and VaD as a vascular disorder of subcortical, cortical, or mixed subcortical and cortical strokes.[1] Over time, however, we have come to better understand the mechanisms and risk factors of these two disorders and now recognize possible common pathophysiologic mechanisms and shared vascular risk factors of these later-life forms of cognitive impairment.[2] For example, common mechanistic linkages for the two disorders may include inflammatory pathways, amyloid deposition, endothelial dysfunction, and angiogenesis.[2-6] A major change in our thinking about these two common disorders occurred with the recognition that stroke and cardiovascular risk factors might also be risks for both AD and VaD.[7-11]

The theme of "little strokes, big trouble" has gained popularity as stroke is a treatable and preventable catastrophe, and it is believed that clinically manifest strokes are far outnumbered by subclinical ones.[12] For example, it has been estimated that there were nine million subclinical brain infarcts and two million subclinical hemorrhages at a time when about 770,000 clinical strokes were diagnosed in the United States.[12] The subclinical brain infarcts are often small, deep ones and may be harbingers of additional stroke risk and cognitive impairment.[13,14] Furthermore, there may be a substantial interaction between cerebrovascular and AD pathologies, with greater cognitive impairment when both are present than with either one of the disorders alone.[15] Prior work by our group and others has suggested the importance of reduced thalamic volumes in relation to the presence of cognitive impairment in either stroke or AD patients.[16,17]

In this chapter, I review prospects for the prevention of cognitive impairment by prevention of stroke. I will discuss contemporary definitions of vascular forms of cognitive impairment and AD, the public health impact of these disorders, stroke and cardiovascular risk factors that may be shared by the two disorders, and potential opportunities for the prevention of dementia and cognitive decline based on stroke prevention.

DEFINITION OF KEY TERMS AND A SHIFT IN THINKING ABOUT COGNITIVE IMPAIRMENT

Alzheimer Disease

AD has been traditionally defined as an amnestic disorder with deterioration of language, visuospatial deficits, progression of loss of higher-level activities of daily living followed by loss of basic activities of daily living, and behavioral disturbances such as mood change, apathy, psychosis, and agitation.[18] The initial symptom typically may be inability to retain recently acquired information with memory for remote events relatively spared.[19] With disease progression there is impairment of language, abstract reasoning, and executive function or decision making associated with difficulty at work, in social situations, or in household activities.[19] Delusions and psychosis may occur, and the latter manifestation during the early stage of diagnosis may be suggestive of dementia with Lewy bodies.

Vascular Cognitive Impairment

The term vascular cognitive impairment (VCI) was conceived to include a spectrum of severity from prodrome (vascular cognitive impairment, no dementia [VCIND]) to full-blown manifestations of cognitive impairment, VaD, and the pathological spectrum from pure AD through degrees of vascular comorbidity or mixed disease, to pure VaD.[20,21] Currently there are research definitions of VCI, and validation of these definitions is being studied.[15] It has been recommended that diagnostic criteria to characterize cognitive impairment associated with vascular disease include two key factors: (1) demonstration of the presence of a cognitive disorder by neuropsychological testing, and (2) history of clinical stroke or presence of vascular disease by neuroimaging.[21] Evidence of stroke and cognitive impairment may be linked via a clinically manifest presentation or a more occult one. The definition of VCI captures a possible spectrum of disease and therefore allows for the occurrence of AD brain changes (mixed dementia or cognitive impairment) to occur concomitantly. It is recognized that it may be difficult to separate the presence of AD in patients with stroke and cognitive impairment.

Shift in Thinking About Cognitive Impairment

In the context of this chapter, we sometimes use the terms dementia or cognitive impairment. These terms are referred to as some studies do not provide information according to specific dementia or cognitive impairment subtype, but use these terms to indicate the presence of dementia or cognitive impairment. The term dementia, however, has been criticized as being too categorical, exclusive, and arbitrary.[20] The term generally has been used in the context of a threshold effect. In actuality, cognitive impairment may be better defined in relation to a continuum that affects different cognitive domains at different rates depending on cause.[20] It may be important, therefore, to shift our thinking to the earliest stages or prestages of cognitive impairment as an opportunity to prevent the occurrence or progression of cognitive impairment. Use of the term VCI takes advantage of the latter opportunity as it implies a vascular component and the existence of treatable or preventable factors.[20] In addition, a shift in thinking to causes of cognitive impairment rather than its effects provides the potential for prevention and treatment of such disorders.

MAGNITUDE OF THE PUBLIC HEALTH IMPACT OF VASCULAR COGNITIVE IMPAIRMENT AND ALZHEIMER DISEASE

AD is estimated to be the most common cause of dementia in developed regions.[19] There are about 17 million persons worldwide with AD and five million in the United States. It is believed that the incidence of AD increases from 1% between the ages of 60 and 70 years to 6% to 8% by age 85 years and older, and the proportion of persons 80 years or older with the disorder approaches 30%.[19] Billions of dollars are spent annually in the United States for the care of AD patients,[18] and these costs are expected to rise as the proportion of elderly individuals increases.

AD has been considered to be the most common form of nonreversible dementia, and this has been especially true among predominantly white populations in developed regions.[22] VaD may be considered, on the other hand, the second most common form of dementia. Because stroke is common in the elderly, and cognitive impairment risk and prevalence increase with age, the potential for a substantial contribution of stroke to cognitive impairment exists. In a Framingham Study publication, for example, a nested case-control study paradigm among 212 subjects who were free of dementia in January 1982 and sustained a first stroke after that date, and 1060 age- and sex-matched, dementia-free and stroke-free controls showed that dementia developed in 19.3% of cases and 11.0% of controls.[23] Overall, occurrence of stroke doubled the risk of dementia, and adjustment of factors such as age, sex, education, and individual stroke risk factors did not diminish the risk. In a subsequent publication from the Framingham Study, it was shown that the lifetime risk of stroke in middle-aged adults was one in six or more, a statistic equal to or greater than the lifetime risk of AD. In addition, blood pressure, a modifiable factor, was a significant risk for stroke in these persons.[24]

It has been estimated that up to almost two-thirds of persons experiencing a stroke have some degree of cognitive impairment, up to one-third will have frank dementia, and up to about one-third of those with substantial cognitive impairment who eventually have brain necropsy will have significant vascular pathology.[15] Furthermore, populations such as those in certain Asian countries who are at high risk of stroke may be more likely to develop cognitive impairment related to stroke.[25] These observations suggest that the contribution of stroke to cognitive impairment previously may have been underestimated based on disparate study methods and definitions, challenges in accurately defining cognitive impairment subtypes, and lack of proper neuropathologic validation studies.

From an economic standpoint, stroke is a very costly public health problem. In the United States alone, direct and indirect costs annually total about $70 billion.[26] Given the potential for a high frequency of some form of VCI in patients with stroke, it is anticipated that VCI probably contributes substantially to the overall public health economic burden of stroke, although precise cost estimates are not available.

STROKE AND CARDIOVASCULAR RISK FACTORS AND LINKAGE TO VASCULAR COGNITIVE IMPAIRMENT AND ALZHEIMER DISEASE

Stroke has been and continues to be a highly preventable disease.[27-30] It is well suited for prevention as it has many modifiable risk factors that have been well tested in clinical trials to reduce stroke risk.[31] In the final two sections of this chapter, I discuss stroke and cardiovascular factors that may heighten risk of stroke, AD, and VCI, and prospects for the prevention of dementia and cognitive impairment.

Nonmodifiable, and Well-Documented and Modifiable Risk Factors for Stroke

Table 14–1 is a list of nonmodifiable and well-documented/modifiable risk factors for stroke.[31,32] These factors have been reviewed in detail in other chapters in this text and set the stage for a discussion of shared risks for stroke, VCI, and AD. Other factors that have been considered less well-documented/potentially modifiable risks for stroke include such factors as metabolic syndrome, alcohol abuse, hyperhomocysteinemia, drug abuse, hypercoagulable states, oral contraceptive use, recent infections and inflammatory disease, migraine, sleep-disordered breathing, and lipoprotein-associated phospholipase A_2.[31,32]

Stroke and Cardiovascular Risk Factors That Have Been Linked to Dementia and AD

As previously mentioned, AD and vascular forms of cognitive impairment were once considered very differently from a mechanistic standpoint and from the viewpoint of risks.[9,10] More recently, it has been observed that there may be shared stroke risk factors for AD and VCI.[7,9] The Rotterdam Study was one of the early systematic inquiries of a population-based, prospective cohort study to elucidate vascular risk factors for dementia,[33] and Sparks was one of the first to point out a possible relationship between AD neuropathological changes, coronary artery disease, and hypertension.[34-36] Then a number of epidemiological studies began to report associations between various vascular risk factors and dementia, cognitive impairment, and AD. Table 14–2 lists various stroke and cardiovascular risk factors that have been

Table 14–1. Nonmodifiable, and Well-Documented and Modifiable Risk Factors for Stroke[31,32]

Nonmodifiable Risk Factors for Stroke
Age
Race/ethnic group (eg, black, Asian, Hispanic ancestry)
Well-Documented and Modifiable Risk Factors
Hypertension
Cigarette smoking
Diabetes mellitus
Heart disease (eg, atrial fibrillation, coronary heart disease, heart failure)
Peripheral artery disease
Asymptomatic carotid stenosis
Sickle cell disease
Dyslipidemia
Dietary Factors (eg, high sodium and low potassium intake)
Obesity and physical inactivity
Postmenopausal hormone replacement therapy

From Gorelick PB, Ruland S. Cerebral vascular disease. *Disease-a-Month*. 2010;56:33-100l; and Goldstein LB, Adams R, Alberts MJ, et al. Primary prevention of ischemic stroke: a guideline from the American Heart Association/American Stroke Association Stroke Council. *Stroke*. 2006;37: 1583-1633.

Table 14–2. Stroke and Cardiovascular Risk Factors Linked to Dementia, Cognitive Impairment, or Alzheimer Disease[2,5,9]

Discretionary Factors
Cigarette smoking
Saturated fat intake
Obesity
Physical inactivity
Traditional and Other Factors
Atrial fibrillation
Diabetes mellitus
Hypertension
Hypercholesterolemia
Hyperhomocysteinemia
Metabolic syndrome
Systemic markers of inflammation
Alcohol consumption (heavy)
Cigarette smoking
Myocardial infarction

From Gorelick PB. Role of inflammation in cognitive impairment: results of observational epidemiological studies and clinical trials. *Ann NY Acad Sci*. 2010;1207:155-162; Casserly I, Topol E. Convergence of atherosclerosis and Alzheimer's disease: inflammation, cholesterol, and misfolded proteins. *Lancet*. 2004;363:1139-1146; and Gorelick PB. Risk factors for vascular dementia and Alzheimer disease. *Stroke*. 2004;35(Suppl I):2620-2622.

linked to dementia, cognitive impairment, or AD.[2,5,9] Although white matter changes (eg, leukoaraiosis), lacunar infarcts, brain atrophy, and other neuroimaging findings may be important for conferring risk or progression of cognitive impairment,[21] these factors are beyond the scope of this review, which is limited to possible stroke and cardiovascular risks.

Stroke and Cardiovascular Risk Factors That Have Been Linked to VCI

Exploratory epidemiological studies of stroke and cardiovascular risk factors for VCI have been somewhat limited.[37-39] Most of the research efforts in the field of dementia and cognitive impairment have been geared toward AD. The study of VCI has been challenged by a number of methodological issues,[21] and the exclusion of AD in these cases may be problematic. As we observe in Table 14–3, putative risks for VCI overlap or are similar to those of stroke and AD (see Tables 14–1 and 14–2 for comparison).[40,41] Therefore, as we consider common causes of dementia and cognitive impairment in later life, we should be considering shared risks and possible common mechanistic pathways. By shifting the paradigm upstream to possible early mechanistic pathways for these disorders, our opportunities for the prevention of these disorders may be heightened.[2]

We now discuss possible pathophysiologic mechanisms of key vascular risk factors in relation to dementia, cognitive impairment, AD, and VCI.

Mechanistic Considerations

We now focus on possible mechanisms of four key stroke and cardiovascular risks that may play an important role in the causation of dementia, cognitive impairment, AD, and VCI. These factors include hypertension, diabetes mellitus, dyslipidemia, and inflammation.

HYPERTENSION

Iadecola and Davisson provide a thoughtful review of hypertension, cerebrovascular dysfunction, and cognitive impairment.[42] They emphasize that high blood pressure alters the structure of cerebral blood vessels and disrupts vasoregulatory mechanisms that ensure blood supply to brain. These mechanisms may render

Table 14–3. Stroke and Cardiovascular Risk Factors Which May Be Linked to Vascular Cognitive Impairment[40,41]

Atrial fibrillation
Alcohol consumption (heavy)
Cigarette smoking
Diabetes mellitus
High blood pressure
High cholesterol
Myocardial infarction

Table 14–4. Functional and Morphological Alterations Related to Hypertension That May Lead to Brain Injury and Dementia or Cognitive Impairment[42]

Functional Alterations	Morphological Alterations
Functional hyperemia	Atherosclerosis
Endothelial-dependent vasodilation	Lipohyalinosis
Autoregulation	Hypertrophy/remodelling
Blood-brain barrier exchange	Wall stiffening

From Iadecola C, Davisson RL. Hypertension and cerebrovascular dysfunction. *Cell Metab.* 2008;7: 476-484.

the brain vulnerable to not only to ischemic injury, but also to AD. Specific mechanisms are listed in Table 14–4.[42] Other mechanisms by which dementia or cognitive impairment may occur in persons with raised blood pressure include cerebrovascular injury to strategic areas of the brain involved in cognition, occurrence of smaller brain size and presence of hallmark brain AD neuropathologic changes, renin-angiotensin system inhibition of acetylcholine release by angiotensin II, endothelial injury potentiating amyloid deposition, and clustering of risk factors (eg, metabolic syndrome).[43]

DIABETES MELLITUS

Several provocative mechanisms exist whereby diabetes mellitus may be associated with cognitively impairing processes[43]: role of insulin-degrading enzyme in degradation of amyloid B-protein,[44] decreased insulin signaling, lower brain insulin levels and insulin resistance in association with brain toxins in AD patients,[45] inadequate production of acetylcholine,[46] and advanced glycation end-products (AGE), which may promote atherosclerosis and AD brain changes.[47]

DYSLIPIDEMIA

Mechanisms by which dyslipidemia may be linked to cognitive impairment include membrane cholesterol regulation promotion of amyloidogenic processing, promotion of oxidative stress in AD brains by oxysterols, and APO E e4-associated mechanisms.[43,48-50]

INFLAMMATION

Inflammation plays a key role in the atherosclerotic process,[51] and an inflammatory response has been observed in the neuropathologic cascade of the formation of amyloid neuritic plaques.[2] In AD the brain immune response is thought to be mediated by microglial cells.

Recent Studies of Stroke and Cardiovascular Risk Factors in Relation to Dementia, Cognitive Impairment, AD, and VCI

Table 14–5 provides a summary of results of recent epidemiologic studies that have shown associations between vascular risk factors and dementia, cognitive impairment,

Table 14–5. Recent Epidemiologic Studies of Stroke and Cardiovascular Risk Factors in Relation to Dementia, Cognitive Impairment, AD, and VCI

I. Observational Epidemiological Studies (2010): Main Findings by Vascular Risk Category

Nutrition/Diet/Obesity

1. *Washington Heights-Inwood Columbia Aging Project*: Dietary pattern higher in salad dressing, nuts, fish, tomatoes, poultry, cruciferous vegetables, fruits, and dark and green leafy vegetables, and a lower intake of high-fat dairy products, red meat, organ meat, and butter was associated with lower risk of AD.[52]
2. *The Rotterdam Study*: Higher intake of foods rich in vitamin E were associated with a modest reduction of the long-term risk of dementia and AD.[53]
3. *Framingham Offspring Cohort*: Visceral fat in healthy middle-aged adults is associated with lower brain volume.[54]
4. *Epidemiologie de l'Oseoporose Study*: Inadequate weekly vitamin D dietary intake was associated with cognitive impairment.[55]

Inflammation/Metabolic Syndrome

1. *Systematic Evaluation and Alteration of Risk Factors for Cognitive Health Study*: Low-grade inflammation as measured by high-sensitivity C-reactive protein was associated with cerebral microstructural damage on high-field MRI, predominantly affecting frontal pathways and executive function.[56]
2. *Adult Changes in Thought Study*: Greater use of nonselective nonsteroidal anti-inflammatory drugs was associated with neuritic plaque accumulation.[57]

Diabetes Mellitus

1. *Leukoaraiosis and Disability Study*: Diabetes and white matter changes are independent predictors of cognitive decline in initially nondisabled elderly.[58]
2. *Hisayama Study*: Hyperinsulinemia and hyperglycemia associated with insulin resistance accelerates neuritic plaque formation in combination with APOE e4.[59]
3. *Vantaa 85+ Study*: Presence of diabetes doubled the incidence of dementia, AD, and VaD and was associated with more vascular pathology.[60]

Infarction

1. *Framingham Offspring Study*: Among middle-aged adults, brain infarction with incident stroke was independently associated with increased risk of stroke and dementia, whereas white matter hyperintensities were associated with an increased risk of stroke, amnestic mild cognitive impairment, dementia, and death.[61]

II. Clinical Trials (2010): Main Findings by Vascular Risk Category

Lipids

1. *Atorvastatin in Alzheimer's Dementia*: Intensive lipid lowering with atorvastatin in patients with mild to moderate AD who were taking donepezil over 72 weeks did not benefit cognition when compared to placebo.[62]
2. *Health in Men Study*: Vitamin supplementation with daily doses of B_{12}, folic acid, and B_6 did not improve cognition in men ≥75 years of age who had hypertension.[63]
3. *Prospective Study of Pravastatin in the Elderly at Risk*: Among elderly patients with diabetes mellitus but no dementia, there was accelerated brain atrophy with increased decline in cognition compared to those without diabetes mellitus.[64]

(Continued)

Table 14–5. Recent Epidemiologic Studies of Stroke and Cardiovascular Risk Factors in Relation to Dementia, Cognitive Impairment, AD, and VCI (*Continued*)

III. Select Epidemiological Studies and Clinical Trials (2008/2009)
Diabetes Mellitus
1. *Washington Heights-Inwood Columbia Aging Project*: In relation to hippocampal dysfunction, blood glucose levels were inversely and selectively correlated with dentate gyrus cerebral blood volume, whereas blood glucose levels were selectively and inversely correlated with total recall, and CA1 dysfunction was associated with cerebral infarcts in an area noted to be vulnerable to transient hypotension.[65]
2. *SMART Study*: Type 2 diabetes was associated with diffuse cerebral atrophy, leukoaraiosis, and lacunar infarcts, but not large infarcts.[66]
Coronary Artery Bypass Grafting (CABG)
1. *Case series of coronary heart disease patients with on-pump CABG, off-pump procedures, and medically managed community controls*: All 3 groups showed similar declines in cognitive function over a 6-year time period and on-pump CABG patients were not cognitively worse.[67]
Hypertension
1. *Cardiovascular Health Study*: Centrally acting angiotensin-converting enzyme inhibitors were associated with a reduction in cognitive decline.[68]
2. *HYVET-COG*: Among those 80 years and older who were treated with indapamide with or without perindopril vs placebo, there was no effect in this clinical trial on dementia risk.[69]
Homocysteine, Folic Acid, and Vitamin B$_{12}$
1. *Three-City Study*: No correlation was found between B$_{12}$ and cognition, but there was a correlation between low folate and cognition, and hyperhomocysteinemia when folate levels were low.[70]
Nutrition/Diet/Obesity
1. *Framingham Study*: Circulating leptin was associated with reduced risk of dementia and AD and with higher total cerebral brain volume and lower temporal horn volume, although the latter measure did not reach statistical significance.[71]

AD, or VCI.[52-71] This summary of results is not an exhaustive one, but rather addresses select papers published in 2008/2009 and 2010. For additional reviews of vascular factors, the reader is referred to other recent publications.[2,21,43,72]

PREVENTION OF DEMENTIA AND COGNITIVE DECLINE: PRACTICAL AND RESEARCH CONSIDERATIONS

There has been substantial interest in the prevention of or slowing of progression of the major forms of cognitive impairment of later life. As discussed above, it has become clear that a number of vascular factors are shared risks for both AD and VCI. Therefore, it may be advantageous to study persons in early stages of or at high risk for cognitive impairment to determine if modification of vascular risk factors may lead to reduction in AD or VCI risk. When prevalence of a risk factor and relative risk for a disease are taken into account, a calculation called the population attributable risk can be made, which provides an estimate of the contribution of various risks to a specific disease. In the case of VCI, it has been estimated that hypertension, current cigarette smoking, and low-density lipoprotein (LDL) cholesterol might be important factors to target for modification in cognitive impairment as these factors may explain 66%, 17%, and 37% of VCI, respectively.[40]

Thus far, however, a number of clinical trials primarily or nonprimarily designed to reduce the risk of cognitive impairment by modification of vascular risks or prevention of strokes has not resulted in significant preservation of cognition.[69,73-79] Additional studies are ongoing such as the Aspirin in Reducing Events in Elderly (ASPREE) and Systolic Blood Pressure Intervention Trial (SPRINT)-MIND studies.[80,81] I now summarize a recent statement from the US National Institute of Health about the status of vascular risk factors in relation to preservation of cognition.

National Institutes of Health Statement on Prevention of Alzheimer Disease and Cognitive Decline

Based in part on a contemporary systematic literature review of factors that might reduce the risk of dementia or cognitive decline, the National Institutes of Health (NIH) issued a summary paper from a consensus conference that addressed the possible role of cardiovascular (CV) risk factors on cognitive decline or dementia.[82,83] The review was designed to summarize evidence about putative risk and protective factors for cognitive decline in older persons and the possible role of interventions to prevent cognitive decline.[82] English-language publications were selected among those from 1984 through October 27, 2009. Observational studies with 300 or more participants and randomized controlled trials (RCTs) with 50 or more subjects who were age 50 years or older, from general populations, and followed for at least one year were included for analysis. In addition, relevant systematic reviews were studied. An overall rating system of quality of evidence was used to rate studies (GRADE: Grading of Recommendations Assessment, Development, and Evaluation). A total of 127 observational epidemiological studies, 22 RCTs, and 16 systematic reviews were analyzed and included information about nutritional factors, medical factors and medications, socioeconomic or behavioral factors, toxic exposures, and genetics.[82]

For observational studies, it was concluded that current tobacco use, presence of apolipoprotein E e4 genotype, and diabetes were likely to be associated with cognitive decline, as were depressive symptoms and metabolic syndrome. Other factors that were thought to be probably associated with a lower risk of cognitive decline included participation in cognitive or physical activity, other leisure activities, and dietary factors including a Mediterranean diet or vegetable or omega-3 fatty acid intake. There was no consistent association for the following factors: hypertension, hyperlipidemia, homocysteine, or obesity.[82] In relation to RCTs and CV-related factors, only two factors had an effect on cognitive decline—cognitive training and physical exercise—but there was limited to absent RCT data on many of the factors, and there was high-quality evidence for only one factor: cognitive training.[82] The NIH Consensus Panel went on to conclude that there was no current substantial evidence to suggest any association that a modifiable factor reduced risk for AD or cognitive decline in older persons; the quality of evidence was generally low and in relation to therapeutic interventions inadequate to conclude that there could be delayed onset of AD or reduction of cognitive decline; inconsistent and varied methodological assessments prevented provision of clear and concise answers; and research recommendations to bridge gaps in our knowledge were needed and summarized (see Appendix available at www.annals.org).[83]

SUMMARY

Given the many shared vascular risk factors associated with stroke, VCI, and AD, and potential shared mechanistic pathways for these disorders, it makes sense for us to develop well-designed RCTs to study the influence of vascular risk factors on the prevention of cognitive impairment or reduction of cognitive decline in appropriate high-risk groups.[2,84] Such efforts will likely and eventually lead to fewer strokes and possibly a reduction in the risk of major subclasses of dementia and rates of cognitive decline associated with these disorders. An upstream mechanistically based approach to the reduction of cognitive impairment and cognitive decline with the proper intervention administered in the proper time window is needed. This will likely require long-term study, as intervention in midlife may be required. Hypertension and elevated LDL cholesterol may be important targets for such study.

REFERENCES

1. Gorelick PB, Nyenhuis DL, Garron DC, Cochran E. Is vascular dementia really Alzheimer's disease or mixed dementia? *Neuroepidemiology.* 1996;15:286-290.
2. Gorelick PB. Role of inflammation in cognitive impairment: results of observational epidemiological studies and clinical trials. *Ann NY Acad Sci.* 2010;1207:155-162.
3. Iadecola C, Gorelick PB. Converging pathogenic mechanisms in vascular and neurodegenerative dementia. *Stroke.* 2003;34:335-337.
4. Vagnucci AH, Li WW. Alzheimer's disease and angiogenesis. *Lancet.* 2003;361:605-608.
5. Casserly I, Topol E. Convergence of atherosclerosis and Alzheimer's disease: inflammation, cholesterol, and misfolded proteins. *Lancet.* 2004;363:1139-1146.
6. Wu Z, Guo H, Chow N, et al. Roles of the MEOX2 homeobox gene in neurovascular dysfunction in Alzheimer disease. *Nat Med.* 2005;11:959-965.
7. Gorelick PB, Erkinjuntii T, Hofman A, Rocca WA, Skoog I, Winblad B. Prevention of vascular dementia. *Alzheimer Dis Assoc Disord.* 1999;13(Suppl 3):S131-S139.
8. Gorelick PB. Can we save the brain from the ravages of midlife cardiovascular risk factors? *Neurology.* 1999;52:1114-1115.
9. Gorelick PB. Risk factors for vascular dementia and Alzheimer disease. *Stroke.* 2004;35(Suppl I): 2620-2622.
10. Gorelick PB. William Feinberg Lecture: cognitive vitality and the role of stroke and cardiovascular disease risk factors. *Stroke.* 2005;36:875-879.
11. Craft S. The role of metabolic disorders in Alzheimer disease and vascular dementia. *Arch Neurol.* 2009;66:300-305.
12. Hachinski V. World Stroke Day 2008. "Little strokes, big trouble." *Stroke.* 2008;39:2407-2408.

13. Vermeer SE, Longstreth WT, Koudstaal PJ. Silent brain infarcts: a systematic review. *Lancet Neurol.* 2007;6:611-619.

14. Pantoni L. Leukoaraiosis: from an ancient term to an actual marker of poor prognosis. *Stroke.* 2008;39:1401-1403.

15. Hachinski V, Iadecola C, Petersen RC, et al. National Institute of Neurological Disorders and Storke-Canadian Stroke Network vascular cognitive impairment harmonization standards. *Stroke.* 2006;37:2220-2241.

16. Stebbins GT, Nyenhuis DL, Wang C, et al. Gray matter atrophy in patients with ischemic stroke with cognitive impairment. *Stroke.* 2008;39:785-793.

17. de Jong LW, van der Hiele K, Veer IM, et al. Strongly reduced volumes of putamen and thalamus in Alzheimer's Disease. MRI Study. *Brain.* 2008;131(12):3277-3285.

18. Cummings JL. Alzheimer's disease. *N Engl J Med.* 2004;351:56-67.

19. Mayeux R. Early Alzheimer's disease. *N Engl J Med.* 2010;362:2194-2201.

20. Hachinski V. Shifts in thinking about dementia. *JAMA.* 2008;300:2172-2173.

21. Gorelick PB, Scuteri A, Arnett D, et al. Vascular contributions to cognitive impairment and dementia. *Stroke.* 2011;42(9):2672-2713.

22. Rocca WA, Hofman A, Brayne C, et al. The prevalence of vascular dementia in Europe: facts and fragments from 1980-1990 studies. *Ann Neurol.* 1991;30:817-824.

23. Ivan CS, Seshadri S, Beiser A, et al. Dementia after stroke. The Framingham Study. *Stroke.* 2004;35:1264-1269.

24. Seshadri S, Beiser A, Kelly-Hayes M, et al. The lifetime risk of stroke. Estimates from the Framingham Study. *Stroke.* 2006;37:345-350.

25. White L, Petrovitch H, Ross W, et al. Prevalence of dementia in older Japanese-American Men in Hawaii. The Honolulu-Asia Aging Study. *JAMA.* 1996;276:955-960.

26. Lloyd-Jones D, Adams R, Carnethon M, et al. Heart disease and stroke statistics—2009 update. *Circulation.* 2009;119:e21-e181.

27. Gorelick PB. Stroke prevention. *Arch Neurol.* 1995;52:347-355.

28. Gorelick PB, Sacco RL, Smith DB, et al. Prevention of a first stroke. A review of guidelines and a multidisciplinary consensus statement from the National Stroke Association. *JAMA.* 1999;281:1112-1120.

29. Gorelick PB. The future of stroke prevention by risk factor modification. *Handb Clin Neurol.* 2009;94:1261-1276.

30. Spence JD. Secondary stroke prevention. *Nat Rev Neurol.* 2010;6:1-10.

31. Gorelick PB, Ruland S. Cerebral vascular disease. *Disease-a-Month.* 2010;56:33-100.

32. Goldstein LB, Adams R, Alberts MJ, et al. Primary prevention of ischemic stroke: a guideline from the American Heart Association/American Stroke Association Stroke Council. *Stroke.* 2006;37:1583-1633.

33. Ruitenberg A. *Vascular factors in dementia. Observations in the Rotterdam Study.* Thesis. Ipskamp, Enschede: Print Partners; 2000:3-149.

34. Sparks DL, Lui H, Scheff SW, Coyne CM, Hunsaker JC. Temporal sequence of plaque formation in the cerebral cortex of non-demented individuals. *J Neuropathol Exper Neurol.* 1993;52:135-142.

35. Sparks DL, Scheff SW, Lui H, Landers TM, Coyne CM, Hunsaker JC. Increased incidence of neurofibrillary tangle (NFT) in non-demented individuals with hypertension. *J Neurol Sci.* 1995;131:162-169.

36. Sparks DL. Coronary artery disease, hypertension, ApoE, and cholesterol: a link to Alzheimer's disease? *Ann NY Acad Sci.* 1997;826:128-146.

37. Gorelick PB, Chatterjee A, Patel D, et al. Cranial computed tomographic observations in multi-infarct dementia. *Stroke.* 1992;23:804-811.

38. Gorelick PB, Brody JA, Cohen D, et al. Risk factors for dementia associated with multiple cerebral infarcts. A case-control analysis in predominantly African-American hospital-based patients. *Arch Neurol.* 1993;50:714-720.

39. Gorelick PB, Freels S, Harris Y, Dollear T, Billingsley M, Brown N. Epidemiology of vascular and Alzheimers' dementia among African Americans in Chicago, Illinois: baseline frequency and comparison of risk factors. *Neurology.* 1994;44:1391-1396.

40. Gorelick PB. Prevention (Chapter 23). In: Bowler J, Hachinski V (eds). *Vascular Cognitive Impairment. Preventable Dementia.* New York: Oxford University Press; 2003:308-320.

41. Gorelick PB. Status of risk factors for dementia associated with stroke. *Stroke.* 1997;28:459-463.

42. Iadecola C, Davisson RL. Hypertension and cerebrovascular dysfunction. *Cell Metab.* 2008;7: 476-484.
43. Testai FD, Gorelick PB. Cerebrovascular disease/cognitive function (Chapter 5e). In: Baliga R, Bakris G (eds). *Hypertension.* New York: Oxford University Press; (submitted).
44. Steen E, Terry BM, Rivera EJ, et al. Impaired insulin and insulin-like growth factor expression and signaling mechanisms in Alzheimer's disease—is this type 3 diabetes? *J Alzheimers Dis.* 2005;7:63-80.
45. De Felice FG, Wu D, Lambert MP, et al. Alzheimer's disease-type neuronal tau hyperphosphorylation induced by A beta oligomers. *Neurobiol Aging.* 2008;29:1334-1347.
46. Rivera EJ, Goldin A, Fulmer N, Tavares R, Wands JR, de la Monte SM. Insulin and insulin-like growth factor expression and function deteriorate with progression of Alzheimer's disease: link to brain reductions in acetylcholine. *J Alzheimers Dis.* 2005;8:247-268.
47. Takeuchi M, Kikuchi S. Sasaki N, et al. Involvement of advanced glycation end-products in Alzheimer's disease. *Curr Alzheimer Res.* 2004;1:39-46.
48. Wahrie S, Das P, Nyborg AC, et al. Cholesterol-dependent gamma-secretase activity in buoyant cholesterol-rich membrane microdomains. *Neurobiol Dis.* 2002;9:11-23.
49. Chang JY, Liu LZ. Neurotoxicity of cholesterol oxides on cultured cerebellar granule cells. *Neurochem Int.* 1998;32:317 323.
50. Herz J, Chen Y. Reelin, lipoprotein receptors and synaptic plasticity. *Nat Rev Neurososci.* 2006;7: 850-859.
51. Gorelick PB. Stroke prevention therapy beyond antithrombotics. Unifying mechanisms in ischemic stroke pathogenesis and implications for therapy. An invited review. *Stroke.* 2002;33:862-875.
52. Gu Y, Nieves JW, Stern Y, Luchsinger JA, Scarmeas N. Food combination and Alzheimer disease risk. A protective diet. *Arch Neurol.* 2010;67:699-706.
53. Devore EE, Grodstein F, van Rooij FJA, et al. Dietary antioxidants and long-term risk of dementia. *Arch Neurol.* 2010;67:819-825.
54. Debette S, Beiser A, Hoffmann U, et al. Visceral fat is associated with lower brain volume in healthy middle-aged adults. *Ann Neurol.* 2010;68:136-144.
55. Annweiler C, Schott AM, Rolland Y, Blain H, Herrmann FR, Beaucher O. Dietary intake of vitamin D and cognition in older women. A large population-based study. *Neurology.* 2010;75:1810-1816.
56. Wersching H, Duning T, Lohmann H, et al. Serum C-reactive protein is linked to cerebral microstructural integrity nad cognitive function. *Neurology.* 2010;74:1022-1029.
57. Sonnen JA, Larson EB, Walker RL, et al. Nonsteroidal anti-inflammatory drugs are associated with increased neuritic plaques. *Neurology.* 2010;75:1203-1210.
58. Verdelho A, Madureira S, Doleiro C, et al. White matter changes and diabetes predict cognitive decline in the elderly. The LADIS Study. *Neurology.* 2010;75:160-167.
59. Matsuzaki T, Sasaki K, Tanizaki Y, et al. Insulin resistance is associated with the pathology of Alzheimer disease. The Hisayama Study. *Neurology.* 2010;75:764-770.
60. Ahtiluoto S, Polvikoski T, Peltonen M, et al. Diabetes, Alzheimer disease, and vascular dementia. *Neurology.* 2010;75:1195-1202.
61. Debette S, Beiser A, DeCarli C, et al. Association of MRI markers of vascular brain injury with incident stroke, mild cognitive impairment, dementia, and mortality. The Framingham Offspring Study. *Stroke.* 2010;41:600-606.
62. Feldman HH, Doody RS, Kivipelto M, et al. Randomized controlled trial of atorvastatin in mild to moderate Alzheimer disease. LEADe. *Neurology.* 2010;74:956-964.
63. Ford AH, Flicker L, Alfonso H, et al. Vitamins B_{12}, B_6, and folic acid for cognition in older men. *Neurology.* 2010;75:1540-1547.
64. van Elderen SGC, de Roos A, de Craen AJM, et al. Progression of brain atrophy and cognitive decline in diabetes mellitus. A 3-year follow-up. *Neurology.* 2010;75:997-1002.
65. Wu W, Brickman AM, Luchsinger J, et al. The brain in the age of old: the hippocampal formation is targeted differentially by diseases of late life. *Ann Neurol.* 2008;64:698-706.
66. Tiehuis AM, van der Graaf Y, Visseren FL, et al. Diabetes increases atrophy and vascular lesions on brain MRI in patients with symptomatic arterial disease. *Stroke.* 2008;39:1600-1603.
67. Selnes OA, Grega MA, Bailey MM, et al. Do management strategies for coronary artery disease influence 6-year cognitive outcomes? *Ann Thorac Surg.* 2009;88:445-454.

68. Sink KM, Leng X, Williamson J, et al. Angiotensin-converting enzyme inhibitors and cognitive decline in older adults with hypertension. *Arch Intern Med.* 2009;169(13):1195-1202.

69. Peters R, Beckett N, Forette F, et al. Incident dementia and blood pressure lowering in the Hypertension in the Very Elderly Trial Cognitive function assessment (HYVET COG): a double-blind, placebo controlled trial. *Lancet Neurol.* 2008;7:683-689.

70. Vidal J-S, Dufouil C, Ducros V, Tzourio C. Homocysteine, folate and cognition in a large community-based sample of elderly people—the 3C Dijon study. *Neuroepidemiology.* 2008;30:207-214.

71. Lieb W, Beiser AS, Vasan RS, et al. Association of plasma leptin levels with incident Alzheimer disease and MRI measures of brain aging. *JAMA.* 2009;302:2565-2572.

72. Gorelick PB, Bowler JV. Advances in vascular cognitive impairment. *Stroke.* 2010;41:e93-e98.

73. Aisen PS. Schafer KA, Grundman M, et al. Effects of rofecoxib of naproxen vs placebo on Alzheimer disease progression. A randomized controlled trial. *JAMA.* 2003;289:2819-2826.

74. ADAPT Research Group. Naproxen and celecoxib do not prevent AD in early results from a randomized controlled trial. *Neurology.* 2007;68:1800-1808.

75. ADAPT Research Group. Cognitive function over time in the Alzheimer's Disease Anti-inflammatory Prevention Trial (ADAPT). Results of a randomized, controlled trial of naproxen and celecoxib. *Arch Neurol.* 2008;65:896-905.

76. Kang JH, Cook N, Manson J, Buring JE, Grodstein F. Low dose aspirin and cognitive function in the women's health study cognitive cohort. *BMJ.* 2007;334:987.

77. Price JF, Stewart MC, Deary IJ, et al. Low dose aspirin and cognitive function in middle aged to elderly adults: randomized controlled trial. *BMJ.* 2008;337:a1198.

78. Bentham P, Gray R, Sellwood E, Hills R, Crome P, Faftery J. Aspirin in Alzheimer's disease (AD2000): a randomized open-label trial. *Lancet Neurol.* 2008;7(1):41-49.

79. Diener HC, Sacco RL, Yusuf S, et al. Effects of aspirin plus extended-release dipyridamole versus telmisartan on disability and cognitive function after recurrent stroke in patients with ischemic stroke in the Prevention Regimen for Effectively Avoiding Second Strokes (PRoFESS) trial: a double-blind, active and placebo-controlled study. *Lancet Neurol.* 2008;7:875-884.

80. Nelson M, Reid C, Beilin LJ, et al. Rationale for a trial of low-dose aspirin for the primary prevention of major adverse cardiovascular events and vascular dementia in the elderly: Aspirin in Reducing Events in the Elderly (ASPREE). *Drugs Aging.* 2003;20(12):897-903.

81. NIH News. NIH launches multicenter clinical trial to test blood pressure strategy. http://public.nhlbi.nih.gov/newsroom/home/GetPressRelease.aspx?id=2667 (accessed November 2, 2009).

82. Plassman BL, Williams JW Jr, Burke JR, Holsinger T, Benjamin S. Systematic review: factors associated with risk for the possible prevention of cognitive decline in later life. *Ann Intern Med.* 2010;153:182-193.

83. Daviglus ML, Bell CC, Berrettini W, et al. National Institutes of Health State-of-the-Science Conference statement: preventing Alzheimer disease and cognitive decline. *Ann Intern Med.* 2010;153:176-181.

84. Pantoni L, Gorelick PB. Advances in Vascular Cognitive Impairment. *Stroke.* 2011;42(2):291-293.

Minimizing Adverse Effects of Cardiovascular Drugs

15

J. David Spence

INTRODUCTION

It is important to minimize adverse effects of drugs in order to maximize compliance. There is evidence that drug classes with fewer adverse effects have better long-term persistence with therapy.[1] Minimizing numbers of pills to the extent possible will also aid patients to take their prescribed medications reliably.

An important, avoidable cause of noncompliance is misinformation. Pharmacists often provide lists of "side effects" that are worse than useless, because they are not a list of causally related adverse effects; rather, they are a list of all symptoms known to humankind, whether caused by cancer, a hangover, a flulike illness, or whatever. Such lists are all the same, and all include symptoms such as fatigue, headache, nausea, vomiting, dizziness, diarrhea, constipation, and so on. Wait a minute: diarrhea and constipation on the same list? Does this make sense? Patients will study such lists whenever they have a symptom, highlight the offending item on the list with a yellow highlighter, and bring it to a clinic as documentary proof of causality. This problem is known to the branch of philosophy called Logic as the "post hoc ergo propter hoc fallacy" (because A preceded B, it caused B.) Some patients become very fixed in their ideation, believing that they are somehow special and that all drugs disagree with them.

One solution can be a blinded N of 1 crossover trial (discussed below), with capsules containing placebos alternating with capsules containing active drug; unfortunately, some patients are so fixed in their ideation that this is not convincing. In such patients, if resistant hypertension is the result of noncompliance, surgical options such as adrenalectomy for primary aldosteronism or renal bypass,[2] or new approaches such as renal nerve ablation[3] or carotid baroreceptor stimulation[4] may be needed.

At the same time as these lists are contributing to nonpersistence by providing information that is misleading (although intended to be helpful), physicians are becoming increasingly pressured by high workloads and may find it easier to "switch than fight." That is, they may find it easier to switch to another drug rather than spend time explaining to the patient that the symptom is unlikely to be causally related to the drug, or devise a rational approach to analyzing causality, such as a blinded "n of 1" trial (see below). Unfortunately, switching the drug reinforces the patient's belief that the original drug was causing the symptoms. In my Hypertension Clinic, I saw patients on almost a monthly basis who were referred because they were "allergic to all antihypertensive drugs." Scrutiny of the list they brought in might reveal that they had cough from six different angiotensin-converting enzyme (ACE) inhibitors, thought they had cough from several angiotensin receptor blockers (ARBs) (meaning that the cough was probably due to asthma or another cause), "dizziness" on eight different medications (meaning that they had postural hypotension from several alpha-blockers), and vertigo from their Meniere disease while taking several other drugs from different classes.

What we really need for patients is a list of the symptoms that occur more often with active drug than with placebo, and a focus on the important adverse effects for each drug.

ANTIHYPERTENSIVE DRUGS

Sometimes, to minimize adverse effects, it is important to tailor the therapy to the physiology of the underlying cause of the hypertension, as described below and in Chapter 6. For example, patients whose adverse effects (such as postural hypotension, fatigue, muscle cramps) are due to potassium depletion from kaliuretic diuretics will do better with aldosterone antagonists if they have primary hyperaldosteronism, drugs that effectively block the renin/angiotensin/aldosterone (RAAS) system if they have secondary hyperaldosteronism, or amiloride if they have variants of Liddle syndrome. Potassium supplements are less effective than blocking the underlying cause of potassium depletion; they do not restore intracellular potassium unless given with magnesium.[5,6] An important and little-recognized issue is that the key problem is not hypokalemia; it is depletion of intracellular potassium. A normal serum potassium does not exclude significant depletion of intracellular potassium.[7] Acid urine in the face of systemic alkalosis is a more sensitive indicator of potassium depletion.[7]

ADVERSE EFFECTS BY DRUG CLASS

Blood Pressure Medications

ANGIOTENSIN-CONVERTING ENZYME INHIBITORS

These drugs do not only block the conversion of angiotensin I to angiotensin II; as shown in Figure 15–1, they also block the breakdown of bradykinin. It is probably the elevation of bradykinin levels that causes cough (in about 8% of patients).

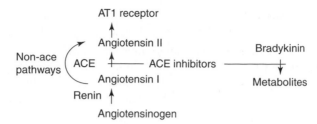

Figure 15–1. Angiotensin-converting enzyme (ACE) inhibitors also raise bradykinin levels. ACE inhibitors not only block ACE, they also block the breakdown of bradykinin. Most of the adverse effects, and possibly most of the action of ACE inhibitors, is due to increased levels of bradykinin, which increases the release of nitric oxide (NO) via cyclic guanosine monophosphate (GMP). ACE inhibitors can be thought of as being similar to long-acting nitrates.

Angioedema (which occurs in fewer than 1 out of 1000 patients) results from elevation of bradykinin levels in susceptible individuals with abnormal bradykinin metabolism.[8] Renal failure may result from blockade of the RAAS system, as discussed in Chapter 6. Besides these class effects that are common to all ACE inhibitors, captopril, because it is a thiol, may cause a morbiliform rash and dysgeusia.

BETA-BLOCKERS

β-Adrenergic blockers will cause bradycardia, will aggravate asthma, and may aggravate congestive heart failure. Atenolol and nadolol, because they are renally excreted, will accumulate in patients with impaired renal function, including the elderly. This may actually aggravate systolic hypertension, because the slower heart rate results in an increased stroke volume; a large stroke volume dumped into a stiff aorta widens the pulse pressure and may actually increase systolic pressure.

Adverse effects from blockade of β_2 receptors, including bronchospasm, cold extremities, reduced muscle blood flow with impaired exercise capacity, insulin release, and lipid metabolism, will be worse with nonselective beta-blockers such as propranolol, nadolol, and timolol. Penetration into the central nervous system, with adverse effects such as vivid dreams and even hallucinations, is greatest with propranolol and pindolol. Pindolol and oxprenolol, which stimulate β_2 receptors while blocking β_1 receptors, may minimize bronchospasm but cause tremors. Metoprolol is a poor choice[9] because it is short acting, so it must be taken more than once a day; it is also impossible to dose correctly because it is metabolized by CYP2D6, the prototype drug for fast metabolizers and slow metabolizers (due to copy number variation). The range of blood levels achieved with a given dose is 150-fold.[9] Because metoprolol is short acting, it is also more likely to provoke rebound hypertension and angina when doses are missed, for example, during nausea from cholecystitis. The beta-blocker that is least likely to cause rebound hypertension is pindolol,[10] probably because it is so tightly bound to receptors that it takes almost a week to lose its effect.

CALCIUM CHANNEL BLOCKERS

The principal adverse effects of these drugs differ by subclass. Dihydropyridines such as nifedipine, felodipine, and amlodipine cause ankle swelling; rarely they may also cause flushing or headache. Amlodipine, because it is longer acting, is less likely to cause edema or flushing. The principal adverse effect of verapamil is constipation; rarely it may aggravate heart failure. The principal adverse effect of diltiazem is bradycardia; rarely it may also aggravate heart failure. The notion that nifedipine and other short-acting dihydropyridines increase the risk of cardiovascular events was a myth resulting from failure to understand that patients who were taking nifedipine were taking it mainly for angina.[11] However, nifedipine, especially "sublingual" nifedipine, should not be used to lower blood pressure acute stroke, as it cannot be taken back once given, and it may aggravate ischemia by dropping the blood pressure too low.[12]

HYDROCHLOROTHIAZIDE

Depletion of potassium and magnesium can lead to fatigue, myalgia, cramps, postural hypotension, and impotence; most of these can be avoided with salt restriction and/or the addition of a potassium/magnesium-sparing diuretic such as amiloride or spironolactone, or an ACE inhibitor or ARB. Which approach is most effective will depend on the renin/aldosterone profile, as discussed in Chapter 6. Potassium supplements don't actually work: they increase urinary potassium but do not restore intracellular potassium unless magnesium is also given.[13]

Thiazides also aggravate gout and diabetes; gout may be avoided by using xanthine oxidase inhibitors such as allopurinol. Higher doses of thiazides cause more adverse effects without a proportional benefit; therefore, low doses such as hydrochlorothiazide 12.5 mg daily are optimal[14]; this is probably particularly important for patients with diabetes and insulin resistance. Indapamide probably does not avoid the metabolic adverse effects of thiazides. Although clorthalidone may be more efficacious at lowering blood pressure, it is so long acting that it causes more depletion of potassium and other ions. Of all the antihypertensive drug classes, diuretics are the most likely to be causally related to adverse effects; preventing depletion of potassium, magnesium, and so on, as discussed above, may minimize this problem. It should be said that most impotence attributed to blood pressure medication is probably from other causes (loss of self-esteem, loss of feelings of control, marital difficulties, etc.).

Potassium/Magnesium-Sparing Diuretics

The principal adverse effect of these drugs is that they may cause hyperkalemia. In addition, amiloride may cause heartburn, and spironolactone causes mastalgia and gynecomastia (mainly in men); occasionally it also causes nausea.

Angiotensin II Antagonists (ARBs)

These drugs (eg, losartan, irbesartan, candesartan, valsartan, telmisartan) are of the first antihypertensive class with fewer adverse effects than placebo (they reduce headache compared with placebo). This probably explains why they have the best long-term adherence among antihypertensive drug classes.[1] However, they can cause trouble by their intended effect of blockade of angiotensin II: They may cause hyperkalemia, and, as do ACE inhibitors, they will aggravate renal failure in patients with bilateral renal artery stenosis (sometimes in patients with heart failure in whom renal artery stenosis is unrecognized). The same is probably true of the new renin inhibitor aliskiren. As discussed in Chapter 6, about a third of patients with congestive heart failure have renal artery stenosis[15]; the secondary hyperaldosteronism undoubtedly adversely affects the heart failure.

Alpha-Blockers

These drugs are the most likely to cause postural hypotension. If they are being used because of prostatic symptomatology, finasteride and related drugs may eventually help the patient get off alpha-blockers, but this takes months to work. Taking longer-acting alpha-blockers (doxazosin), taking the medication at bedtime, and avoiding potassium depletion from diuretics (as described above) may help with postural hypotension. Elevating the head of the bed on blocks may also be helpful.

Clonidine

Clonidine is probably the most likely of all the antihypertensive drugs to cause severe rebound hypertension; for this reason it should seldom be used. Rare indications for clonidine are discussed in Chapter 6.

Antiplatelet Agents

Acetylsalicylic acid (ASA) can aggravate ulcers in the duodenum and cause gastrointestinal (GI) bleeding; in most cases this can be prevented by eradicating *Helicobacter pylori* with antibiotics. Proton pump inhibitors may also reduce GI bleeding. If the patient has not had ulcers but has had erosive gastritis, the stomach problems from ASA or nonsteroidal anti-inflammatory drugs (NSAIDs) are best prevented with misoprostol. ASA can also aggravate gout, and in high doses will cause tinnitus. Low doses of ASA are best, in any case, because low doses are sufficient to impair the function of platelets (which lack nuclei, so cannot recover from ASA), whereas high doses prolong the inhibition of prostacycline production by nucleated endothelial cells.

Clopidogrel is a prodrug, converted to its active form by CYP2C19, so its activation is blocked by proton pump inhibitors (because they inhibit CYP2C19), except for pantoprazole.[16] Ticlopidine causes a severe drop in the white blood cell count in approximately 1% of patients; it probably should not be used. Dipyridamole/ASA is no better than clopidogrel[17] but causes more adverse effects such as headache and flushing.

Drugs for Lowering Cholesterol

These drugs are discussed in Chapter 9.

BLINDED N OF 1 CROSSOVER TRIAL

Whether an adverse drug effect is causally related to the symptom being experienced by the patient can usually be determined from previous experience with the drug. Most causally related adverse drug effects are known, as described above. Occasionally, however, a patient may be convinced that an unlikely symptom is caused by a needed medication; in those circumstances a randomized blinded N of 1 crossover trial may be needed.

This involves persuading your local pharmacy (or perhaps the hospital pharmacy) to prepare two bottles of capsules; in one bottle the capsules contain cornstarch placebo, in the other crushed tablets of the patient's medication. Ask the pharmacy to label the bottles "A" and "B," after tossing a coin to determine which will be placebo and which active, and send you the code.

Ask the patient to take one capsule daily, alternating between bottles, and record the date of which pill was taken and the symptoms on a sheet of paper, and then bring in the results after 12 days on each treatment (assuming the symptom attributed to the drug onsets and offsets within a day—longer crossover periods may rarely be needed). Break the code, count how many days the symptoms occurred on active drug versus placebo, and then look at Table 15–1 to determine whether the differences are statistically significant.

For example, if there are adverse drug reactions on 7 of 12 days on active drug and 2 days or fewer on placebo, the difference is significant and the symptoms probably are causally related to the active drug. If there is no significant difference between placebo and active drug, then the symptoms are probably unrelated.

Table 15–1. Blinded N of 1 Crossover Study to Test If Symptoms Attributed to a Drug Are Causally Related

A. Scoring Sheet Circle Yes (Y) or No (N) for each box that represents each time period on each drug		
Day	**Adverse Effect on Placebo**	**Adverse Effect on Active**
1	Y N	Y N
2	Y N	Y N
3	Y N	Y N
4	Y N	Y N
5	Y N	Y N
6	Y N	Y N
7	Y N	Y N
8	Y N	Y N
9	Y N	Y N
10	Y N	Y N
11	Y N	Y N
12	Y N	Y N
Total Ys		

(Continued)

Table 15-1. Blinded N of 1 Crossover Study to Test If Symptoms Attributed to a Drug Are Causally Related (*Continued*)

B. Statistical Testing	
Number of days with symptoms on active versus placebo that represent significant differences ($P < .05$)	
Active Drug	**Placebo**
4 days	0 days
5	0
6	1 or fewer days
7	2 or fewer
8	3 or fewer
9	4 or fewer
10	5 or fewer
11	6 or fewer
12	8 or fewer

Unfortunately, some patients are so fixed in their ideation that they may not even be convinced by this kind of demonstration.

CONCLUSION

Intensive medical therapy markedly reduces the risk of stroke, but to be effective the therapy must be continued. When a patient stops a drug that reduces risk by half, the result is a doubling of risk. Finding ways to help the patient continue with needed medication is an important part of stroke prevention.

REFERENCES

1. Marentette MA, Gerth WC, Billings DK, Zarnke KB. Antihypertensive persistence and drug class. *Can J Cardiol.* 2002;18:649-656.
2. Spence JD. Treatment options for renovascular hypertension. *Exp Opin Pharmacother.* 2002;3: 411-416.
3. Esler MD, Krum H, Sobotka PA, Schlaich MP, Schmieder RE, Bohm M. Renal sympathetic denervation in patients with treatment-resistant hypertension (the Symplicity HTN-2 trial): a randomised controlled trial. *Lancet.* 2010;376:1903-1909.
4. Scheffers IJ, Kroon AA, Schmidli J, et al. Novel baroreflex activation therapy in resistant hypertension: results of a European multi-center feasibility study. *J Am Coll Cardiol.* 2010;56:1254-1258.
5. Dyckner T, Wester PO. Ventricular extrasystoles and intracellular electrolytes before and after potassium and magnesium infusions in patients on diuretic treatment. *Am Heart J.* 1979;97:12-18.
6. Dyckner T, Wester PO. Effects of magnesium infusions in diuretic induced hyponatraemia. *Lancet.* 1981;1:585-586.
7. Brater DC, Morrelli HF. Digoxin toxicity in patients with normokalemic potassium depletion. *Clin Pharmacol Ther.* 1977;22:21-33.
8. Blais CJr, Rouleau JL, Brown NJ, et al. Serum metabolism of bradykinin and des-Arg9-bradykinin in patients with angiotensin-converting enzyme inhibitor-associated angioedema. *Immunopharmacology.* 1999;43:293-302.
9. Spence JD. Polypill: for Polyanna. *Intl J Stroke.* 2008;3:92-97.

10. Rangno RE, Langlois S. Comparison of withdrawal phenomena after propranolol, metoprolol, and pindolol. *Am Heart J.* 1982;104:473-478.

11. Kloner RA. Nifedipine in ischemic heart disease. *Circulation.* 1995;92:1074-1078.

12. Spence JD, Paulson OB, Strandgaard S. Hypertension and stroke. In: Messerli FH (ed.). *The ABCs of Antihypertensive Therapy.* 2nd ed. New York: Lippincott Williams & Wilkins; 2000:279-296.

13. Dyckner T, Wester PO. Effects on muscle electrolytes of potassium and magnesium infusions, spironolactone medication and operation in a case of primary aldosteronism. *Acta Med Scand.* 1979; 206:137-140.

14. Tweeddale MG, Ogilvie RI, Ruedy J. Antihypertensive and biochemical effects of chlorthalidone. *Clin Pharmacol Ther.* 1977;22:519-527.

15. MacDowall P, Kalra PA, O'Donoghue DJ, Waldek S, Mamtora H, Brown K. Risk of morbidity from renovascular disease in elderly patients with congestive cardiac failure. *Lancet.* 1998;352:13-16.

16. Juurlink DN, Gomes T, Ko DT, et al. A population-based study of the drug interaction between proton pump inhibitors and clopidogrel. *CMAJ.* 2009;180:713-718.

17. Sacco RL, Diener HC, Yusuf S, et al. Aspirin and extended-release dipyridamole versus clopidogrel for recurrent stroke. *N Engl J Med.* 2008;359:1238-1251.

Section 3

When the Stroke Wasn't Prevented

Treatment of Acute Stroke: Medical and Interventional Therapy

16

Alastair M. Buchan
Joyce S. Balami
Francesco Arba

TOPICS

INTRODUCTION

Treatment of acute stroke involves accurate neurological examination; general care management (particularly control of physiological variables); imaging techniques to determine type of stroke; treatment strategies to reperfuse the ischemic area or measures to reduce growth of primary intracerebral hemorrhage (hemostatic therapy); protection of the vulnerable, yet salvageable, ischemic penumbra (neuroprotectant therapy); and possibly surgery.

Neuroimaging is vital to enable rapid differentiation of ischemic from hemorrhagic stroke. The choice of brain imaging modality lies between computed tomography (CT) and magnetic resonance imaging (MRI). However, noncontrast head CT remains the most widely used imaging technique and has been described as the "cardiogram of the brain" (Figure 16–1A).[1]

The early CT signs of infarction include loss of differentiation between the cortical gray and subjacent white matter, loss of the insular ribbon or obscuration of the sylvian fissure, swelling of the cortical gyri with sulcal effacement, blurring of the internal capsule, and hyperdense artery sign, particularly involving the middle cerebral artery (MCA) (Figure 16–2). The Alberta Stroke Program Early CT Score (ASPECTS) system helps to quantify early ischemic changes in brain tissue supplied by the anterior circulation (Figure 16–1B).[2] Similarly, the posterior circulation Acute Stroke Prognosis Early CT Score (pc-ASPECTS) is a predictive scale for quantifying ischemic changes in the posterior circulation.[3]

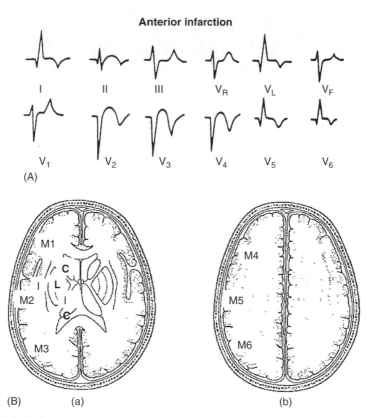

Figure 16–1. (A) ECG equivalent; (B) ASPECTS (Middle cerebral artery territory). MCA territory divided into 10 areas of interest: Figure (a) = slice through the lentiform nuclei and Figure (b) = slice 10 mm higher through the lateral ventricles.

Areas of Interest

Slice (a):
C = caudate
L = lentiform
I = insula
IC = internal capsule
M1, M2, M3 = cortical regions

Slice (b)
M4, M5, M6 = cortical regions

The Score:
Subcortical structures are allotted 3 points (C, L, and IC) and MCA cortex is allotted 7 points (insular cortex, MI,M2, M3, M4, M5, and M6).
10 = normal scan. No change detected.
0 = complete MCA infarct involving all of the MCA territory
(Image from Barber et al: ASPECTS Study group[2])

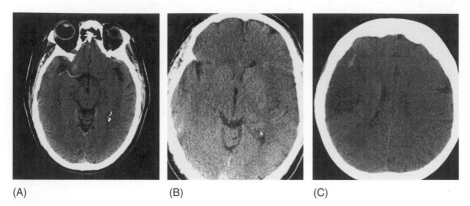

(A)   (B)   (C)

Figure 16–2. CT signs of ischemic stroke: (A) CT showing hyperdense right MCA sign; (B) CT showing loss of left insular ribbon; (C) CT showing loss of gray-white differentiation of the left insular cortex, cortical sulcal effacement, and focal parenchymal hypoattenuation.

Diffusion-weighted imaging (DWI) is particularly sensitive to the early phase of cerebral ischemia within minutes of stroke onset and provides an estimate of the ischemic core. Perfusion-weighted imaging (PWI) provides information about the ischemic penumbra and may be used in selected patients with ischemic stroke (eg, unclear time of onset, late admission) to aid the decision on whether such patients could benefit from treatment if there is a large perfusion-diffusion mismatch (Figure 16–3A).[4]

The cornerstone of acute ischemic stroke (AIS) treatment is rapid recanalization of the occluded blood vessel through dissolving (thrombolysis) or removing the obstructed blood clot (mechanical thrombectomy) and preventing further clot propagation, thereby restoring cerebral blood flow. Currently, there are only three Food and Drug Administration (FDA) approved acute interventions for acute ischemic treatment: thrombolysis by intravenous (IV) recombinant human tissue-type plasminogen activator (rt-PA) and mechanical clot removal with either the Merci Retriever or Penumbra Stroke System.

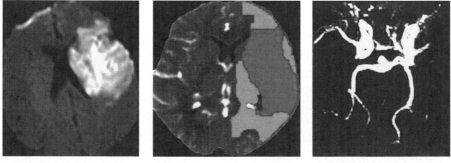

(A)   (B)   (C)

Figure 16–3. MRI Images: (A) Diffusion-weighted imaging (DWI); (B) MRI-mismatch; (C) MRA.

ISCHEMIC STROKE

Thrombolysis

Thrombolytics are pharmacological agents that can break up clots obstructing the flow of blood in an occluded blood vessel. Thrombolytic agents can be administered intravenously, intra-arterially, or through combined intravenous and intra-arterial routes. The basis for using thrombolytics is that the majority of ischemic strokes (about 80%) result from thromboembolic or atherothrombotic processes.

RATIONALE FOR THROMBOLYSIS

One of the immediate goals of AIS therapy is to salvage the ischemic penumbra (ie, tissue at risk that might be salvageable) through recanalization of the occluded cerebral blood vessel. Because "time is brain," timely recanalization of a vascular occlusion might result in the restoration of cerebral perfusion, salvaging threatened ischemic tissue and resulting in improved clinical outcome.[5] Therefore the goal of acute revascularization should not be just to open an occluded vessel, but to open it quickly, as delayed revascularization minimizes the benefit and likely increases risk. This was demonstrated by a meta-analysis of 53 studies that revealed that successful recanalization is strongly associated with a four- to five-fold increase in the odds of improved functional outcome and a four- to five-fold reduction in the odds of death after AIS.[5] Similarly, the RECANALISE study[6] and the recent reanalysis of International Management of Stroke trials[7] have suggested better clinical outcomes with timely recanalization.

Recanalization can be achieved through various treatment modalities with different recanalization rates. For example, the recanalization rate with IV thrombolysis was 46.2%; with intra-arterial (IA) thrombolysis was 63.2%; with combined IV/IA thrombolysis was 67.5%, which was not significantly different from IA alone ($P = .45$); and was 83.6% with mechanical thrombolysis.[5] Likewise, recanalization rates differ across different vessels; for instance, the recanalization rate for middle cerebral artery/anterior cerebral artery vessels was demonstrated to be 61%, and for vertebral and basilar artery vessels was 66.2%, with internal carotid artery (ICA) vessels having the lowest recanalization rate at 49.8% (Table 16–1).[5] Recanalization (either spontaneous or related to thrombolytic or interventional therapies) is less likely with ICA obstruction.[5] ICA obstruction has been shown to predict poorer clinical outcome compared to MCA obstruction after IV rt-PA therapy.[8]

Studies have shown that the likelihood of recanalization depends not only on the location of the occluded vessels (ICA vs M2), but also on the volume of infarction and early hypoattenuation on brain CT scan as quantified by ASPECT score.[9-11]

INTRAVENOUS THROMBOLYSIS

Although the first reported case describing the use of thrombolysis for stroke management appeared in the literature in 1958,[12] it was not until the advent of the era of CT and other neuroimaging modalities that the potential of thrombolysis could be investigated formally.

Table 16–1. Recanalization Rates for Different Treatment Modalities and Types of Vessels

Treatment Modality	Recanalization Rate (%)
Intravenous thrombolysis (IV)	46.2
Intrarterial thrombolysis (IA)	63.2
Intravenous + intrarterial	67.5
Mechanical thrombolysis	83.6
Type of Vessel	
Anterior circulation (MCA or ACA)	61
Posterior circulation	66.2
Internal carotid	49.8

ACA, anterior cerebral artery; IA, intra-arterial; IV, intravenous; MCA, middle cerebral artery.

In 1992, a multicenter clinical trial of the use of IV rt-PA in acute stroke was performed with a total of 139 patients. The results of this trial, which were analyzed by angiogram before and after administration of rt-PA, demonstrated that the site of occlusion, time to recanalization, and time to treatment are important variables in acute stroke intervention with rt-PA.[10]

Following this, the National Institute of Neurological Disorders and Stroke (NINDS) Study Group first established the benefit of IV rt-PA for the treatment of AIS in a randomized, double-blind trial of 624 patients in 1995.[13] The positive results from the NINDS rt-PA trial, which turned out to be a landmark trial, have not only revolutionized stroke management but have also reinvigorated the enthusiasm in stroke care.

Intravenous thrombolysis with IV rt-PA (alteplase) for the treatment of AIS within three hours of symptom onset was approved by the US FDA in 1996, based on the results of the NINDS and the rt-PA Stroke Study Group trial.[13] Subsequently, other countries have followed suit, with Canada in 1999, Germany in 2000, both the United Kingdom and Australia in 2003, and other countries eventually.

Intravenous rt-PA is the only approved thrombolytic agent for treatment of AIS. However, strict time constraints have limited the use of IV rt-PA to less than 10% of eligible patients with AIS, despite the evidence of its benefit in selected patients as shown by several large trials.[13-17] In 2009, the American Heart Association/American Stroke Association extended the time window for treatment of AIS with IV rt-PA from 3 to 4.5 hours after the onset of stroke symptoms. This was based on the results from part 3 of the European Collaborative Acute Stroke Study (ECASS III).[18] ECASS III, a high-quality trial in 821 patients, showed that treatment with IV rt-PA within 3 to 4.5 hours of the onset of ischemic stroke reduced the risk of death or dependency at three months (47.6% vs 54.8%, $P = .04$, number needed to treat [NNT] 14) despite an increase in any intracranial hemorrhage (27% vs 17.6% using the NINDS definition, $P = .001$, NN to harm 10) and in symptomatic intracranial hemorrhage (7.9% vs 3.5%, $P = .006$, NN to harm 22).

The ECASS III results confirmed the meta-analysis of six major randomized, placebo-controlled IV rt-PA stroke trials: the ATLANTIS I and II (Alteplase Thrombolysis for Acute Noninterventional Therapy in Ischemic Stroke), ECASS I and II (European Cooperative Acute Stroke Study), and NINDS I and II.[19] The analysis showed that the odds of a favorable outcome (modified Rankin score 0-1, Barthel score 95-100, and National Institutes of Health Stroke Scale [NIHSS] 0-1) increased as the time between stroke onset and treatment decreased (odds ratio [OR] for benefit of rt-PA compared with placebo: 2.8 [95% confidence interval {CI}, 1.8-9.5] for treatment within 90 minutes; 1.6 [95% CI, 1.1-2.2] for treatment between 91 and 180 minutes; 1.4 [95% CI, 1.1-1.9] for 181-270 minutes and 1.2 [95% CI, 0.9-1.5] for 271-360 minutes) (Table 16–2). The result showed a benefit up to three hours from the onset of stroke symptoms and suggested a potential benefit beyond three hours for some patients. However, there seemed to be no clear benefit from treatment over 270 minutes (4.5 hours) after symptom onset.

Further evidence of the benefit of IV rt-PA beyond three hours comes from the Safe Implementation of Treatments in Stroke International Stroke Thrombolysis Registry (SITS-ISTR), which compared stroke patients who were treated within either 3 hours or 3 to 4.5 hours after symptom onset.[20] There was no significant difference between groups in the rate of symptomatic intracerebral hemorrhage (adjusted OR for those in whom treatment was started after three hours compared with under three hours 1.32; 95% CI, 1.00-1.75; $P = .052$); independent at three months (adjusted OR 0.93; 95% CI, 0.84-1.03); or mortality at three months (adjusted OR 1.15; 95% CI, 1.00-1.33; $P = .053$). Overall, the results suggest that

Table 16–2. Pooled Analysis of NINDS, ECASS I and II, and ATLANTIS, Shown With ECASS III

Time Window		Adjusted OR	(95% CI)	
0-90		2.81	(1.75-4.50)	
91-180		1.55	(1.12-2.15)	
181-270	Pooled	1.40	(1.05-1.85)	
	ECASS III	1.42	(1.02-1.98)	
271-360		1.15	(0.90-1.47)	

Odds ratio (95% CI): 0.10 — 1.00 — 10.00

ECASS III: rt-PA within 3 to 4.5 hours after stroke reduced the risk of death or dependency at 90 days (47.6% vs 54.8%; $P = .04$; NNT 14) despite an increase in intracranial hemorrhage (27% vs 17.6%, using the NINDS definition; $P = .001$; NN to harm 10) and in symptomatic intracranial hemorrhage (7.9% vs 3.5%; $P = .006$; NN to harm 22).

Table 16–3. Pooled Analysis of Eight Trials (NINDS, ATLANTIS, ECASS [Including ECASS III], and EPITHET Trials)

Onset-to-Treatment Time	OR (95% CI)	P value	Estimated NNT
0-90 min	2.55 (1.44-4.52)	.0013	4.5
91-180 min	1.64 (1.12-2-40)	.0116	9.0
181-270 min	1.34 (1.06-1-68)	.0135	14.1
271-360 min	1.22 (0.92-1.61)	.1628	21.4
0-360 min	1.40 (1.20-1.63)	< .0001	12.6

Lees KR, Bluhmki E, von Kummer R, et al. Time to treatment with intravenous alteplase and outcome in stroke: an updated pooled analysis of ECASS, ATLANTIS, NINDS, and EPITHET trials. *Lancet.* 2010;375:1695-1703.

there might be a benefit for treatment with rt-PA 3 to 4.5 hours after stroke onset, although this is likely to be less than for those treated earlier.

The recently updated pooled analysis of eight trials (NINDS, ATLANTIS, ECASS [including ECASS III], and EPITHET trials) consisting of 3670 patients demonstrated that treatment with thrombolysis up to 4.5 hours from stroke onset enhances the chance of favorable outcome. However, the analysis showed that the greatest benefit comes from earlier treatment, because net benefit diminishes rapidly, and it becomes undetectable beyond 4.5 hours (Table 16–3).[21] However, IV rt-PA might be less effective for treating large vessel occlusions as a consequence of large clot burden. For instance, the recanalization rate may be as low as 6% for internal carotid artery terminus, 30% for middle cerebral artery trunk, and 30% for basilar occlusions.[9,10] Even if recanalization is achieved with rt-PA, reocclusion with neurological deterioration has been reported to occur in more than 30% of treated patients.[22,23]

MECHANISM OF ACTION

rt-PA is a serine protease with a half-life of three to five minutes; it converts plasminogen to plasmin as a result of fibrin enhancement. At pharmacological concentrations, rt-PA binds to fibrin within the thrombus, forming an active lytic complex. Its main mechanism of action is to lyse a clot that is occluding a cerebral vessel, thereby reperfusing distal ischemic brain tissue and preventing or limiting the area of cell death and tissue necrosis (Figure 16–4). However, bleeding is a common adverse event due to its intensive fibrinolytic activity.[24] Table 16–4 summarizes the guidelines for the use of rt-PA in AIS.

COMPLICATIONS OF IV RT-PA

(See Table 16–5.)

Arterial Reocclusion

Arterial reocclusion after successful thrombolysis is an important potential complication of treatment with rt-PA. The short half-life of rt-PA with the limited penetration of the clot, because of strong binding with surface fibrin, may delay

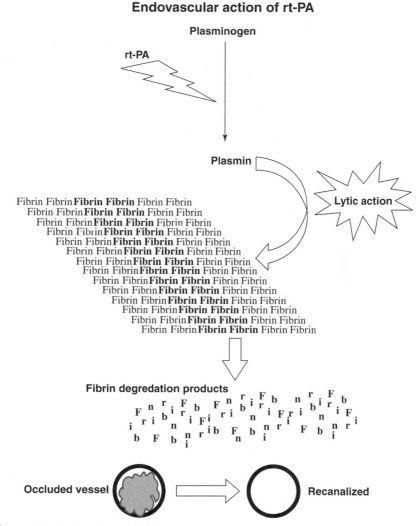

Figure 16–4. How thrombolysis works.

recanalization and increase the risk of recurrent occlusion. The clinical mark of arterial reocclusion is neurological deterioration after initial improvement following thrombolytic treatment with intravenous rt-PA. Early arterial reocclusion has been recognized as a cause of poor outcome. In the NINDS trial, 13% of patients experienced an early clinical deterioration after an initial improvement, which in the absence of intracranial hemorrhage may represent reocclusion of the recanalized vessel.[25]

Reocclusion has been documented by transcranial Doppler (TCD) monitoring within two hours after IV rt-PA in up to 34% of patients with middle cerebral occlusion, and accounted for 14% of clinical worsening after initial improvement.[22,26]

Table 16–4. Guidelines for the Use of Alteplase in Acute Ischemic Stroke

Dose
The recommended dose of rt-PA for AIS is 0.9 mk/kg (maximum dose of 90 mg).
A bolus dose of 10% is administered over 1 min and the remainder is infused over
60 min.

Procedures PRIOR to t-PA Infusion
• History and physical exam consistent with an acute ischemic stroke
• Pretreatment CT scan of the head, axial with 5-mm cuts, window at 80, level at 40
• Pretreatment tests: FBC, U+E, glucose, clotting, ECG (results not required prior to rt-PA
  infusion)
• Compatibility with the inclusion criteria and contraindications

Procedures for rt-PA Infusion and Subsequent Management
• Infuse rt-PA (Alteplase) in a 0.9-mg/kg (maximum 90-mg) continuous IV infusion over
  60 min, with 10% of total dose as a bolus at the start of the infusion (over 2-3 min)
• Monitor in an acute care setting (A & E) for signs of neurological change or bleeding
• BP Q15 min × 2 h/Q30 min × 6 h/Q1 h × 16 h
• Neurovitals Q1 h for the first 12 h, then Q2 h for the next 12 h
• Stroke assessment Q1 h × 6 h, then Q3 h × 48 h
• Daily neurological evaluations after the first 24 h
• NBM × 3 h postinfusion, then reassess
• Bedrest × 24 h postinfusion, then reassess
• Maintain BP <185/110 mm Hg
• If clinical deterioration:
  1. Discontinue infusion
  2. Immediate CT scan
  3. Prepare fibrinogen and platelets
• Repeat CT after 18-24 h in all cases
• No IV heparin or antiplatelet agents until repeat CT scan. Antiplatelet agents and/or
  heparin may be started after this period if the repeat CT is free of hemorrhage.

Inclusion Criteria
• Acute ischemic stroke with a clearly defined time of onset
• Likely disabling with no significant improvement or recovery
• Treatment initiated within 3 h of symptom onset

Absolute Contraindications (DO NOT TREAT)
• Any intracranial hemorrhage
• BP >185/110 mm Hg after 2 attempts to reduce BP
• Surgery or trauma within the last 14 d
• Active internal bleeding
• Hematology abnormalities OR coagulopathy INR >1.7, APTT >40, or platelets
  <100,000 mm^3
• Arterial puncture at a noncompressible site within the last 7 d

Relative Contraindications (STOP & RETHINK)
• Any of the following IN ISOLATION: hemianopia, neglect, dysarthia, ataxia, or sensory
  symptoms
• Pretreatment CT scan showing:
  • Hypodensity, which could represent evolving infarction >3 h old
• Mass effect, edema

Table 16–4. Guidelines for the Use of Alteplase in Acute Ischemic Stroke (*Continued*)

- Tumor, aneurysm, or AVM
- Intracranial surgery or intraspinal surgery <2 mo
- Any non-neurological surgery (including minor surgery) within the past 6 wk
- Stroke or head injury in the preceding 3 mo
- History of GI or urinary tract hemorrhage in prior 21 d
- Previous history of CNS bleeding
- Glucose <2.7 or 22.2 mmol/L
- Seizure at stroke onset
- Possibility of pregnancy (requires negative pregnancy test)
- Endocarditis or acute pericarditis
- Serious underlying medical illness, including liver failure, dementing illness, or serious surgical risk (eg, abdominal aortic aneurysm)
- Greater than **90 min** delay post–CT scan
- Decreased level of consciousness, not arousable with minimal stimulus (unless likely to be due to basilar occlusion)

In a case series of 142 patients with a documented MCA occlusion by TCD, early reocclusion with clinical worsening was reported in up to 12% of MCA stroke patients treated with IV rt-PA. In addition to the worse in-hospital clinical course, patients with reocclusion had a poorer long-term outcome than patients with a sustained recanalization, and the outcome was similar to patients with persistent occlusion.[27]

The independent predictors of arterial reocclusion after IV rt-PA–induced recanalization include stroke severity on admission and the presence of severe ipsilateral carotid artery disease.[27,28] Similarly, it has been shown that partial recanalization frequently preceded reocclusion.[22,28] This is because partial and possibly stepwise or slow recanalization patterns imply a residual clot, which may provide an adequate surface to fibrinogen deposit, promoting reocclusion.[27]

Measures to prevent reocclusion are not well studied. In a small therapeutic pilot study patients with immediate thrombotic reocclusion after successful thrombolysis were treated with IV abciximab. In this study the administration of abciximab, a platelet glycoprotein IIb/IIIa antagonist, successfully dissolved the thrombus in all four patients leading to reperfusion of the reoccluded artery.[28]

Table 16–5. Complications of Intravenous rt-PA

Complications	Rate (%)
Arterial reocclusion	12-14
Hemorrhagic transformation	2.4-6.4
Angioedema	1-5
Systemic bleeding	0.4
Secondary embolization	Less than 0.1

Reocclusion may be prevented by the administration of heparin or antiplatelet drugs.

Hemorrhagic Complication

Intracerebral Hemorrhage   Symptomatic intracerebral hemorrhage (sICH) is one of the most unfavorable and feared complications after IV rt-PA therapy. Based on radiological appearance or on clinical parameters, hemorrhagic transformation (HT) can be graded by either the NINDS or ECASS classification. The NINDS classifies HT into two types: hemorrhagic cerebral infarction, defined as CT findings of acute infarction with punctate or variable hypodensity and hyperdensity, with an indistinct border within the vascular territory; and intracerebral hematoma, defined as CT findings of a typical homogeneous, hyperdense lesion with a sharp border with or without edema or mass effect within the brain.[29] However, ECASS classified HT (Figure 16–5) into hemorrhagic infarction (HI)

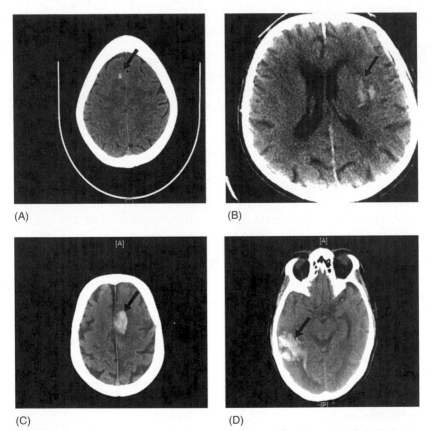

(A)   (B)

(C)   (D)

Figure 16–5.   CT images of hemorrhagic transformation post rt-PA therapy (ECASS Classification): (A) HI-1 (small petechiae); (B) HI-2 (confluent petechiae); (C) PH-1 (haematoma in <30% of the infracted area, with a mild mass effect); (D) PH-2 (haematoma in >30% of the infracted area with a significant mass effect.

and parenchymal hemorrhages (PH), with each class further divided into two types: H1-1, defined as small petechiae along the margins of the infarcted area, and HI-2, defined as confluent petechiae within the infarcted area but with no mass effect; PH-1, defined as hematoma in less than 30% of the infarcted area with mild mass effect, and PH-2, defined as hematoma in more than 30% of the infarcted area with a notable mass effect.[30] Similarly, it can be classified simply using associated symptoms (symptomatic with a ≥4-point deterioration in the NIHSS, or asymptomatic) or duration from thrombolysis (early, ie, <24 hours; or late, ie, >24 hours from thrombolysis).[26]

In NINDS 6.4% of rt-PA–treated patients developed sICH compared with 0.6% who received placebo.[13] In the ECASS trial with IV rt-PA given up to six hours from symptom onset, sICH was found in 20%, compared with 70% on placebo.[16] In ECASS III sICH was noted to be 2.4% in the treated group compared with 0.2% in the placebo group ($P = .008$). In the pooled data of the large randomized IV rt-PA stroke trials, consisting of 2775 patients, the rate of significant intracerebral hemorrhage was 5.9% in those treated with rt-PA compared with 1.1% in the placebo group ($P < .0001$).[19] A meta-analysis of 15 published case series of 2639 patients treated with rt-PA for AIS in general clinical practice showed a symptomatic hemorrhagic rate of 5.2%.[31]

The prognosis of patients with sICH is poor: in the NINDS trial, 75% of patients with sICH were dead at three-month follow-up.[29] Although thrombolysis with rt-PA increases the risk of hemorrhage, it requires 100 patients to be treated with rt-PA to get one significant adverse outcome.[22]

Hemorrhagic complications from thrombolytic therapy may represent the effects of fibrinogen depletion, platelet dysfunction due to circulating fibrin degradation products, and/or reperfusion therapy. rt-PA seems to have some neurotoxic properties, including activation of metalloproteinases, which may result in increased blood-brain barrier (BBB) permeability leading to cerebral hemorrhage.[24] rt-PA provides an exogenous source of excessive plasmin to the ischemic brain, which may worsen brain edema by proteolytic action and by upregulating matrix metalloproteinase (MMP)-9.[32] MMP-9 and plasmin are important molecules that mediate BBB breakdown by degrading vascular extracellular matrix.[32-34] Moreover, reperfusion can exacerbate damage to neurons and vasculature due to the oxygen "surge" and free radical production.[35] Reactive oxygen species (ROS) are generated soon after vessel occlusion, as well as in later stages of ischemic reperfusion (eg, by inflammatory cells) and are the fundamental mediators of reperfusion injury.[36] ROS cause cellular injury via peroxidation of cell membrane lipids[37] and hydrolysis of phospholipids releasing arachidonic acid, which causes nonspecific opening of the BBB.[38] Brain hemorrhage following reperfusion could be devastating particularly, where BBB alterations appear to precede the hemorrhage.[39]

The risk of t-PA–related symptomatic intracerebral hemorrhage is low after early and complete recanalization of occluded blood vessels with restoration of blood flow,[40] and delayed recanalization or persistent occlusion despite treatment with rt-PA have been associated with increased risk for sICH.[40]

The predictors of thrombolysis-related intracerebral hemorrhage include severe stroke, signs of mass effect, brain edema, hypodensity or extensive early infarct change on pretreatment brain imaging, high serum glucose values, and older age.[29,30,41] Other risk factors include diabetes mellitus, previous stroke, and a low platelet count.[42]

Stroke Severity Stroke severity is a major predictor of sICH because of the associated large or increased volume of ischemic brain at risk for hemorrhagic transformation. Stroke severity as measured by means of the NIHSS in the NINDS trial was one of the major risk factors associated with ICH (OR 1.8; 95% CI, 1.2-2.9).[29] Although stroke severity is a risk factor for hemorrhagic complication with a need for caution, patients with severe stroke may still benefit from treatment, as shown in a post hoc analysis of the NINDS[29,43] and the pooled analysis of the NINDS, ECASS, and ATLANTIS trials.[19]

Early CT Changes In the NINDS trial, patients with CT findings of edema and mass effect had a 31% rate of sICH rate, compared with 6% without these findings. Edema and/or mass effect on head CT independently predicted sICH in multivariate analysis (OR 7.8; 99% CI, 2.2-27.1).[29] Similarly, the ECASS-II study showed a significant association between EICs (Early ischemic changes) and sICH.[44] In a large multicenter rt-PA stroke survey of 1205 patients treated in routine clinical practice with IV rt-PA, early ischemic CT changes, particularly if involving more than 33% of the MCA territory, was found to be associated with an increased risk of sICH.[45] However, in another NINDS reanalysis, using the Alberta Stroke Program Early CT Scale (ASPECTS), it was found that patients with subtle and clear EICs (ASPECTS 7) in more than one-third of the MCA territory did not have higher rates of sICH.[46]

Age Older stroke patients are prone to developing intracerebral hemorrhage after thrombolysis due to factors such as impaired rate of rt-PA clearance, higher frequency of transformation in cardioembolic than atherosclerotic infarcts, and possible age-associated microangiopathy (either cerebral amyloid angiopathy or hypertensive microangiopathy) and leukoaraiosis.[47] Age has been identified as a risk factor for sICH in the ECASS-II[44] and in the pooled analysis of major intravenous rt-PA trials[19] except for the NINDS trial, which excluded patients older than 80 years, although the NINDS post hoc analysis showed that age was not a significant independent predictor of sICH.[29] Similarly, a Canadian prospective multicenter cohort found a similar rate of sICH between 270 patients aged 80 years and above and 1135 younger patients, all treated with rt-PA (4.4% vs 4.6%).[48]

Hyperglycemia Hyperglycemia has been shown to be a significant risk factor for sICH.[45,49] Glucose may accelerate blood-brain barrier disruption by increasing MMP-9 expression.[50,51] Hyperglycemia-mediated increase in MMP-9 can cause neuronal damage by an increase in cerebral edema. In addition, hyperglycemia may be responsible for a procoagulant state that can further compromise blood supply to the penumbral areas in AIS.[50]

A retrospective analysis of 138 patients with acute stroke treated with rt-PA showed how the rate of hemorrhage sharply increased above a glucose level of 8.4 mmol/L, resulting in a 25% rate of symptomatic hemorrhage.[49]

Stroke Subtype   Cardioembolic stroke has been shown to be a stroke subtype associated with increased risk for hemorrhagic complication. Atrial fibrillation was associated with sICH in the NINDS trial and in ECASS I, but only in univariate analyses.[29,52]

Systemic Bleeding   Systemic bleeding due to IV rt-PA appears to be relatively uncommon with about 0.4% of patients reported to have major systemic bleeding, usually at the site of femoral puncture for acute angiography.[53,54] Systemic bleeding is usually mild and occurs in the form of oozing from IV cannulated sites, gum bleeding, and ecchymoses, particularly under automated blood pressure cuffs. Major bleeding could be from the genitourinary or gastrointestinal systems, and depending on the severity of the bleeding there might be a need to discontinue rt-PA therapy.

Rarely, acute stroke patients may bleed into the pericardium, leading to life-threatening tamponade after treatment with rt-PA, particularly in those with mild or undetected myocardial or pericardial disease prior to thrombolytic therapy.[55] Recent myocardial ischemia is an independent significant risk factor for hemopericardium and life-threatening tamponade after treatment with thrombolytic drugs in patients with AIS.[56,57]

There is no specific intervention recommended for the management of ischemic stroke patients with asymptomatic hemorrhagic transformation. However, it is recommended that patients with hemorrhage secondary to thrombolytic therapy be treated with infusion of platelets and cryoprecipitate that contains factor VIII to rapidly correct the systemic fibrinolytic state created by rt-PA.[58,59] Similarly, surgical management is recommended for patients presenting with lobar clots greater than 30 mL and within 1 cm of the surface; evacuation of supratentorial ICH by standard craniotomy might be considered.[58,59]

Secondary Embolization

Secondary embolism from thrombolysis with IV rt-PA could result from the therapeutic fragmentation of the original occluding thrombus. For example, when a myocardial infarction (MI) thrombus is broken up by an IV rt-PA, the resulting smaller particles may be large enough to lodge and occlude downstream M2 or M3 branches.

Similarly, thrombolysis with rt-PA for cardiac thrombus could potentially accelerate breakup of the cardiac thrombus and cause secondary embolism. However, there are limited studies that have evaluated the risk-to-benefit ratio of thrombolytic therapy with rt-PA in stroke patients with cardiac thrombus. There are reports of recurrent cerebral embolus, embolic myocardial infarction, and lower limb embolism following therapy with IV rt-PA for ischemic stroke.[60-62]

Angioedema

Orolingual angioedema is one of the rare complications of rt-PA occurring in 1% to 5% of patients treated with rt-PA following AIS.[63-65] It is usually mild and transient, contralateral to the ischemic hemisphere, and the risk of developing angioedema may be associated with lesions in the frontal and insular cortex as well.[65] Additionally, the use of angiotensin-converting enzyme (ACE) inhibitor therapy may increase the risk of developing angioedema.[63,65-67] Plasmin is converted from plasminogen; it cleaves bradykinin from high-molecular-weight kininogen. Together with an ACE inhibitor–mediated decrease in bradykinin metabolism and with an increase in neurokinin levels, this may provide an explanation for the increased risk.[68]

Severe, acute orolingual angioedema is a rare but potentially life-threatening situation, as it may cause partial airway obstruction that may require urgent airway management.[65,69,70] CT of the tongue can distinguish hematoma from angioedema in this setting.[66] Management of such patients includes stopping the drug infusion, administering antihistamines and corticosteroids, and intubating patients who develop stridor.

INTRA-ARTERIAL THROMBOLYSIS

Intra-arterial thrombolysis (IAT) is another method for administering thrombolytic agents with theoretical advantages over IV thrombolysis. The major potential advantage of IAT compared with systematic administration is that microcatheter techniques allow direct access to the occluded vessel, and by penetrating the thrombus with the microcatheter the thrombolytic agent can be infused into the thrombus. This allows a smaller dose, but higher drug concentration delivery into the thrombus with reduced systemic side effects and a higher recanalization rate of the occluded vessel. In addition, the use of IAT may extend the time window out to six hours after symptom onset. However, IAT is still reserved for specialized centers.

In 1998, Hacke et al reported the earliest series of successful recanalization in patients with basilar artery occlusion by infusing urokinase into the occluded basilar artery. This resulted in recanalization in 44% of patients, and 50% of them made good recovery, whereas those patients without recanalization died.[71] Then, in 1998, del Zoppo et al successfully completed the first randomized, double-blind controlled trial of intra-arterial Pro-urokinase in Acute Cerebral Thromboembolism (PROACT-I).[72] The PROACT-I, a phase 2 trial evaluating the safety and recanalization efficacy of intra-arterial local delivery of recombinant pro-urokinase (rpro-UK) with heparin versus heparin alone in acute ischemic stroke, enrolled 40 patients with angiographically documented proximal middle cerebral occlusion within six hours of symptom onset. Recanalization rates were 58% in the rpro-UK group and 14% with placebo ($P = .017$). Early symptomatic ICH occurred in 15.4% with rpro-UK and 7.1% in the placebo group, but this difference was not significant. Similarly, there were good outcomes in 30.8% of the treatment group versus 21.4% in the placebo group, but the results did reach statistical significance.

In the PROACT-II trial, the phase 3 clinical trial, with IA pro-urokinase given within six hours of a stroke, a total of 189 stroke patients were randomized with 121 treated by rpro-UK and heparin, and 59 patients were treated with heparin alone. The trial demonstrated 66% recanalization in the treatment arm compared with 18% in the "heparin-only" arm ($P < .001$). Equally, 40% of those who received intra-arterial thrombolysis had favorable outcome (modified Rankin scale [mRS] 0-2) at 90 days when compared with 25% of those in the heparin control group (OR 2.13; 95% CI, 1.02-4.42; $P = .04$). However, mortality was similar between the groups and the risk of intracranial hemorrhage within 24 hours of stroke onset was higher in the thrombolysis group than in the control group (10% vs 2%).[73] The increased risk of ICH was attributed to the longer time window, up to six hours, in patients treated with IAT as well as greater baseline stroke severity compared with other studies (median NIHSS of 17 in PROACT, 14 in NINDS, and 11 in ECASS 2).

In another study, it was shown that in selected patients with AIS with potentially salvageable brain tissue, as defined by CT perfusion or MRI mismatch, treatment with IAT beyond six hours of symptom onset is feasible and safe with no increase in the risk of ICH or death.[74] IAT for appropriate patients within six hours of symptom onset is now a class II level of evidence intervention for AIS.

A recent meta-analysis of five randomized trials of IA thrombolysis with 395 subjects demonstrated the potential benefits of IA thrombolysis. The analysis showed substantially increased recanalization rates (65% vs 18%, OR 6.4) with good outcome, defined as an mRS score of 0 to 2 (43% vs 28%, OR 2.10) and an excellent clinical outcome defined as an mRS score of 0 to 1 (31% vs 18%, OR 2.1) compared with control (generally IV heparin) in AIS. Although the risk of symptomatic intracerebral hemorrhage was increased with IA thrombolysis (9% vs 2%), there was no increase in mortality (21% vs 24%, OR 0.8; 95% CI, 0.5-1.4).[75] The majority of these favorable results from intra-arterial thrombolytics originate from studies with rpro-UK. Unfortunately, rpro-UK is currently not available for routine clinical use, and IA thrombolysis with rt-PA is not substantiated by randomized controlled trials (RCTs), only observational and non-randomized data. Although the FDA has not approved intra-arterial rt-PA and urokinase for the treatment of acute ischemic stroke, some specialist centers have adopted protocols for using such treatments in specific cases.[76-78]

Complications of Intra-arterial Thrombolysis

The complications of IAT include intracerebral hemorrhage, subarachnoid hemorrhage (SAH), procedural complications, arterial intracranial embolization, arterial perforation, and secondary embolization.

Hemorrhage   Symptomatic ICH is also one of the most feared and major complications of intra-arterial thrombolytic therapy as it is for IV thrombolysis, with a reported frequency between 6% and 15%.[72,73,77,79,80] The microcatheter contrast injections used during IA thrombolysis have been shown to be an independent risk factor for hemorrhagic complication.[81,82]

Postulated mechanisms for this risk include increased contrast extravasation and pressure transmission. Contrast extravasation after IAT is a potential marker of blood-brain barrier permeability, possibly directly toxic, and based on several studies may be a risk factor for HT.[83] Extravasated contrast medium on CT scan[83] and early venous filling on angiography during IA reperfusion[84] are radiological signs, which may be markers of symptomatic hemorrhage.

Additionally, lesion location may be associated with hemorrhagic complications.[51] For example, internal carotid artery occlusion (versus middle cerebral artery; OR

4.196; 95% CI, 1.229-14.325) was an independent predictor of total hemorrhage in the IMS I trial after controlling for baseline NIHSS score. Atrial fibrillation was another independent predictor of total hemorrhage in the IMS I trial.

The other independent predictors of hemorrhagic complication are similar to those of IV thrombolysis, which include stroke severity as defined by higher NIHSS score, high blood glucose level, longer time to recanalization, and lower platelet count.[85]

Procedural Complication Intra-arterial stroke therapy has been associated with a 5% to 7% risk for clinically significant procedural complications such as groin hematoma, arterial perforation, etc.[72,73]

INTRAVENOUS VERSUS INTRA-ARTERIAL THROMBOLYSIS

In the SYNTHESIS pilot RCT trial that compared IAT to intravenous thrombolysis (IVT) with rt-PA in AIS, rapid initiation of IAT was demonstrated to be a safe and feasible alternative to IVT. Although almost twice as many patients on IAT as those on IVT survived without residual disability, there was no significant difference in the rate of other serious adverse events.[86] SYNTHESIS expansion is currently ongoing to help verify whether IAT is more effective than standard therapy with IV rt-PA. Another randomized trial comparing standard IV rt-PA with a combined IV and IA approach (IMS-III) is also in progress.[87]

COMBINED INTRAVENOUS–INTRA-ARTERIAL THROMBOLYSIS

Combination therapy, also known as bridging therapy (BT), is another approach to improved vessel recanalization through the early use of intravenous thrombolysis followed by local intra-arterial thrombolysis. Bridging therapy has the potential of combining the advantages of each treatment modality: the wide availability of early rapid IV thrombolysis and the potentially higher recanalization rates of IA rt-PA, thus allowing for better rates of recanalization and clinical outcome for patients with AIS. Several studies have evaluated the feasibility, safety, and efficacy of this combined approach in patients with acute stroke.

The first pilot study of combined therapy was the Emergency Management of Stroke (EMS) Bridging trial, a placebo-controlled multicenter study, which randomly assigned 35 patients within three hours of symptom onset to either two-third dose IV rt-PA (0.6 mg/kg) followed by IA rt-PA (maximum of 20 mg for 2 hours) or placebo followed by IA rt-PA.[88] Although recanalization of middle cerebral artery occlusions was greater with combined IV/IA therapy (82%) than with IA therapy alone (50%), with lower NIHSS at 90 days, there was a significantly higher mortality in the treatment group (29% vs 5.5%; $P = .06$), but the risk of symptomatic intracerebral hemorrhage in both groups was similar.

The Interventional Management of Stroke (IMS-I) study was another multicenter open-labeled trial performed to further test the feasibility and safety of combined IV/IA-rtPA therapy.[89] The study enrolled 80 patients who were treated with 0.6 mg/kg IV rt-PA followed by cerebral angiography and infused intra-arterial tissue plasminogen (up to 22 mg over two hours) in cases with arterial occlusive lesions.[89] The median times for IV and IA administration of drugs were 140 and

212 minutes, respectively. Comparisons were made to patients in the NINDS rt-PA trial (matched for stroke severity), as there was no control group.

The combination therapy was found to be feasible with safety similar to IV rt-PA alone, and the 90-day mortality rate in the IMS subjects (16%) was lower, but not significantly different from the mortality rate of the placebo (24%) or rt-PA–treated subjects (21%) in the NINDS rt-PA Stroke Trial. Outcomes in the IMS subjects were also significantly better at three months than the placebo subjects of NINDS.[89] The rate of symptomatic intracranial hemorrhage in the IMS study was similar to that in the IV rt-PA–treated patients in the NINDS trial.

The findings from IMS-I were subsequently confirmed in the IMS-II study,[90,91] which found a benefit with combined treatment for Barthel Index and Global Test Statistics at 90 days and similar rates for symptomatic intracerebral hemorrhage. Furthermore, complications related to angiography and treatment in the IMS-II trial were less than 4%. Encouragement from these findings led to IMS-III, a randomized, multicenter clinical trial, which is in progress and may help assess whether combined IV/IA therapy is superior to standard IV therapy alone when initiated within three hours of symptom onset.[87]

Similarly, IA thrombolytic treatment after full-dose IV rt-PA administration might be an acceptable treatment option for patients with diffusion-weighted imaging (DWI)/perfusion-weighted imaging (PWI) mismatch.[92] However, chemical thrombolysis is limited by the low rate of complete recanalization and increased rate of intracranial hemorrhage (ICH).

Delayed Thrombolysis up to Six Hours

Although the clinical benefit from thrombolysis gradually diminishes as stroke onset to treatment time increases, a useful clinical benefit remains possible. The ECASS III trial, which confirmed clinical benefit within 4.5 hours of stroke onset (OR 1.34; 95% CI, 1.02-1.76; $P = .04$), also showed a wider 95% CI at six hours (0.9-1.5 for 271-360 minutes in the meta-analysis),[18] suggesting the possibility for a potential benefit from thrombolytic therapy even beyond 4.5 hours.

MRI perfusion/diffusion mismatch can help select patients who have remaining salvageable tissue and might benefit from delayed treatment. Although DWI allows visualization of ischemic regions within minutes of stroke onset and provides an estimate of the ischemic core, PWI provides information about the ischemic penumbra (ie, tissue at risk that might be salvageable). It has been proposed that in patients who awake with symptoms or when time of onset is unknown, PWI could help determine if they could benefit from thrombolytic therapy.

Perfusion CT is an alternative imaging modality that might be comparable to MRI despite the known limitations of CT with regard to brain coverage to identify ischemic brain tissue at risk and to aid with the decision on whether to use thrombolysis.[93-95]

Evidence of the potential benefit for IV rt-PA up to six hours in patients with tissue at risk as defined by MRI comes from a multicenter German nonrandomized trial with comparison made with the pooled data from the NINDS, ATLANTIS, and ECASS I and II that evaluated ischemic stroke treatment with rt-PA or placebo within six hours.[96] The trial, which selected 174 patients based on MRI screening criteria, demonstrated a more favorable outcome in the MRI-selected rt-PA patients (48% [95% CI, 39-54]) compared with pooled placebo (33% [95% CI, 31-36]; $P < .001$) and pooled rt-PA patients (40% [95% CI, 37-42]; $P = .046$). The rate of symptomatic intracerebral hemorrhage in MRI-selected rt-PA patients (3% [95% CI, 0-5]) was lower than in the pooled rt-PA group (8% [95% CI, 7-10]; $P = .012$) and comparable to the pooled placebo group (2% [95% CI, 1-3]; $P = .392$).

Data from both the Diffusion and perfusion imaging Evaluation For Understanding Stroke Evolution (DEFUSE)[97,98] and Echoplanar Imaging Thrombolytic Evaluation Trial (EPITHET)[99] randomized studies, designed to determine whether IV rt-PA given three to six hours after symptom onset would reduce infarct growth in patients with PWI/DWI mismatch, demonstrated strong associations between recanalization, reperfusion, reduced infarct growth, and favorable clinical response in patients with a PWI/DWI mismatch.

A meta-analysis of five trials (DIAS I, DIAS II, EPITHET, DEFUSE, and DEDAS) including a total of 502 mismatch patients thrombolyzed beyond three hours showed how delayed thrombolysis among patients selected according to mismatch imaging is associated with increased reperfusion/recanalization.[100] However, delayed thrombolysis in mismatch patients was not confirmed to improve clinical outcome, with a significant risk of symptomatic intracerebral hemorrhage and possibly increased mortality.

The ongoing Third International Stroke Trial (IST-3)[87] aims to evaluate the safety and efficacy of treatment with rt-PA within six hours of onset of acute ischemic stroke.

MANAGEMENT OF PHYSIOLOGICAL VARIABLES BEFORE THROMBOLYSIS

Hypertension

Admission high blood pressure is an independent predictor for poor outcome after stroke/thrombolysis.

Elevated pretreatment blood pressure is independently associated with an increased likelihood of sICH.[101] The retrospective analysis of the Safe Implementation of Thrombolysis in Stroke—International Stroke Thrombolysis Register (SITS-ISTR) demonstrated a strong linear association between systolic blood pressure (SBP) and risk of sICH.[102] A multicenter study of transcranial Doppler monitoring of recanalization after intravenous thrombolysis showed how pretreatment SBP of 185 mm Hg was associated with markedly high rates of persisting occlusion and partial recanalization.[103]

The reasons for lowering BP poststroke include preventing further vascular damage, averting early recurrent stroke, and reducing the risk of HT of the infarction and the formation of brain edema. However, aggressive treatment of BP may lead to neurological worsening by reducing perfusion pressure to the ischemic area of the brain.[104] This has led to ongoing controversy regarding optimal blood pressure management in the hyperacute phase after stroke. In the recently concluded Scandinavian Candesartan Acute Stroke Trial[105] using the angiotensin-receptor blocker candesartan for treatment of acute stroke, there was no evidence of a beneficial effect of careful blood pressure–lowering treatment with candesartan in patients with acute stroke and raised blood pressure.[105] Although within the first seven days blood pressure was significantly lowered in the candesartan group compared with the placebo group (mean BP 147/82 mm Hg [standard deviation {SD} 23/14] vs 152/84 mm Hg [SD 22/14]), there was no difference at 6 months in the risk of the composite vascular endpoint between the treatment group and placebo (120 events vs 111 events [adjusted hazard ratio {HR} 1.09; 95% CI, 0.84-1.41; P = .52]). Similarly, there was no difference in terms of the secondary endpoint (death from any cause). There was even a higher risk of poor functional outcome in the candesartan group (adjusted common OR 1.17; 95% CI, 1.00-1.38; P = .048).

This was studied in the Controlling Hypertension and Hypotension Immediately Post-Stroke (CHHIPS)[106] pilot trial of blood pressure treatment in patients with acute stroke (excluding rt-PA–treated patients and those with intracranial hemorrhage). Although the trial showed that BP can be safely reduced with labetalol or lisinopril after acute stroke, there was no significant difference in the primary outcome (death or dependency [mRS >3]) at two weeks (61% vs 59%) or in early neurological deterioration (NIHSS score of ≥4 points) at 72 hours (6% vs 5%) between the active treatment (labetalol or lisinopril) and placebo. The authors commented that the study might have been underpowered to detect smaller but clinically significant changes between groups in this primary outcome. However, there was a reduction in mortality by half at six months (10% with active treatment vs 20% with placebo) that was of borderline statistical significance.[106]

The results of the ongoing Efficacy of Nitric Oxide in Stroke (ENOS)[87] and Valsartan Efficacy on Modest Blood Pressure Reduction in Acute Ischemic Stroke (VENTURE)[87] may provide an answer to the controversy regarding management of hypertension in the setting of acute stroke.

Although the management of blood pressure in the setting of AIS is controversial, it is recommended that thrombolytic agents should only be administered to patients with systolic blood pressure less than 185 mm Hg and diastolic blood pressure less than 110 mm Hg at the time of treatment to avoid hemorrhagic transformation.[104] Elevated blood pressure could be treated with intravenous agents; agents such as labetalol that are easily titrated and have minimal vasodilatory effects on cerebral blood vessels are preferred.

Hyperglycemia

Hyperglycemia is one of the most important predictors of bad outcome in patients with acute stroke, either with or without treatment with IV rt-PA. It decreases the recanalization rate, increases the risk of hemorrhage, and reduces the probability of good functional outcome.[107,108]

It has been suggested that acute rather than chronic hyperglycemia delays reperfusion of the ischemic penumbra in stroke patients treated with rt-PA[107] and the detrimental effect of acute hyperglycemia is higher after early than after delayed or no reperfusion.[109] Transcranial Doppler monitoring to assess recanalization after intravenous thrombolysis showed that hyperglycemia was an independent predictor of poor outcome at three months in patients who recanalized, but not in patients with permanent occlusion.[110] This finding may reflect the observation that early recanalization is associated with a larger penumbral area susceptible to the adverse effects of hyperglycemia.[109]

A study of MRI to measure infarct progression in patients receiving intravenous thrombolysis showed significant increase in infarct volume in patients with high glucose level compared to normoglycemic patients ($P < .05$).[111]

Hyperglycemia greater than 140 mg/dL (7.7 mmol/L) before reperfusion with IV rt-PA has been shown to be an independent risk factor for failure of recanalization[107] and has been associated with diminished neurological improvement, greater infarct size, and worse clinical outcome at three months after treatment.[109]

In several thrombolysis trials, hyperglycemia was found to be associated with hemorrhagic events and poor clinical outcome, a finding that was reconfirmed in a reanalysis of the NINDS rt-PA Stroke Study.[112]

In a cohort of IV rt-PA–treated stroke patients from the multicenter Canadian Alteplase for Stroke Effectiveness Study (CASES),[113] admission glucose level greater than 8.0 mmol/L was found to be independently associated with increased risk of death (adjusted risk ratio 1.5 [95% CI, 1.2-1.9]), sICH (1.69 [0.95-3.00]) and a poor functional outcome at 90 days (0.7 [0.5-0.9]). Similarly, in the SITS-ISTR registry of IV rt-PA-treated patients, blood glucose greater than 120 mg/dL was associated with significantly higher odds for mortality (OR 1.24; 95% CI, 1.07-1.44; $P = .004$) and lower odds for independence (OR 0.58; 95% CI, 0.48-0.70; $P < .001$), and blood glucose from 181 to 200 mg/dL was associated with an increased risk of sICH (OR 2.86; 95% CI, 1.69-4.83; $P < .001$).[114]

These findings suggest that ultra-early glycemic control before thrombolysis may improve outcomes, and correction with rapidly acting insulin is recommended when the blood glucose is greater than 180 mg/dL.[104]

Other Thrombolytic Agents

To date, the only approved treatment for AIS is intravenous recombinant tissue plasminogen activator (alteplase, rt-PA). Although the time window, which was a limitation for treatment with rt-PA, has been extended, there remain concerns regarding adverse bleeding risk.

The limited fibrin specificity of rt-PA and its possible neurotoxic effects have fueled the search for other plasminogen activators that display greater fibrin dependence and selectivity but lack detrimental effects within the central nervous system. Development of an alternative thrombolytic therapy that might be easier and safer to administer could lead to wider acceptance and use of thrombolytic therapy for stroke. Although other thrombolytic agents have failed to show benefit over rt-PA, there is still ongoing research in search of an alternative agent with potentially improved half-life, higher target specificity, and better safety profile.

DESMOTEPLASE

Desmoteplase (recombinant plasminogen activator α-1) is a plasminogen activator derived from the saliva of the vampire bat, *Desmodus rotundus*. The high fibrin specificity, the lack of activation by β amyloid,[115,116] and the absence of neurotoxicity[117] make desmoteplase a promising thrombolytic drug. It is considered more fibrin specific than rt-PA and may allow an expanded time window of up to nine hours post–symptom onset.[118]

Desmoteplase showed promising results in two phase 2 trials: the DIAS (Desmoteplase in Acute Ischemic Stroke) and DEDAS (Dose Escalation study of Desmoteplase in Acute Ischemic Stroke).[119,120] In these two studies, doses of 90 µg/kg and 125 µg/kg desmoteplase administered up to nine hours after stroke onset in patients who were selected by PWI/DWI mismatch on MRI demonstrated improved safety profiles, superior reperfusion, and improved clinical outcome at 90 days compared with placebo.

The follow-up study DIAS II, a phase 3 trial that included 186 patients to confirm the results of the DIAS/DEDAS studies, did not show a benefit of desmoteplase given three to nine hours after the onset of stroke on clinical outcome at 90 days.[121] However, subsequent analysis revealed multiple errors in the methodology.[121] DIAS-3 and DIAS-4 are currently under way and may demonstrate effectiveness in acute stroke.[87]

TENECTEPLASE

Tenecteplase (TNK) is a third-generation modified form of rt-PA, with longer half-life, greater fibrin specificity, and more resistance to plasminogen activator-1 than rt-PA.[122] Tenecteplase has been approved for use in myocardial infarction, in which it is associated with fewer systemic bleeding complications than rt-PA.[123]

A pilot dose-escalation safety study of TNK in patients with AIS demonstrated safety and tolerability of TNK with no observed symptomatic intracranial hemorrhages among 75 patients treated with doses ranging from 0.1 to 0.4 mg/kg within three hours of symptom onset.[124] Patients treated with 0.1 mg/kg had better neurological improvement at 24 hours than patients treated with the higher dose of 0.4 mg/kg, suggesting the possibility of an inverse dose response. The three-month outcomes were similar to those of patients treated with rt-PA in the NINDS rt-PA Stroke Trial.

Based on these encouraging results, a follow-up, phase 2B/3, randomized, multicenter, double-blind trial of intravenous tenecteplase versus standard-dose rt-PA in patients with AIS within three hours of onset was conducted. Unfortunately, the trial was prematurely terminated during phase 2B due to slower than expected enrollment after only 112 patients had been randomized at eight clinical centers between 2006 and 2008.[125] Despite the limited number of patients recruited, symptomatic intracranial hemorrhage rates were highest in the 0.4-mg/kg tenecteplase group and lowest in the 0.1-mg/kg tenecteplase group. Also, there were no statistically significant differences in the 90-day outcomes between the tenecteplase and rt-PA groups. However, because of the termination of the trial, no convincing evidence can be extracted of tenecteplase as a potential new thrombolytic agent for treatment of AIS or about the promise of future study of tenecteplase.

Another trial that compared patients receiving TNK between three and six hours to patients treated with rt-PA within three hours demonstrated that the TNK group had more reperfusion and major neurological improvement at 24 hours and less ICH than the rt-PA group.[126] The TNK patient group was selected based on MR or CT perfusion imaging criteria.

Reteplase, a recombinant peptide with longer plasma half-life than rt-PA, is currently undergoing testing in combination with abciximab in the ROSIE and ROSIE-CT trials (CATALIST TRIAL).[87]

PLASMIN

Plasmin is a direct-acting thrombolytic agent that possesses a distinctly different mode of action than plasminogen activators,[127] and preclinical studies suggest that catheter-delivered plasmin achieves thrombolytic efficacy without causing bleeding, as first formulated in 2001 by Marder et al.[128] In contradistinction to plasminogen activators, which risk bleeding at any effective thrombolytic dose, plasmin is tolerated without bleeding at several-fold greater amounts than those needed for thrombolysis.

Plasmin was shown to be safe in a current trial in patients with peripheral arterial or graft occlusion, and efforts are now directed toward therapy of stroke caused by cerebral artery occlusion.

A phase 1 safety and dose-finding study of intra-arterial plasmin has been initiated for patients with ischemic MCA stroke at 8.5 hours or earlier after onset, with focal deficit and a rather broad National Institute of Health Stroke Scale score of 4 to 25.[87]

MICROPLASMIN

Microplasmin is another direct-acting thrombolytic agent assessed for treatment of ischemic stroke in human trials. Microplasmin used IV in MCA ischemic stroke showed a trend toward better recanalization compared with placebo,[129] and the phase 2A results of IA microplasmin in basilar artery stroke are not published.[130,131]

Clot Retrieval

The need for a wider therapeutic window with favorable outcome to facilitate an increase in the proportion of acute stroke patients who receive treatment has led to the advancement of endovascular intervention for AIS. Mechanical clot removal is achieved through placement of a minimally invasive catheter into the femoral artery and guided into the cerebral vasculature and into the clot. It has the theoretical advantage of avoiding the systematic bleeding risk associated with thrombolytic drugs. However, the use of mechanical devices is highly labor and capital intensive and is limited to specialist centers. The mechanical clot removal devices include the Merci Retriever, Penumbra Stroke System, Solitaire Stent, and the Phenox devices, but only the Merci and Penumbra are FDA approved.

Mechanical thromboembolectomy (MT) offers the potential of faster recanalization in a higher proportion of patients, with improved outcome. This is in addition to being a promising alternative for patients who are ineligible for thrombolytic therapy or in cases of failed recanalization after thrombolytic therapy.

THE MERCI RETRIEVER SYSTEM

The MERCI (Mechanical Embolus Removal in Cerebral Ischemia) clot removal system is an embolectomy device approved by the FDA in 2004 as a tool for the removal of blood clots from brain blood vessels (Figure 16–6A). The device has a flexible tapered wire with helical loops that can be embedded in the thrombus

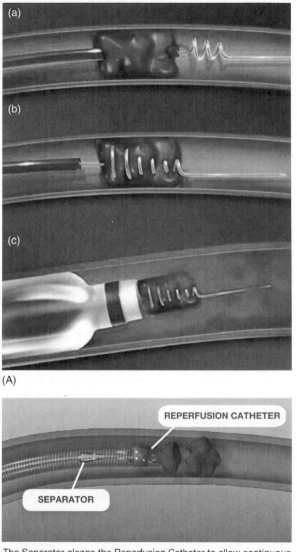

Figure 16–6. Mechanical devices: (A) MERCI device; (B) Penumbra device. (Reproduced with permission from Grunwald IQ, Wakhloo Ak, Walter S, et al. Endovascular stroke treatment today. *AJNR Am J Neuroradiol.* 2011;Feb32(2):238-243 [Page 241, Fig 2])

for retrieval. The Merci retrieval device is passed through the thrombus followed by deployment of a corkscrew-like coil distal to the thrombus. The retriever goes through the clot and utilizes a reperfusion catheter to aspirate the clot and a separator to extract any residual clot that was not initially aspirated.[132]

Mechanical thrombectomy with the Merci devices is a promising alternative treatment for patients with AIS who have either failed or are ineligible for IV rt-PA within eight hours of initial symptom onset. In addition the Merci retrieval system may have a higher recanalization rate for intracranial internal carotid artery (ICA) occlusion, which generally has a poor prognosis with poor response to intravenous thrombolysis.

The Mechanical Embolus Removal in Cerebral Ischemia (MERCI) and Multi MERCI are trials that evaluated the safety and efficacy of thrombectomy in the treatment of intracranial arterial occlusions within eight hours of stroke onset.[132,133] In the MERCI trial, only patients ineligible for IV rt-PA were included, and the Multi MERCI enrolled patients even if they had received rt-PA but failed to recanalize on subsequent angiogram. In addition, the Multi MERCI also included a newer version of the retriever device (L5) in addition to the older models (X5 and X6). Higher rates of recanalization were associated with a newer-generation thrombectomy device compared with first-generation devices, but these differences did not achieve statistical significance.[133]

In the MERCI trial, of 151 patients (141 of whom could be treated) with proximal (internal carotid, middle cerebral, or vertebrobasilar) arterial occlusions treated within six hours of onset of symptoms (mean 4.3 hours to catheterization), recanalization was achieved in 48% of those in whom the device was deployed, with 28% having asymptomatic intracerebral hemorrhage and 8% having symptomatic hemorrhages. Good neurological outcomes (modified Rankin scale [mRS] score 2) were more frequent at 90 days in patients with successful recanalization compared with patients with unsuccessful recanalization (46% vs 10%; relative risk [RR] 4.4; 95% CI, 2.1-9.3; $P < .0001$). Mortality was lower in those who were successfully recanalized than the patients with unsuccessful recanalization (32% vs 54%; RR 0.59; 95% CI, 0.39-0.89; $P = .01$).[132]

In the Multi MERCI trial, of 164 patients, treatment with the newer-generation (L5 Retriever) device within eight hours of stroke onset resulted in successful recanalization in 75 of 131 (57.3%) treatable vessels and in 91 of 131 (69.5%) after adjunctive therapy (intra-arterial tissue plasminogen activator, mechanical). Favorable clinical outcomes (mRS 0-2) occurred in 36% and mortality was 34%; both outcomes were significantly related to vascular recanalization. Symptomatic intracerebral hemorrhage was 9.8%. Procedural complications occurred in 9.8% of patients and were clinically significant in 5.5%.

Although the Multi MERCI findings support the results of the MERCI trial by demonstrating how recanalization was associated with increased survival and improved outcome, neither trial had a control arm, and as such no conclusion can be made to show that thrombectomy improves stroke outcomes. Mechanical embolectomy with the MERCI device is undergoing further analysis in the Magnetic Resonance and Recanalization of Stroke Clots Using Embolectomy (MR RESCUE).[87]

The pooled analysis of MERCI and Multi MERCI Part I trials showed that patients with ICA occlusions can achieve a relatively high revascularization rate.[134] The pooled analysis, which identified 80 patients with acute stroke from intracranial ICA occlusion, demonstrated that 53% had successful ICA recanalization with the Merci Retriever alone, and 63% had ICA recanalization with the use of the Merci Retriever plus adjunctive endovascular treatment. Good clinical outcome, defined by a modified Rankin Scale of 0 to 2 at 90 days, occurred in 39% of patients with ICA recanalization (n = 19 of 49) and in 3% of patients without ICA recanalization (n = 1 of 30) (P < .001; one patient was lost to follow-up for 90-day modified Rankin Scale). The 90-day mortality was 30% in the recanalized group compared with 73% in the nonrecanalized group (P < .001). However, no statistically significant differences for symptomatic hemorrhage were observed between the recanalized (6%) and nonrecanalized (16.7%) groups (P = .14).[134]

A retrospective analysis of data from the MERCI and Multi MERCI trials that assessed the difference in clinical outcomes between mechanical revascularization of the MCA M2 occlusion and the MCA M1 among patients with AIS treated by mechanical thrombectomy with the Merci family of retriever devices suggests a higher rate of recanalization among patients with MCA M2 occlusions than MCA M1 occlusions.[135]

The pooled analysis from the data consisting of 178 patients, 84.3% with M1 lesions and 15.7% with isolated M2 lesions, treated in the MERCI and Multi MERCI trials demonstrated how patients with isolated M2 occlusions had a higher rate of revascularization with fewer numbers of passes, and a trend toward shorter mean procedure time than patients with M1 occlusions. Although there were no statistically significant differences found in the rate of clinically significant procedural complications, symptomatic hemorrhage, favorable outcome at 90 days, or 90-day mortality between M2 and M1 groups, the M2 outcomes were numerically better than those in M1 subjects.[135] However, recanalization using the Merci Retriever System is not always successful. For instance, the Merci Retriever System failed to achieve recanalization in a large proportion of stroke patients (43%-54%) treated up to eight hours after symptom onset.[132,133]

The Merci device has the same logistic limitations as intra-arterial thrombolytic therapy but offers the possibility of treatment for selected patients who cannot be given a thrombolytic drug (eg, patients who have undergone a recent operation or invasive procedure).

The MERCI clot retrieval system was associated with a 6% to 8% rate of symptomatic intracerebral hemorrhage[132,134] and clinically significant procedural complications in around 5.5% to 7% of patients.[132,133] The procedural complications include embolization, dissection, SAH, vessel perforation, and groin hemorrhage.

PENUMBRA

The Penumbra system is one of the new generation of mechanical devices approved by the US FDA in 2008, specifically for the revascularization of large intracranial vessel occlusion in acute stroke (Figure 16–6B).[136] The Penumbra device was designed to mechanically disrupt intravascular thrombus and aspirate clot fragments through a reperfusion catheter. By working on the proximal surface of the occlusion, there is no need for navigation beyond the clot, and the device is able to remove the thrombus. The Penumbra device also uses an aspiration platform containing multiple devices that are size matched to the specific neurovascular anatomy, allowing clots to be gently aspirated out of intracranial vessels.[137]

Results from the Pivotal trial indicated that although the Penumbra system has a high rate of revascularization (80%), it has a lower than expected rate of good functional outcome (25%).[137] A post-trial, retrospective case review of 157 patients treated with the Penumbra system revealed that the revascularization rate and safety profile of the device are comparable to those reported in the Pivotal trial. Patients who were successfully revascularized with the Penumbra system had significantly better functional outcomes than those who were not.[138] In this review of treatment with the Penumbra system, 87% of the treated vessels were revascularized to thrombolysis in myocardial infarction (TIMI) 2 (54%) or 3 (33%) as compared with 82% reported in the Pivotal trial. Clinically significant procedural complications occurred in 5.7%, and the all-cause mortality rate was 20%. Forty-one percent of patients had an mRS score of 2 or below at three-month follow-up compared with only 25% in the Pivotal trial.[138]

Similarly, the Penumbra system has been shown to have a high potential for treating acute thromboembolic occlusions of the large cerebral arteries, which are often resistant to recanalization, according to a retrospective review.[139] The retrospective analysis, which involved case series of 27 patients with severe AIS, all of whom received standard thrombectomy treatment as monotherapy or in combination with thrombolysis or IC stent placement, showed a recanalization to TICI 2 or 3 in 25 patients (93%). None of the patients developed sICH, 13 patients (48%) had an mRS score of less than 2 at 90 days, and the 90-day all-cause mortality was 11%. There was a significant correlation between complete vessel recanalization and favorable outcome.[139]

Angioplasty and Stenting

Angioplasty and stenting of intracranial lesions is another interventional technique that has been used for acute stroke management (Figure 16–7). The WINGSPAN Stent System (Boston Scientific Corporation, Natick, MA) is approved by the FDA for this purpose, but its use is more for secondary stroke prevention, not acute reperfusion. The major advantages of the use of self-expanding stents compared with other interventional techniques for acute stroke management include a higher rate of recanalization and the potential to achieve immediate recanalization.

However, an important disadvantage with the use of stenting for acute stroke treatment is that the clot is only pressed to the vessel wall and not removed from the occluded vessel, which could lead to early rethrombosis. Other concerns include late in-stent stenosis and the use of aggressive antiplatelet therapy after placement.

The use of self-expandable stents in the setting of AIS was first reported by Levy et al.[140] The first prospective trial of stent-assisted recanalization in AIS demonstrated a 100% recanalization rate in 20 patients with a reasonable safety profile.[141] Subsequent studies have reported positive outcomes with self-expanding stents (SES) for AIS as well as being feasible and safe in patients with acute intracranial occlusions.[142,143] Additionally, excellent outcomes with SES in patients with acute intracranial occlusions in whom other recanalization methods have failed have been reported from case series.[140,142,144]

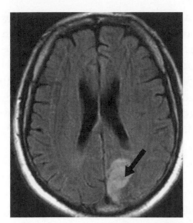
(A)

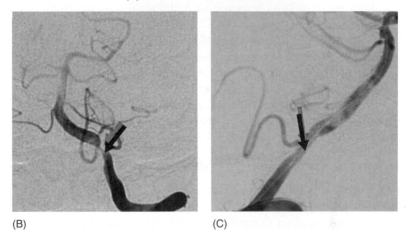
(B)   (C)

Figure 16–7. Angioplasty and stenting: (A) MRI of cerebellar infarct; (B) Angiogram demonstrating vertebral artery stenosis; (C) Post-stent of vertebral artery stenosis.

Recanalization rates of 79% to 90% have been reported with stenting, mainly for vessel occlusions resistant to other therapies.[140,145] Similarly, stents have been used to recanalize occluded or severely stenosed cervical arteries to increase blood flow to the cerebral arteries in acute stroke patients.[142,146-148] However, it has been suggested that randomized controlled trials to prove the safety and efficacy in a large number of patients are needed.[142]

Transcranial Ultrasound

Doppler ultrasound was first applied to patients in the 1960s.[149] However, successful insonation of the middle cerebral artery was only described in 1982[150] after the revolution that sufficient ultrasound could pass through the skull to allow recording from intracerebral vessels. Since then transcranial Doppler (TCD) has been rapidly evolving from a simple diagnostic imaging tool to one with a broad spectrum of clinical applications, particularly in patients with cerebrovascular disease.

The main advantages of TCD are that it is noninvasive, it is relatively cheap, it can be used at the bedside, and it allows monitoring both in acute emergency settings as well as for prolonged periods with a high temporal resolution, thereby making it ideal for studying dynamic cerebrovascular responses.[151] The ability of TCD to monitor blood flow in a blood vessel over prolonged periods of time, with the potential of showing microembolic signals in AIS, carotid artery disease, atrial fibrillation, and during angiography is another important advantage of TCD. However, TCD is highly operator dependent, and between 7% and 20% of acute stroke patients, particularly elderly patients and those from certain ethnic groups such as blacks and Asians, do not have an adequate acoustic window,[152,153] thus hindering its widespread use. A new TCD technology, power motion mode Doppler (PMD-TCD), is thought to improve window detection and simplifies the operator dependence of TCD by providing multigate flow information simultaneously in the power M-mode display.[154,155]

TCD has been shown to have diagnostic, therapeutic, and prognostic applications in patients with cerebrovascular disease, and has become an important and valuable tool for evaluating stroke mechanisms and planning and monitoring treatment, as well as for determining stroke prognosis.

TCD provides noninvasive real-time monitoring of arterial occlusion and recanalization during rt-PA treatment.[156] It can be used to quickly determine if occlusion is present or persistent, and whether recanalization has been achieved.[152,156-160]

Ultrasound-Guided Thrombolysis (Uss)

Ultrasound-enhanced thrombolysis represents a new therapeutic approach that holds promise for improving recanalization rates and outcome. Ultrasound energy may have a biological effect that enhances the thrombolytic properties of fibrinolytic agents. Experimental evidence suggests that the use of ultrasound, particularly in the low MHz-kHz frequency range, can substantially enhance the thrombolytic effect of IV rt-PA.

The mechanism of ultrasound-enhanced thrombolysis includes reversible alteration of the fibrin structure and microcavity formation in the shallow layers of thrombus, allowing increased penetration of rt-PA into the clot and enhancing flow with microstreaming and vessel dilation.[22,27,161,162]

An initial pilot study established how complete recanalization and dramatic clinical recovery from stroke occurred during transcranial Doppler monitoring of blood flow after rt-PA infusion (Alexandrov Stroke 2000). Among the 40 stroke patients studied, recanalization was complete in 12 (30%) patients and partial in 16 (40%) patients. There was dramatic recovery as defined by NIHSS score of 3 points or less, in eight (20%) patients, all with complete recovery. Encouragement from the pilot study led to a phase 2 randomized trial with a predetermined sample size to evaluate rates of recanalization and clinical recovery with IV rt-PA administered with or without continuous monitoring with transcranial Doppler ultrasonography.[163] In this Combined Lysis of Thrombolysis in Brain Ischemia Using

Transcranial Ultrasound and Systemic rt-PA (CLOT-BUST) trial, continuous 2-MHz transcranial Doppler (TCD) ultrasonography applied for two hours augmented the rate of rt-PA–induced arterial recanalization. Complete recanalization or dramatic clinical recovery within two hours after the administration of rt-PA occurred in 49% of those receiving TCD compared with 30% in the controlled group ($P = .03$). However, CLOT-BUST was not powered to evaluate the efficacy of ultrasound-enhanced thrombolysis in improving functional outcome.

A meta-analysis of randomized with nonrandomized studies of ultrasound-enhanced thrombolysis in ischemic stroke has shown that the likelihood of complete recanalization was higher in patients receiving the combination of TCD with rt-PA compared with patients treated with rt-PA alone (pooled OR 2.99; 95% CI, 1.70-5.25; $P = .0001$).[164]

The Interventional Management of Stroke (IMS)-II trial evaluated IV versus IV/IA rt-PA along with the EKOS MicroLysus catheter (Bothell, WA) by directly exposing the clot to low-power Uss. The recanalization rate of grades 2 and 3 in EKOS-treated subjects in IMS-II was 45.5% versus 30% in the IMS I–treated subjects ($P = .26$).[90]

The administration of microbubbles, which are small microspheres filled with air or gas, has also been shown to further safely accelerate ultrasound-enhanced thrombolysis in acute stroke. A pilot study in 111 patients showed enhanced recanalization and a trend toward better short- and long-term outcome with a combination of microbubbles and Uss compared with Uss/rt-PA and rt-PA alone.[165]

Laser Therapy for Stroke Treatment

The NeuroThera Laser System (NTS) uses an infrared laser technology that involves photobiostimulation. Possible mechanisms include improving energy metabolism and enhancing cell viability, and may also involve prevention of apoptosis in the ischemic penumbra and enhancement of neurorecovery mechanisms.[166] Transcranial laser therapy (TLT) is a noninvasive technology that uses near-infrared laser energy delivered transcranially to modulate biochemical changes within neural cells.

The NeuroThera Effectiveness and Safety Trial-1 (NEST-1),[166] a randomized controlled trial of 120 patients aged 40 to 85 years, showed the efficacy and reasonable safety of laser therapy for the treatment of ischemic stroke in humans when initiated within 24 hours of stroke onset.

The trial showed that 70% of patients in the active treatment group had successful outcomes versus 51% of the control, as measured prospectively on the bNIH ($P = .035$ stratified by severity and time to treatment; $P = .048$ stratified only by severity). Similarly, 59% of patients had successful 90-day outcomes compared with 44% for controls as measured by a binary mRS score of 0 to 2 ($P = .034$). In addition, more patients in the active treatment group had successful outcomes than controls as measured by the change in mean NIHSS score from baseline to 90 days ($P = .021$). The rate of serious adverse effects was 25.3% for the active group and 36.6% for the control group. However, the mortality rate did not differ significantly: 8.9% for the treatment group compared with 9.8% for the control.

The NeuroThera Laser System (NEST-2),[167] a double-blind, randomized, and sham-controlled (placebo) phase 3 trial, enrolled 660 stroke patients up to 90 years of age within 24 hours of stroke; 331 received TLT and 327 received sham therapy. The trial included patients with moderate to severe stroke (NIHSS ranging from 7-22), but excluded patients who had received thrombolytic therapy with rt-PA or those with evidence of hemorrhagic infarct.

In NEST-2, the TLT group achieved a favorable outcome in 120 (36.3%) patients compared with 101 (30.9%) patients in the sham group ($P = .094$) within 90 days. The difference of 5.4% did not reach statistical significance. Similarly, there was no difference between the mortality rates and serious adverse events between the two groups.

However, a post hoc analysis of 434 patients considered to have moderate to moderately severe stroke impairment, with a baseline NIHSS of less than 16, showed that a significantly favorable 90-day outcome in 51.6% of events was 37.8% and 41.8% for TLT and sham, respectively. However, "no serious adverse events were directly attributable to transcranial laser treatment." Similarly, there was no difference in the mortality rate, which was 17.5% in the TLT group and 17.4% in the sham group. Although TLT demonstrated safety for the treatment of ischemic stroke when initiated within 24 hours of stroke onset, it did not meet formal statistical significance for efficacy.[168] The pooled analysis of the NEST-1 and NEST-2 trials demonstrated a significantly improved success rate in stroke patients treated with laser therapy. A further phase 3 (NEST-3)[87] double-blind, randomized, sham-controlled trial is planned. This may provide further information on the safety and efficacy of TLT with the NeuroThera Laser System for the treatment of AIS between 4.5 and 24 hours of stroke onset.[168]

Neuroprotection

Another approach to AIS therapy is neuroprotection, which offers the promise of limiting infarct tissue damage. This concept of neuroprotection is to preserve brain cells that remain under ischemic stress within the penumbral region where the cells are still capable of being salvaged.[169] The assumption here is that the infarcted area of damage will not be salvaged, but that the penumbra (ie, the tissue at risk) can be salvaged. It has been demonstrated that if left untreated, the penumbra region can become part of the infarcted area.[170] This is because the sudden deprivation of oxygen and glucose to neuronal tissues can cause a series of pathological cascades, leading to neuronal death. The various mechanisms that might be responsible for ischemic damage, especially in the penumbral zones, include excessive activation of glutamate receptors, abnormal recruitment of inflammatory cells, excessive production of free radicals, accumulation of intracellular calcium cations, and initiation of pathological apoptosis. Accordingly, it has been suggested that each mechanism along the ischemic cascade offers a potential target for therapeutic intervention, and disrupting these mechanisms could protect the brain from further injury.[171] Neuroprotective agents have the potential to interfere with these biochemical cascades of events that can lead to cell death. Some neuroprotective agents can target one or more mediators of neuronal damage, such as excitatory neurotransmitters and their receptors, free radicals, secondary mediators of neuronal damage, temperature, hyperoxygenation, inflammation, and other potential targets.[172-175]

A large number of neuroprotective agents that aim to salvage ischemic tissue, limit infarct size, prolong the time window for reperfusion therapy, or minimize postischemic reperfusion injury or inflammation have demonstrated varying degrees of effectiveness for treating acute stroke in animal models.

The various neuroprotection agents include neurotransmitter agonists and antagonists (for γ-aminobutyric acid [GABA], 5HT, glycine), ion channel antagonists, Na$^+$/Ca^{2+} transport blockers, ROS scavengers, neurotrophic factors, neural stem cells, and others.[171,176] However, despite the benefits of these neuroprotective drugs in preclinical studies, there has been a failure of translation to clinical settings. None of these agents have been translated to successful human use, with the exception of NXY-059 (SAINT I trial),[177] which followed many of the STAIR guidelines.[178] Unfortunately, the follow-up SAINT II trial failed to duplicate the results of SAINT-I.[179] NXY-059 is a potent free radical–trapping agent that targets some of the biochemical abnormalities at the cellular level that contribute to cell death. It has been extensively tested in both small and large animal models of focal ischemic stroke, and has been shown to reduce the size of an infarct and preserve brain function after AIS.[176]

The SAINT trials were based on the evidence that free radicals play a major role in damaging the endothelium and that tissue oxidation is a major cause of brain injury after ischemic stroke. SAINT I revealed that the use of NXY-059 within six hours of onset of ischemic stroke significantly improved the primary outcome (reduced disability at 90 days) compared with placebo, but it did not significantly improve the functional outcome.[177] The post hoc analysis of the data also showed that treatment with NXY-059 significantly reduced the rate of intracranial hemorrhage among patients thrombolyzed with rt-PA.[180]

However, SAINT II, a phase 3 study with a larger sample, was neutral for the primary and all secondary outcomes including the failure to reduce the rate of hemorrhagic transformation with NXY-059 after thrombolysis.[179] Similarly, the pooled analysis of the SAINT I and II trials failed to show any neuroprotectant effect of NXY-059 in the treatment of AIS within six hours of symptom onset, and likewise for the subgroups and the prevention of rt-PA–associated hemorrhage.[181]

These disappointments created a great deal of pessimism regarding the future of neuroprotection trials and cast doubt on the neuroprotection hypothesis. Some have even suggested that the initially favorable result in SAINT I was likely a chance finding and that the idea of neuroprotection as a form of treatment for acute stroke should be abandoned.

Another clinical study with erythropoietin (EPO) as a neuroprotectant failed to show any benefit in patients with AIS, possibly due to increased risk of mortality in a subgroup.[87] The REGENESIS study, evaluating EPO and human chorionic gonadotropin (hCG) in combination, may provide further answers.

Why Have Trials Failed?

Although more than 1000 drugs have been investigated, only around 100 have reached clinical trials.[182] Despite evidence of utility in animal models, there has

Table 16–6. Translational Problems From Animal Studies to Clinical Settings

Animal Models	Human Studies
Homogeneous	Heterogeneous
Younger models	Older patients
Non–multiple stroke mechanism	Multiple stroke mechanism
Ischemic penumbra targeted	Not always possible to target ischemic penumbra
Short time window	Longer time window
Infarct volume as outcome	Function as outcome
Effective compounds	Ineffective compounds/small sample number
Possible limited flaws in animal studies	Flaws in clinical trials

been poor translation in humans. There are several reasons for the failure of translation of experimental studies into the clinical setting (Table 16–6). First, because stroke does not represent a single homogeneous category of injury, it is hardly cured by a single approach.[183] Stroke results in the activation of a number of pathways that independently lead to cell death. Second, current research focuses on neurons, but other types of cells are actively involved in stroke progress. In humans, stroke affects mostly the white matter, and in rats and mice (the most commonly used species in preclinical studies), there is very little white matter compared to humans.[184] Third, current animal studies are on young animals, which do not truly mimic the clinical setting.[185,186] More than 80% of all strokes occur in people aged 65 or over with possible multiple comorbidities, and the risk of stroke and the likelihood of a poor outcome increases with age.[187,188] Aging is associated with significant structural and functional alterations in the brain[189] and the response of the central nervous system to stroke differs as a function of age.[185] The Stroke Therapy Academic Industry Roundtable now recommends that aged animals be considered in preclinical studies.[178] The other reasons for the failure of translation from animal studies to clinical settings may be due to factors such as flaws in clinical trial designs, small sample sizes, choice of ineffective compounds, treatment time window, dosing, failure to achieve adequate plasma levels of study medications, and analysis.[171,190-192] It has also been suggested that early success in the preclinical studies may have prematurely pushed numerous agents into clinical trials.[171]

Some Promising New Approaches

Some recent and ongoing studies are focusing on the use of albumin, magnesium, minocycline, and statins as potential new approaches to neuroprotection.

ALBUMIN

Further optimism about the role of neuroprotection was generated from the positive results of the pilot study ALIAS (Albumin in Acute Stroke), which confirm that high-dose albumin (ALB) therapy is safe and that it may be neuroprotective after ischemic stroke.[193] The only ALB-related side effect noted during the study was mild or moderate pulmonary edema and it was effectively managed with diuretics. The results have led to a large randomized, multicenter phase 3 trial of albumin therapy, which is ongoing—the ALIAS (Albumin in Acute Stroke) trial.[87] This study may provide further definitive answers as to whether high-dose ALB therapy confers neuroprotection in patients with AIS treated within five hours of symptom onset.

The proposed mechanisms of action include amelioration of brain swelling, enhancing blood flow to subocclusive microvascular lesions, maintaining vascular patency, and preventing reocclusion after successful thrombolysis.[193]

NTx-265

NTx-265 is a therapeutic regimen of two approved and clinically well-defined drugs, human chorionic gonadotropin (hCG) and erythropoietin alfa (EPO), for the treatment of acute stroke. The basis for using NTx-265 is to stimulate the growth and differentiation of new neurons, thus replacing the ischemic brain cells damaged by the stroke. The ongoing study, REGENESIS-LED, is designed to assess the neurological outcome in AIS patients treated with NTx-265 compared with placebo, as well as the safety and tolerability of NTx-265.[87]

MINOCYCLINE

Minocycline, a semisynthetic tetracycline, has been shown to offer the potential for neuroprotection in acute stroke. The possible mechanism of action includes its anti-inflammatory effect and reduction of microglial activation and matrix metalloproteinase, as well as nitric oxide production and inhibition of apoptotic cell death.[194] In an open-label evaluator study, acute stroke patients treated with minocycline had significantly better outcomes compared with placebo.[194] In Minocycline to Improve Neurological Outcome in Stroke (MINOS), a dose-finding study, minocycline was shown to be safe and well tolerated up to doses of 10 mg/kg intravenously, alone and in combination with tissue plasminogen activator.[195]

The Neuroprotection with Minocycline Therapy for Acute Stroke Recovery Trial (NeuMAST), a multicenter randomized, double-blind, placebo-controlled trial, is in progress. The focus of this trial is to determine if minocycline, when administered within 3 to 48 hours after AIS onset, reduces neurological deficit and improves functional outcome at 90 days poststroke compared with placebo.[87]

MAGNESIUM

Magnesium is an ion-channel blocker that is known to block calcium-mediated glutamine reuptake into neuronal axons. The Field Administration of Stroke Therapy–Magnesium (FAST-MAG) Pilot Trial, an open-label, single-arm study, was performed to examine the feasibility, safety, and achievable time savings of paramedic initiation of magnesium sulfate neuroprotective therapy for patients with acute stroke identified in the field.[196] This is on the background that previous human neuroprotective clinical trials have failed due to delayed time of delivery of neuroprotective agents in clinical settings, as compared to animal studies.[196] The trial enrolled 20 patients with a mean age of 74 (range 44-92), and patients were shown to have received paramedic-administered magnesium at an average of 26 minutes (95% CI, 15-64) after symptom onset versus in-hospital–initiated magnesium (historic controls) 139 minutes (95% CI, 66-300; $P < .0001$) after symptom onset. The results demonstrated improvement in 20% of the cases and deterioration in 7%, with no change in 73%. Good functional outcome at 3 months as defined by modified Rankin scale (mRS) score of 2 or below occurred in 69% of patients. The mortality rate was 20% and no serious adverse events were associated with field therapy initiation. The encouraging results have led to a large phase 3 clinical trial aimed at evaluating the effectiveness and safety of field-administered magnesium sulphate neuroprotective therapy in improving the long-term functional outcome of stroke patients identified in the field.[87]

STATINS

Hydroxymethylglutaryl-coenzyme A (HMG-CoA) reductase inhibitors (statins) are the most widely used cholesterol-lowering drugs for stroke prevention. The Stroke Prevention by Aggressive Reduction in Cholesterol Levels (SPARCL) trial established the role of high-dose statins in secondary prevention. In addition to reducing ischemic stroke,[197] there is evidence supporting that statins are also neuroprotective.[198] The main proposed neuroprotective mechanism elicited by statins seems to be related to an increase in nitric oxide bioavailability that regulates cerebral perfusion and improves endothelial function. The other mechanisms include antioxidant properties, atherosclerotic plaque stabilization, and anti-inflammatory benefits.[198] The Neuroprotection with Statin Therapy for Acute Recovery Trial (NeuSTART II) is a safety study evaluating short-term, high-dose lovastatin use in AIS.[87]

Hypothermia

Hypothermia is another approach to arrest the acute ischemic cascade. The concept comes from the observation that hibernating animals have profound hypothermia to allow them to function at extremely low cerebral blood flow.[169] Induced hypothermia is one of the most promising neuroprotective therapies that has consistently shown benefit against a variety of brain injuries at experimental levels, and it is known to be neuroprotective in the setting of cardiac arrest and anoxic injury in humans.[199,200]

Hypothermia is believed to work by reducing cell death, cerebral reperfusion injury, and edema. Its neuroprotective effect is thought to occur through multiple mechanisms, including decrease in the release of excitatory amino acids, reduction in free radical formation, and reduction in protein kinase C activity.[201,202]

However, there are a number of limitations in applying hypothermia to stroke patients. Stroke patients are generally awake and do not tolerate cooling, which is in contrast to cardiac arrest and brain injury patients. Attaining target temperature and prolonging or maintaining the temperature in stroke patients while awake could be very challenging. Another problem with applying hypothermia to stroke patients is the rebound increased intracranial pressure experienced during rewarming, a phenomenon that is not well studied in laboratory models.[203]

Nonetheless, preliminary human trials have also been encouraging. A small number of clinical studies of therapeutic hypothermia in AIS have shown that mild therapeutic hypothermia is feasible, although not totally without complications, which include hypotension, cardiac arrhythmias, electrolyte derangements, and infections. The complications are related to the degree of cooling and the duration of treatment.[204,205]

Two clinical studies have utilized intravascular cooling devices to cool acute stroke patients. The Cooling for Acute Ischemic Brain Damage (COOL-AID) studies, COOL-AID I (using surface cooling)[206] and COOL-AID II (using endovascular cooling),[207] both demonstrated feasibility but were not powered to answer questions regarding the safety and efficiency of hypothermia for AIS. Whereas COOL-AID I confirmed only the safety and feasibility of the procedure itself,[206] COOL-AID II pointed to possible effectiveness based on MRI (diffusion weighted), which demonstrated a trend toward less growth of the infarct volume in the group of patients who were cooled to 32°C.[207] Most patients tolerated hypothermia, and clinical outcomes were similar in both groups.[207] Complications of endovascular hypothermia included hypotension, cardiac arrhythmias, electrolyte derangements, infections, and deep vein thrombosis. The side effects were thought to be related to the degree of cooling and the duration of treatment.[104]

The Intravascular Cooling in the Treatment of Stroke–Longer TPA window (ICTuS-L) study was a randomized multicenter trial designed to test the combination of IV rt-PA and hypothermia in acute stroke patients. This trial enrolled 58 patients, 28 to hypothermia at 33°C for 24 hours and 30 to normothermia. Of the hypothermic group, 24 patients were also given rt-PA. The catheter-based cooling was well tolerated in patients given rt-PA with no occurrence of brain hemorrhage. There were no differences in 90-day outcomes, although the study was not powered to determine efficacy. Pneumonia was a more frequent complication among the cooled patients.[208]

Other safety and efficacy clinical studies, such as Controlled Hypothermia in Large Infarction (CHILI) and Cooling in Acute Stroke (COAST-II), or combined cytoprotection with hypothermia plus t-PA, caffeine, and ethanol are currently ongoing.[87]

HEMORRHAGIC STROKE

Currently, there is little evidence-based targeted therapy for spontaneous hemorrhagic stroke, in contrast to ischemic stroke, despite it being the most devastating type of stroke. Therefore, management is largely supportive with strategies aimed at limiting hematoma enlargement and preventing associated complications such as seizures.[209]

Hematoma volume has been shown to be the strongest single predictor of mortality and outcome of hemorrhagic stroke. Similarly, early hematoma expansion is the major cause of early neurological deterioration after ICH.[210] The spot sign score has been shown to be a potent predictor of hematoma expansion, as well as an independent predictor of in-hospital mortality and poor outcome among survivors with primary ICH (Figure 16–8).[211]

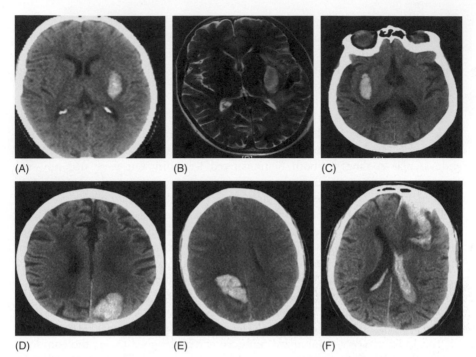

(A)   (B)   (C)

(D)   (E)   (F)

Figure 16–8. Spontaneous hemorrhage: (A) CT image–hemorrhage in the left lentiform nucleus with no resulting significant mass effect; (B) MRI image–hemorrhage in the left lentiform nucleus; (C) CT image–hemorrhage in the right basal ganglia without significant space occupying effect to surrounding structures; (D) CT image–showing a 30 × 46 mm hyperdense intraparenchymal haemorrhage in the left occipital lobe with surrounding vasogenic oedema. There is adjacent sulcal effacement but no significant contralateral shift of the midline structures; (E) CT image–showing a large right parietal-occipital haemorrhage measuring 56 × 33 mm with minimal extension into the right lateral ventricle posterior horn. There is resultant mass effect with adjacent sulcal efface-ment, contralateral shift of the midline structure by 6 mm and effacement of the posterior horn of the right lateral ventricle; (F) Extensive left frontal intra-cerebral hemorrhage extending into the with ventricular system (both lateral, third, and fourth ventricles). There is surrounding low attenuation edema and shift of midline structures.

Optimism was generated for the use of recombinant factor VII (rFVIIa) in patients with ICH after the publication of a phase 2 trial that found a reduction in hematoma volume expansion as well as improvement in neurological outcomes and mortality in rFVIIa-treated patients (18% compared with 29% in the placebo arm).[210] The phase 3 study, the FAST trial, despite showing a significant reduc-tion in hematoma growth in rFVIIa-treated patients, failed to show any functional or survival benefit, in addition to higher arterial thrombotic events.[212] However, a subgroup analysis of the FAST trial suggested a potential benefit in younger patients without known risk factors for poor outcome such as large hematoma vol-ume or significant IVH.[213] Even so, the future role of rFVIIa in the management of patients with ICH remains unclear.

The largest published trial of surgical management of ICH to date, the Surgical Trial in Intracerebral Hemorrhage (STICH), showed no overall benefit from early surgery compared with initial conservative treatment for patients (26% vs 24% favorable outcome, $P = .41$). However, a subgroup analysis found that patients with hematoma within a centimeter of the cortical surface showed a benefit for early surgery, although this did not reach statistical significance ($P = .007$).[214] Pending further data from STICH II, which is in progress and eagerly awaited, the current American Heart Association/American Stroke Association (AHA/ASA) guidelines suggest that surgery might be considered in patients with lobar ICH.[59,215]

A meta-analysis involving 10 trials of surgery for supratentorial ICH has demonstrated a benefit of surgery in primary supratentorial ICH in reducing odds of an unfavorable outcome (death and dependence) at follow-up; however, the authors concluded that more trials were needed to make a definitive conclusion.[216]

In the preliminary analysis of the Minimally Invasive Surgery plus T-PA for Intracerebral Hemorrhage Evacuation (MISTIE) trial, an ongoing open-label evacuation trial designed to determine the optimal dose of t-PA and determine the safety of this approach, suggests that minimally invasive surgery plus rt-PA shows greater clot resolution than medical treatment.[217]

ORGANIZATION OF STROKE CARE—WHAT IT CAN ACCOMPLISH

Organization of stroke care is aimed at improving the level of stroke care, thereby reducing the morbidity and mortality associated with stroke. Evidence-based research has demonstrated the benefits of organized stroke care.[218] However, the organization and implementation of stroke systems of care has become an increasingly complex and challenging task requiring numerous services and disciplines to be engaged. There are huge disparities between countries in the organization of stroke care. Similarly, the organization and provision of stroke services varies at both local and national levels in different countries.

Organized stroke care comprises several components, including prehospital evaluation and services, emergency or immediate specialized hospital treatment, and organized rehabilitation and follow-up evaluation. Emergency medical services systems and related services such as telemedicine, air ambulances, mobile CT, and mobile stroke units are other elements of organized stroke care.[219-222]

The concepts of primary stroke centers (PSCs) and comprehensive stroke centers (CSCs) were first recommended by the Brain Attack Coalition based on expert opinion, because evidence supporting their effect on patient outcome was sparse.[223] The American Stroke Association (ASA), Brain Attack Coalition, and The Joint Commission aligned to identify criteria for certifying "primary stroke centers" with the resources, organization, and expertise to diagnose and manage patients with AIS. In the United States, PSCs maintain personnel, facilities, diagnostic imaging, and infrastructure to evaluate and manage patients with uncomplicated stroke. CSCs maintain processes for the management of complicated stroke cases requiring neuroendovascular interventions and neurocritical care.[104] In the United Kingdom and Scandinavia the systems of stroke care units focus on comprehensive care including rehabilitation, and in Austria and Germany they focus on acute care.[224]

Organized stroke care can (1) help facilitate the rapid recognition of stroke through public awareness and education, thus avoiding delayed transfer to hospital; (2) optimize emergency medical services; and (3) enhance immediate acute management such as neuroimaging, maintenance of physiological homoeostasis, and the timely use of thrombolytic therapy and/or endovascular therapy. The benefits of organized stroke care appear to justify service reorganization as it can improve outcomes and reduce mortality.

Of the various components of organized stroke care, the hospital care system is the most developed and studied. It has been shown to improve outcomes through a variety of processes, including (1) standardized management of care protocols and infrastructure, (2) stroke teams and stroke units, (3) concentration of stroke expertise, (4) monitoring of disease performance measures, and (5) improvements in outcomes through quality-improvement processes.[218,223,225] The use of stroke centers is one approach to coordinating and promoting patient access to the full range of treatments and services associated with stroke prevention, treatment, and rehabilitation. A stroke unit within a stroke center is one component of the hospital care system that has been shown to reduce the risk of death and improve functional outcomes.[223] Evidence-based research has demonstrated how stroke units save lives and significantly improve functional outcomes.[226-229] Patients with acute stroke are more likely to survive, return home, and regain independence if they receive organized inpatient (stroke unit) care. A coordinated multidisciplinary team operating within a discrete ward that can offer a substantial period of rehabilitation if required typically provides this.[230]

Various aspects of care in a stroke unit such as the correction of abnormal physiological variables after stroke (routine hydration and active treatment of fever and hyperglycemia) and early mobilization have been shown to improve stroke care, reduce disability, and improve long-term survival.[104,231,232] Similarly, management on stroke units has been shown to reduce the risk of in-hospital complications (ie, aspiration pneumonia, urinary tract infections, deep venous thrombosis) and reduce the risk of stroke.[104,233] Admission to a stroke unit has been shown to have significant potential benefit across all age ranges.[234,235]

According to the US and European guidelines and the Helsingborg Declaration, all patients with stroke can benefit from treatment in a stroke unit and should be treated in one.[104,236,237] Similarly, a neuroscience intensive care unit and care by a neurointensivist within a comprehensive stroke center is another element of the hospital care system that can reduce length of stay and improve outcomes for critically ill patients with strokes.[225]

REFERENCES

1. Buchan AM. Aspects of stroke imaging. *Can J Neurol Sci.* 2001;28:99-100.
2. Barber PA, Demchuk AM, Zhang J, et al. Validity and reliability of a quantitative computed tomography score in predicting outcome of hyperacute stroke before thrombolytic therapy: ASPECTS Study Group-Alberta Stroke Programme Early CT Score. *Lancet.* 2000;355:1670-1674.

3. Puetz V, Sylaja PN, Coutts SB, et al. Extent of hypoattenuation on CT angiography source images predicts functional outcome in patients with basilar artery occlusion. *Stroke.* 2008;39:2485-2490.

4. Schellinger PD, Fiebach JB, Hacke W. Imaging-based decision making in thrombolytic therapy for ischemic stroke: present status. *Stroke.* 2003;34:575-583.

5. Rha JH, Saver JL. The impact of recanalization on ischaemic stroke outcome. A meta-analysis. *Stroke.* 2007;38:967-973.

6. Mazighi M, Sefaty JM, Labreeucher J, et al. Comparison of intravenous alteplase with a combined intravenous-endovascular approach in patients with stroke and confirmed arterial occlusions (RECANALISE study): a prospective cohort study. *Lancet Neurol.* 2009;8:802-809.

7. Khatri P, Abruzzo T, Yeatts SD, Nicholsn C, Broderick JP, Tomsick TA. Good clinical outcome after ischaemic with successful revascularization is time-dependent. *Neurology.* 2009;73:1066-1072.

8. De Silva DA, Brekenfeld C, Ebinger M, et al. The benefits of intravenous thrombolysis relate to the site of baseline arterial occlusion in the Echoplanar Imaging Thrombolytic Evaluation Trial (EPITHET). *Stroke.* 2010;41(2):295-299.

9. Saqqur M, Uchino K, Demchuk AM, et al. Site of arterial occlusion identified by transcranial Doppler predicts the response to intravenous thrombolysis for stroke. *Stroke.* 2007;38:948-954.

10. del Zoppo GJ, Poeck K, Pessin MS, et al. Recombinant tissue plasminogen activator in acute thrombotic and embolic stroke. *Ann Neurol.* 1992;32:78-86.

11. Hill MD, Rowley HA, Adler F, et al. Selection of acute ischemic stroke patients for intra-arterial thrombolysis with pro-urokinase by using ASPECTS. *Stroke.* 2003;34:19-25.

12. Sussman BJ, Fitch TS. Thrombolysis with fibrinolysin in cerebral arterial occlusion. *JAMA.* 1958;167:1705-1709.

13. Tissue plasminogen activator for acute ischaemic stroke. The National Institute of Neurological Disorders and stroke rt-PA Stroke Study Group. *N Engl J Med.* 1995;333:1581-1587.

14. Clark WM, Wissman S, Albers GW, et al. Recombinant tissue-type plasminogen activator (Alteplase) for ischaemic stroke 3 to 5 hours after symptom onset. The ATLANTIS Study: a randomised controlled trial. Alteplase Thrombolysis for Acute Noninterventional Therapy in Ischemic Stroke. *JAMA.* 1999;282:2019-2026.

15. Albers GW, Clark WM, Madden KP, Hamilton SA. ATLANTIS trial: results from patients treated within 3 hours of stroke onset. Alteplase Thrombolysis for Acute Noninterventional Therapy in Ischemic Stroke. *Stroke.* 2002;33:493-495.

16. Hacke W, Kaste M, Fieschi C, et al. Intravenous thrombolysis with tissue plasminogen activator for acute hemispheric stroke. The European Cooperative Acute Stroke Study (ECASS). *JAMA.* 1995;274:1017-1025.

17. Hacke W, Kaste M, Fieschi C, et al. Randomised double-blind placebo-controlled trial of thrombolytic therapy with intravenous alteplase in acute ischemic stroke (ECASS II). Second European–Australasian Acute Stroke Study investigators. *Lancet.* 1998;352:1245-1251.

18. Hacke W, Kaste M, Bluhmki E, et al. Thrombolysis with alteplase 3 to 4.5 hours after acute ischaemic stroke. *N Engl J Med.* 2008;359:1317-1329.

19. Hacke W, Donnan G, Fieschi C, et al. Association of outcome with early stroke treatment: pooled analysis of ATLANTIS, ECASS, and NINDS rt-PA stroke trials. *Lancet.* 2004;363:768-774.

20. Wahlgren N, Ahmed N, Davalos A, et al. Thrombolysis with alteplase 3-4.5 h after acute ischaemic stroke (SITS-ISTR): an observational study. *Lancet.* 2008;372:1303-1309.

21. Lees KR, Bluhmki E, von Kummer R, et al. Time to treatment with intravenous alteplase and outcome in stroke: an updated pooled analysis of ECASS, ATLANTIS, NINDS, and EPITHET trials. *Lancet.* 2010;375:1695-1703.

22. Alexandrov AV, Grotta JC. Arterial reocclusion in stroke patients treated with intravenous tissue plasminogen activator. *Neurology.* 2002;59:862-867.

23. Ribo M, Alvarez-Sabín J, Montaner J, et al. Temporal profile of recanalization after intravenous tissue plasminogen activator. Selecting patients for rescue reperfusion techniques. *Stroke.* 2006;37:1000-1004.

24. Kaur J, Zhao Z, Klein GM, Lo EH, Buchan AM. The neurotoxicity of tissue plasminogen activator. *J Cereb Blood Flow Metab.* 2004;24:945-963.

25. Grotta JC, Welch KM, Fagan SC, et al. Clinical deterioration following improvement in the NINDS rt-PA Stroke Trial. *Stroke.* 2001;32:661-668.

26. Burgin WS, Alexandrov AV. Deterioration following improvement with tPA therapy: carotid thrombosis and reocclusion. *Neurology.* 2001;56:568-570.

27. Rubiera M, Alvarez-Sabin J, Ribo M, et al. Predictors of early arterial reocclusion after tissue plasminogen activator-induced recanalization in acute ischemic stroke. *Stroke*. 2005;36:1452-1456.

28. Heo JH, Lee KY, Kim SH, Kim DI. Immediate reocclusion following a successful thrombolysis in acute stroke: a pilot study. *Neurology*. 2003;60:1684-1687.

29. The National Institute of Neurological Disorders and Stroke rt-PA Stroke Study Group. Intracerebral haemorrhage after intravenous t-PA therapy for ischaemic stroke. *Stroke*. 1997;28:2109-2118.

30. Larrue V, Von Kummar R, del Zoppo G, et al. Haemorrhagic transformation in acute ischaemic stroke. Potential contributing factors in the European Cooperative Acute Stroke Study. *Stroke*. 1997:28:957-960.

31. Graham GD. Tissue plasminogen activator for acute ischemic stroke in clinical practice. A meta-analysis of safety data. *Stroke*. 2003;34:28-47.

32. Jin R, Yang G, Li G. Molecular insights and therapeutic targets for blood-brain barrier disruption in ischemic stroke: critical role of matrix metalloproteinases and tissue-type plasminogen activator. *Neurobiol Dis*. 2010;38:376-385.

33. Barr TL, Latour LL, Lee KY, et al. Blood-brain barrier disruption in humans is independently associated with increased matrix metalloproteinase-9. *Stroke*. 2010;41(3):e123-e128.

34. Bauer AT, Bürgers HF, Rabie T, Marti HH. Matrix metalloproteinase-9 mediates hypoxia-induced vascular leakage in the brain via tight junction rearrangement. *J Cereb Blood Flow Metab*. 2010;30:837-848.

35. Aronowski J, Strong R, Grotta JC. Reperfusion injury: demonstration of brain damage produced by reperfusion after transient focal ischemia in rats. *J Cereb Blood Flow Metab*. 1997;17:1048-1056.

36. Heo JH, Han SW, Lee SK. Free radicals as triggers of brain edema formation after stroke. *Free Radic Biol Med*. 2005;39:51-70.

37. Awasthi D, Church DF, Torbati D, Carey ME, Pryor WA. Oxidative stress following traumatic brain injury in rats. *Surg Neurol*. 1997;47:575-581; discussion 581-572.

38. Tomimoto H, Shibata M, Ihara M, Akiguchi I, Ohtani R, Budka H. A comparative study on the expression of cyclooxygenase and 5-lipoxygenase during cerebral ischemia in humans. *Acta Neuropathol*. 2002;104:601-607.

39. Del Zoppo GJ, Higashida R, Furlan AJ, Pessin MS, Rowley HA, Gent M. PROACT: a phase II randomized trial of recombinant pro-urokinase by direct arterial delivery in acute middle cerebral artery stroke. *Stroke*. 1998;29:4-11.

40. Saqqur M, Tsivgoulis G, Molina CA, et al. Symptomatic intracerebral hemorrhage and recanalization after IV rt-PA: a multicenter study. *Neurology*. 2008;71:1304-1312.

41. Saver JL. Hemorrhage after thrombolytic therapy for stroke: the clinically relevant number needed to harm. *Stroke*. 2007;38:2279-2283.

42. Tanne D, Kasner SE, Demchuk AM, et al. Markers of increased risk of intracerebral haemorrhage after intravenous recombinant tissue plasminogen activator therapy for acute ischaemic stroke in clinical practice: the multi-center rt-PA stroke survey. *Circulation*. 2005;105:1679-1685.

43. Kwiatkowski T, Libman R, Tilley BC, et al. The impact of imbalances in baseline stroke severity on outcome in the National Institute of Neurological Disorders and Stroke Recombinant Tissue Plasminogen Activator Stroke Study. *Ann Emerg Med*. 2005;45:377-384.

44. Larrue V, von Kummer RR, Muller A, Bluhmki E. Risk factors for severe hemorrhagic transformation in ischemic stroke patients treated with recombinant tissue plasminogen activator: a secondary analysis of the European-Australasian Acute Stroke Study (ECASS II). *Stroke*. 2001;32:438-441.

45. Tanne D, Kasner SE, Demchuk AM, et al. Markers of increased risk of intracerebral hemorrhage after intravenous recombinant tissue plasminogen activator therapy for acute ischemic stroke in clinical practice: the Multicenter rt-PA Stroke Survey. *Circulation*. 2002;105:1679-1685.

46. Demchuk AM, Hill MD, Barber PA, et al. Importance of early ischemic computed tomography changes using ASPECTS in NINDS rtPA Stroke Study. *Stroke*. 2005;36:2110-2115.

47. Derex L, Nighoghossian N. Thrombolysis, stroke-unit admission and early rehabilitation in elderly patients. *Nat Rev Neurol*. 2009;5:506-511.

48. Sylaja PN, Cote R, Buchan AM, Hill MD. Thrombolysis in patients older than 80 years with acute ischaemic stroke: Canadian Alteplase for Stroke Effectiveness Study. *J Neurol Neurosurg Psychiatry*. 2006;77:826.

49. Demchuk AM, Morgenstern LB, Krieger DW, et al. Serum glucose level and diabetes predict tissue plasminogen activator-related intracerebral hemorrhage in acute ischemic stroke. *Stroke*. 1999;30:34-39.

50. Garg R, Chaudhuri A, Munschauer F, Dandona P. Hyperglycemia, insulin, and acute ischemic stroke: a mechanistic justification for a trial of insulin infusion therapy. *Stroke*. 2006;37:267-273.

51. Khatri, P, Wechsler LR, Broderick JP. Intracranial hemorrhage associated with revascularization therapies. *Stroke*. 2007;38:431-440.

52. Fiorelli M, Bastianello S, von Kummer R, et al. Hemorrhagic transformation within 36 hours of a cerebral infarct: relationships with early clinical deterioration and 3-month outcome in the European Cooperative Acute Stroke Study I (ECASS I) cohort. *Stroke*. 1999;30:2280-2284.

53. Hill MD, Buchan AM. Thrombolysis for acute ischemic stroke: results of the Canadian Alteplase for Stroke Effectiveness Study. Canadian Alteplase for Stroke Effectiveness Study (CASES) Investigators. *CMAJ*. 2005;172:1307.

54. Heuschmann PU, Berger K, Misselwitz B, et al. Frequency of thrombolytic therapy in patients with acute ischemic stroke and the risk of in-hospital mortality: the German Stroke Registers Study Group. *Stroke*. 2003;34:1106-1113.

55. Kasner SE, Villar-Cordova CE, Tong D, Grotto JC. Hemopericardium and cardiac tamponade after thrombolysis for acute ischemic stroke. *Neurology*. 1998;50:1853.

56. Kremen SA, Wu MN, Ovbiagele B. Hemopericardium following intravenous thrombolysis for acute ischemic stroke. *Cerebrovasc Dis*. 2005;20:478-479.

57. De Keyser J, Gdovinova Z, Uyttenboogaart M, Vroomen, PC, Luijckx GJ. Intravenous alteplase for stroke: beyond the guidelines and in particular clinical situations. *Stroke*. 2007;38(9):2612-2618.

58. Broderick J, Conolly S, Felmann E, et al. Guidelines for the management of spontanous intracerebral haemorrhage in adults: 2007 update: a guideline from the American Heart Association/American Stroke Association Council. *Stroke*. 2007;38:2001-2023.

59. Morgenstern LB, Hemphill JC III, Anderson C, et al. Guidelines for the management of spontaneous intracerebral hemorrhage: a guideline for healthcare professionals from the American Heart Association/American Stroke Association. *Stroke*. 2010;41(9):2108-2129.

60. Gomez-Beldarrain M, Telleria M, Garcia-Monco JC. Peripheral arterial embolism during thrombolysis for stroke. *Neurology*. 2006;67:1096-1097.

61. Yasaka M, Yamaguchi T, Yonehara T, Moriyasu H. Recurrent embolization during intravenous administration of tissue plasminogen activator in acute cardioembolic stroke: a case report. *Angiology*. 1994;45:481-484.

62. Meissner W, Lempert T, Saeuberlich-Knigge S, Bocksch W, Pape UF. Fatal embolic myocardial infarction after systemic thrombolysis for stroke. *Cerebrovasc Dis*. 2006;22:213-214.

63. Hill MD, Barber PA, Takahashi J, Demchuk AM, Feasby TE, Buchan AM. Anaphylactoid reactions and angioedema during alteplase treatment of acute ischemic stroke. *CMAJ*. 2000;162(9):1281-1284.

64. Hill MD, Buchan AM. Thrombolysis for acute ischemic stroke: results of the Canadian Alteplase for Stroke Effectiveness Study. Canadian Alteplase for Stroke Effectiveness Study (CASES) Investigators. *CMAJ*. 2005;172:1307.

65. Hill MD, Lye T, Moss H, et al. Hemi-orolingual angioedema and ACE inhibitors after ateplase treatment of stroke. *Neurology*. 2003;60:1525-1527.

66. Engelter ST, Fluri F, Buitrago-Tellez C, et al. Life-threatening orolingual angioedema during thrombolysis in acute ischaemic stroke. *J Neurol*. 2005;252:1167.

67. Tan CH, Tang SC, Lin RJ, Jeng JS. Orolingual angio-oedema after alteplase therapy in a stroke patient concurrently using angiotensin II receptor blocker. *J Neurol Neurosurg Psychiatry*. 2010;81(10):1079.

68. Molinaro G, Gervais N, Adam A. Biochemical basis of angioedema associated with recombinant tissue plasminogen activator treatment: an in vitro experimental approach. *Stroke*. 2002;33(6):1712-1716.

69. Wallon D, Girardie P, Bombois S, Lucas C. Angioneurotic orolingual oedema following thrombolysis in acute ischaemic stroke. *BMJ Case Rep*. 2010;18(2).

70. Chodirker WB. Reactions to alteplase in patients with acute thrombotic stroke. *CMAJ*. 2000;163(4): 387-388.

71. Hacke W, Zeumer H, Ferbert A, et al. Intra-arterial thrombolytic therapy improves outcome in patients with acute vertebrobasilar occlusive disease. *Stroke*. 1988;19:1216-1222.

72. Del Zoppo GJ, Higashida RT, Furlan AJ, et al. PROACT: a phase II randomised trial of recombinant pro-urokinase by direct arterial delivery in acute middle cerebral artery stroke. *Stroke*. 1998;29:4-11.

73. Furlan A, Higasshida R, Wechsler L, et al. Intra-arterial prourokinase for acute ischaemic stroke. The PROACT II study: a randomized controlled trail. Prolyse in acute cerebral thromboembolism. *JAMA*. 1999;282:2003-2011.

74. Abou-Chebl A. Endovascular treatment of acute ischemic stroke may be safely performed with no time window limit in appropriately selected patients. *Stroke.* 2010;41;1996-2000.

75. Lee M, Hong KS, Saver JL. Efficacy of intra-arterial fibrinolysis for acute ischemic stroke: meta-analysis of randomized controlled trials. *Stroke.* 2010;41(5):932-937.

76. Sacco RL, Chong JY, Prabhakaran S, Elkind MS. Experimental treatments for acute ischaemic stroke. *Lancet.* 2007;369:331-341.

77. Smith WS. Intra-arterial thrombolytic therapy for acute basilar occlusion: pro. *Stroke.* 2007;38: 701-703.

78. Ahn JY, Han IB, Chung SS, Chung YS, Kim SH, Yoon PH. Endovascular thrombolysis and stenting of a middle cerebral artery occlusion beyond 6 hours post-attack: special reference to the usefulness of diffusion-perfusion MRI. *Neurol Res.* 2006;28:881-885.

79. Jahan R, Duckwiler GR, Kidwell CS, et al. Intraarterial thrombolysis for treatment of acute stroke: experience in 26 patients with long-term follow-up. *Am J Neuroradiol.* 1999;20:1291-1299.

80. Nakano S, Iseda T, Kawano H, Yoneyama T, Ikeda T, Wakisaka S. Parenchymal hyperdensity on computed tomography after intra-arterial reperfusion therapy for acute middle cerebral artery occlusion: incidence and clinical significance. *Stroke.* 2001;32:2042-2048.

81. Khatri P, Broderick JP, Khoury JC, Carrozzella JA, Tomsick TA; the IMS I and II Investigators. Microcatheter contrast injections during intra-arterial thrombolysis may increase intracranial hemorrhage risk. *Stroke.* 2008;39(12):3283-3287.

82. Khatri P, Broderick JP, Khoury JC, Carrozzella J, Tomsick T. Microcatheter contrast injections during intra-arterial thrombolysis increase intracranial hemorrhage risk. *Stroke.* 2006;37:622.

83. Yoon W, Seo JJ, Kim JK, Cho KH, Park JG, Kang HK. Contrast enhancement and contrast extravasation on computed tomography after intra-arterial thrombolysis in patients with acute ischemic stroke. *Stroke.* 2004;35:876-881.

84. Ohta H, Nakano S, Yokogami K, Iseda T, Yoneyama T, Wakisaka S. Appearance of early venous filling during intra-arterial reperfusion therapy for acute middle cerebral artery occlusion: a predictive sign for hemorrhagic complications. *Stroke.* 2004;35:893-898.

85. Kidwell CS, Saver JL, Carneado J, et al. Predictors of hemorrhagic transformation in patients receiving intra-arterial thrombolysis. *Stroke.* 2002;33:717-724.

86. Ciccone A, Valvassori L, Ponzio M, et al. Intra-arterial or intravenous thrombolysis for acute ischaemic stroke. The SYNTHESIS pilot trial. *J Neuro Intervent Surg.* 2010;2:74-79.

87. http://www.strokecenter.org/trials/index.aspx (accessed on March 21, 2011).

88. Lewandoski CA, Frankel M, Tomsick TA, et al. Combined intravenous and intra-arterial therapy of acute ischaemic stroke: emergency management of stroke (EMS) bridging trial. *Stroke.* 1999;30:2598-2605.

89. Broderick J; IMS Study Investigators. Combined intravenous and intraarterial recanalization for acute ischaemic stroke: the Interventional Management of Stroke Study. *Stroke.* 2004;35:904-911.

90. The IMS II Trial Investigators. The interventional management of stroke (IMS) II study. *Stroke.* 2007;38:2127-2135.

91. IMS I and IMS II Trial Investigators. Pooled analysis of the IMS I and IMS II Trials. *Stroke.* 2007;38:505.

92. Yoo DS, Won YD, Huh PW, et al. Therapeutic results of intra-arterial thrombolysis after full-dose intravenous tissue plasminogen activator administration. *Am J Neuroradiol.* 2010;31(8):1536-1540.

93. Wintermark M, Flanders AE, Velthuis B, et al. Perfusion-CT assessment of infarct core and penumbra: receiver operating characteristic curve analysis in 130 patients suspected of acute hemispheric stroke. *Stroke.* 2006;37:979-985.

94. Wintermark M, Meuli R, Browaeys P, et al. Comparison of CT perfusion and angiography and MRI in selecting stroke patients for acute treatment. *Neurology.* 2007;68(9):694-697.

95. Wintermark M, Lev MH. FDA investigates the safety of brain perfusion CT. *Am J Neuroradiol.* 2010;31(1):2-3.

96. Thomalla G, Schwark C, Sobesky J, et al. Outcome and symptomatic bleeding complications of intravenous thrombolysis within 6 hours in MRI-selected stroke patients: comparison of a German multicenter study with the pooled data of ATLANTIS, ECASS, and NINDS tPA trials. *Stroke.* 2006;37:852-858.

97. Albers GW, Thijs VN, Wechsler L, et al. Magnetic resonance imaging profiles predict clinical response to early reperfusion: the diffusion and perfusion imaging evaluation for understanding stroke evolution (DEFUSE) study. *Ann Neurol.* 2006;60:508-517.

98. Olivot JM, Mlynash M, Thijs VN, et al. Relationships between infarct growth, clinical outcome, and early recanalization in diffusion and perfusion imaging for understanding stroke evolution (DEFUSE). *Stroke.* 2008;39:2257-2263.

99. Davis SM, Donnan GA, Parsons MW, et al. Effects of alteplase beyond 3 h after stroke in the Echoplanar Imaging Thrombolytic Evaluation Trial (EPITHET): a placebo-controlled randomised trial. *Lancet Neurol.* 2008;7(4):299-309.

100. Mishra NK, Albers GW, Davis SM, et al. Mismatch-based delayed thrombolysis: a meta-analysis. *Stroke.* 2010;41(1):e25-e33.

101. Tsivgoulis G, Frey JL, Flaster M, et al. Pre-tissue plasminogen activator blood pressure levels and risk of symptomatic intracerebral hemorrhage. *Stroke.* 2009;40(11):3631-3634.

102. Ahmed N, Wahlgren N, Brainin M, et al. Relationship of blood pressure, antihypertensive therapy, and outcome in ischemic stroke treated with intravenous thrombolysis. Retrospective analysis from safe implementation of thrombolysis in Stroke–International Stroke Thrombolysis Register (SITS-ISTR). *Stroke.* 2009;40:2442-2449.

103. Tsivgoulis G, Saqqur M, Sharma VK, Lao AY, Hill MD, Alexandrov AV. CLOTBUST Investigators. Association of pretreatment blood pressure with tissue plasminogen activator-induced arterial recanalization in acute ischemic stroke. *Stroke.* 2007;38:961-966.

104. Adams HP Jr, del ZG, Alberts MJ, et al. Guidelines for the early management of adults with ischemic stroke: a guideline from the American Heart Association/American Stroke Association Stroke Council, Clinical Cardiology Council, Cardiovascular Radiology and Intervention Council, and the Atherosclerotic Peripheral Vascular Disease and Quality of Care Outcomes in Research Interdisciplinary Working Groups. *Stroke.* 2007;38;1655-1711.

105. Sandset EC, Bath PMW, Boysen G, et al. The angiotensin-receptor blocker candesartan for treatment of acute stroke (SCAST): a randomized, placebo-controlled, double-blind trial. *Lancet.* 2011;377:741-750.

106. Potter JF, Robinson TG, Ford GA, et al. Controlling hypertension and hypotension immediately post stroke (CHHIPS): a randomised, placebo-controlled, double blind pilot trial. *Lancet Neurol.* 2009;8:48-56.

107. Ribo M, Molina C, Montaner J, et al. Acute hyperglycemia state is associated with lower tPA-induced recanalization rates in stroke patients. *Stroke.* 2005;36:1705-1709.

108. Gilmore RM, Stead LG. The role of hyperglycemia in acute ischemic stroke. *Neurocrit Care.* 2006;5:153-158.

109. Alvarez-Sabin J, Molina CA, Ribo M, et al. Impact of admission hyperglycemia on stroke outcome after thrombolysis: risk stratification in relation to time to reperfusion. *Stroke.* 2004;35:2493-2498.

110. Alvarez-Sabin J, Molina CA, Montaner J, et al. Effects of admission hyperglycemia on stroke outcome in reperfused tissue plasminogen activator-treated patients. *Stroke.* 2003;34:1235-1241.

111. Els T, Klisch J, Orszagh M, et al. Hyperglycemia in patients with focal cerebral ischemia after intravenous thrombolysis: influence on clinical outcome and infarct size. *Cerebrovasc Dis.* 2002;13:89-94.

112. Bruno A, Levine SR, Frankel MR, et al. NINDS rt-PA Stroke Study Group. Admission glucose level and clinical outcomes in the NINDS rt-PA Stroke Trial. *Neurology.* 2002;58;669-674.

113. Poppe AY, Majumdar SR, Jeerakathil T, et al. Admission hyperglycemia predicts a worse outcome in stroke patients treated with intravenous thrombolysis. *Diabetes Care.* 2009;32(4):617-622.

114. Ahmed N, Dávalos A, Eriksson N, et al. Association of admission blood glucose and outcome in patients treated with intravenous thrombolysis. Results from the Safe Implementation of Treatments in Stroke International Stroke Thrombolysis Register (SITS-ISTR). *Arch Neurol.* 2010;67(9):1123-1130.

115. Kingston IB, Castro MJ, Anderson S. In vitro stimulation of tissue-type plasminogen activator by Alzheimer amyloid beta-peptide analogues. *Nat Med.* 1995;1:138-142.

116. Ellis V, Daniels M, Misra R, Brown DR. Plasminogen activation is stimulated by prion protein and regulated in a copper-dependent manner. *Biochemistry.* 2002;41:6891-6896.

117. Liberatore GT, Samson A, Bladin C, Schleuning WD, Medcalf RL. Vampire bat salivary plasminogen activator (desmoteplase): a unique fibrinolytic enzyme that does not promote neurodegeneration. *Stroke.* 2003;34:537-543.

118. Paciaroni M, Medeiros E, Bogousslavsky J. Desmoteplase. *Expert Opin Biol Ther.* 2009;9:773-778.

119. Hacke W, Albers G, Al-Rawi Y, et al. The desmoteplase in acute ischemic stroke thrombolysis trial with intravenous desmoteplase. *Stroke.* 2005;36:66-73.

120. Furlan AJ, Eyding D, Albers GW, et al. Dose Escalation of Desmoteplase for Acute Ischemic Stroke (DEDAS): evidence of safety and efficacy 3 to 9 hours after stroke onset. *Stroke.* 2006;37: 1227-1231.

121. Hacke W, Furlan AJ, Al-Rawi Y, et al. Intravenous desmoteplase in patients with acute ischaemic stroke selected by MRI perfusion-diffusion weighted imaging or perfusion CT (DIAS-2): a prospective, randomised, double-blind, placebo-controlled study. *Lancet Neurol.* 2009;8:141-150.

122. Tanswell P, Modi N, Combs D, Danays T. Pharmacokinetics and pharmacodynamics of tenecteplase in fibrinolytic therapy of acute myocardial infarction. *Clin Pharmacokinet.* 2002;41:1229-1245.

123. Van de Werf F, Ardissino D, Amstrong PW, et al. Assessment of the Safety and Efficacy of a New Thrombolytic (ASSENT-2) Investigators. Single bolus tenecteplase compared with front-loaded alteplase in acute myocardial infarction: the ASSENT-2 double-blind randomized trial. *Lancet.* 1999;354:716-722.

124. Haley EC Jr, Lyden PD, Johnston KC, Hemmen TM; the TNK in Stroke Investigators. A pilot dose-escalation safety study of tenecteplase in acute ischemic stroke. *Stroke.* 2005;36:607-612.

125. Haley EC Jr, Thompson JLP, Grotto JC, et al. Phase IIB/III trial of tenecteplase in acute ischemic stroke: results of a prematurely terminated randomized clinical trial. Supplemental appendix: the Tenecteplase in Stroke Investigators. *Stroke.* 2010;41(4):707-711.

126. Parsons MW, Miteff F, Bateman GA, et al. Acute ischemic stroke: imaging-guided tenecteplase treatment in an extended time window. *Neurology.* 2009;72(10):915-921.

127. Marder VJ, Novokhatny V. Direct fibrinolytic agents: biochemical attributes, preclinical foundation and clinical potential. *J Thromb Haemost.* 2009;8:433-444.

128. Marder VJ, Landskroner K, Novokhatny V, et al. Plasmin induces local thrombolysis without causing hemorrhage: a comparison with tissues plasminogen activator in the rabbit. *Thromb Harmost.* 2001;86:739-745.

129. Thijs VNS, Peeters A, Vosko MR, et al. Randomized, placebo-controlled, dose-ranging clinical trial of intravenous microplasmin in patients with acute ischemic stroke. *Stroke.* 2009;40:3789-3795.

130. National Institutes of Health. Intra-arterial microplasmin administration in patients with acute intracranial vertebrobasilar artery occlusion (MITI-IA). 2009. Registered at www.clinicaltrials.gov (identifier 00123266).

131. National Institutes of Health. A safety and dose finding study of plasmin (human) administered into the middle cerebral artery of stroke patients. 2010. Registered at www.clinicaltrials.gov (identifier 01014975).

132. Smith WS, Sung G, Starkman S, et al. MERCI Trial Investigators. Safety and efficacy of mechanical embolectomy in acute ischemic stroke: results of the MERCI trial. *Stroke.* 2005;36:1432-1438.

133. Smith WS, Sung G, Saver J, et al. Mechanical thrombectomy for acute ischemic stroke: final results of the multi MERCI trial. *Stroke.* 2008;39:1205-1212.

134. Flint AC, Duckwiler GR, Budzik RF, Liebeskind DS, Smith WS. Mechanical thrombectomy of intracranial internal carotid occlusion: pooled results of the MERCI and Multi MERCI Part I trials. *Stroke.* 2007;38:1274-1280.

135. Shi ZS, Loh Y, Walker G, Duckwiler GR; the MERCI and Multi MERCI Investigators. Endovascular thrombectomy for acute ischemic stroke in failed intravenous tissue plasminogen activator versus nonintravenous tissue plasminogen activator patients: revascularization and outcomes stratified by the site of arterial occlusions. *Stroke.* 2010;41(6):1185-1192.

136. Bose A, Henkes H, Alfke K, et al. Penumbra Phase 1 Stroke Trial Investigators. The Penumbra System: a mechanical device for the treatment of acute stroke due to thromboembolism. *Am J Neuroradiol.* 2008;29:1409-1413.

137. The Penumbra Stroke Trial Investigators. Safety and effectiveness of a new generation of mechanical devices for clot removal in intracranial large vessel occlusive disease. *Stroke.* 2009;40:2761-2768.

138. Tarr D, Hsu K, Alfke R, et al. The POST trial: initial post-market experience of the Penumbra System: revascularization of large vessel occlusion in acute ischemic stroke in the United States and Europe. *J Neurointerv Surg.* 2010;2(4):341-344.

139. Kulcsar Z, Bonvin C, Pereira VM, et al. Penumbra System: a novel mechanical thrombectomy device for large-vessel occlusions in acute stroke. *Am J Neuroradiol.* 2010;31(4):628-633.

140. Levy EI, Mehta R, Gupta R, et al. Self-expanding stents for recanalization of acute cerebrovascular occlusions. *Am J Neuroradiol.* 2007;28:816-822.

141. Levy EI, Siddigui AH, Crumlish A, et al. First Food and Drug Administration-approved prospective trial of primary intracranial stenting for acute stroke. SARIS (Stent-Assisted Recanalization in Acute Ischaemic Stroke). *Stroke.* 2009;40;3552-3556.

142. Brekenfeld C, Schroth G, Mattle H, et al. Stent placement in acute cerebral artery occlusion. Use of a self-expandable intracranial stent for acute stroke treatment. *Stroke.* 2009;40:847-852.

143. Roth C, Papanagiotou P, Behnke S, et al. Stent-assisted mechanical recanalization for treatment of acute intracerebral artery occlusions. *Stroke.* 2010;41(11):2559-2567.

144. Zaidat OO, Wolfe T, Hussain SI, et al. Interventional acute stroke therapy with intracranial self-expanding stent. *Stroke.* 2008;39:2392-2395.

145. Sauvageau E, Samuelson RM, Levy EI, Jeziorski AM, Mehta RA, Hopkins LN. Middle cerebral artery stenting for acute ischemic stroke after unsuccessful Merci retrieval. *Neurosurgery.* 2007;60:701-706.

146. Nedeltchev K, Remonda L, Do DD, et al. Acute stenting and thromboaspiration in basilar artery occlusions due to embolism from the dominating vertebral artery. *Neuroradiology.* 2004;46:686-691.

147. Nedeltchev K, Brekenfeld C, Remonda L, et al. Internal carotid artery stent implantation in 25 patients with acute stroke: preliminary results. *Radiology.* 2005;237:1029-1037.

148. Eckert B, Koch C, Thomalla G, et al. Aggressive therapy with intravenous abciximab and intra-arterial rtPA and additional PTA/stenting improves clinical outcome in acute vertebrobasilar occlusion: combined local fibrinolysis and intravenous abciximab in acute vertebrobasilar stroke treatment (FAST): results of a multicenter study. *Stroke.* 2005;36:1160-1165.

149. Satomura S, Kaneko Z. Ultrasound blood rheograph. In: *Proceedings of the 3rd International Conference on Mecical Electronics.* 1960:254-258.

150. Asslad R, Markwalder T-M, Nornes H. Noninvasive transcranial Doppler ultrasound recording of flow velocity in basal cerebral arteries. *J Neurosurg.* 1982;50:570-577.

151. Yeo LL, Sharma VK. Role of transcranial Doppler ultrasonography in cerebrovascular disease. *Recent Pat CNS Drug Discov.* 2010;5(1):1-13.

152. Alexandrov AV, Burgin WS, Demchuk AM, El-Mitwalli A, Grotto JC. Speed of intracranial clot lysis with intravenous tissue plasminogen activator therapy: sonographic classification and short-term improvement. *Circulation.* 2001;103(24):2897-2902.

153. Alexandrov AV, Bornstein NM. Advances in neurosonology 2005. *Stroke.* 2006;37(2):299-300.

154. Moehring MA, Spencer MP. Power M-mode Doppler (PMD) for observing cerebral blood flow and tracking emboli. *Ultrasound Med Biol.* 2002;28:49-57.

155. Alexandrov AV, Demchuk AM, Burgin WS. Insonation method and diagnostic flow signatures for transcranial power motion (M-mode) Doppler. *J Neuroimaging.* 2002;12:236-244.

156. Alexandrov AV, Demchuk AM, Wein TH, Grotta JC. Yield of transcranial Doppler in acute cerebral ischemia. *Stroke.* 1999;30:1604-1609.

157. Alexandrov AV, Demchuk AM, Felberg RA, et al. High rate of complete recanalization and dramatic clinical recovery during tPA infusion when continuously monitored with 2-MHz transcranial Doppler monitoring. *Stroke.* 2000;31:610-614.

158. Demchuk AM, Christou I, Felberg R, et al. The accuracy and criteria for localizing arterial occlusion with transcranial Doppler. *J Neuroimaging.* 2000;10:1-12.

159. Felberg RA, Okon NJ, El-Mitwalli A, Burgin WS, Grotto JC, Alexandrov AV. Early dramatic recovery during intravenous tissue plasminogen activator infusion: clinical pattern and outcome in acute middle cerebral artery stroke. *Stroke.* 2002;33(5):1301-1307.

160. Burgin WS, Malkoff M, Demchuk AM, et al. Transcranial Doppler ultrasound criteria for recanalization after thrombolysis for middle cerebral artery stroke. *Stroke.* 2000;31:1128-1132.

161. Labiche LA, Malkoff M, Alexandrov AV. Residual flow signals predict complete recanalization in stroke patients treated with tPA. *J Neuroimaging.* 2003;13:28-33.

162. Suchkova V, Siddiqi FN, Carstensen EL, Dalecki D, Child S, Francis CW. Enhancement of fibrinolysis with 40-kHz ultrasound. *Circulation.* 1998;98:1030-1035.

163. Alexandrov AV, Molina CA, Grotta JC, et al. Ultrasound-enhanced systemic thrombolysis for acute ischemic stroke. *N Engl J Med.* 2004;351:2170-2178.

164. Tsivgoulis G, Eggers J, Ribo M, et al. Safety and efficacy of ultrasound-enhanced thrombolysis: a comprehensive review and meta-analysis of randomized and nonrandomized studies. *Stroke.* 2010;41(2):280-287.

165. Molina CA, Ribo M, Rubiera M, et al. Microbubble administration accelerates clot lysis during continuous 2-MHz ultrasound monitoring in stroke patients treated with intravenous tissue plasminogen activator. *Stroke.* 2006;37:425-429.

166. Lampl Y, Zivin JA, Fisher M, et al. Infrared laser therapy for ischemic stroke: a new treatment strategy: results of the NeuroThera Effectiveness and Safety Trial-1 (NEST-1). *Stroke.* 2007;38:1843-1849.

167. Zivin JA, Albers GW, Bornstein N, et al, for the NEST-2 Investigators. Effectiveness and safety of transcranial laser therapy for acute ischemic stroke. *Stroke.* 2009;40:1359.

168. Stemer AB, Huisa BN, Zivin JA. The evolution of transcranial laser therapy for AIS, including a pooled analysis of Nest-1 AND Nest-2. *Curr Cardiol Resp.* 2010;12:29-33.

169. Ly JV, Zavala JA, Donnan GA. Neuroprotection and thrombolysis: combination therapy in acute ischaemic strokle. *Exp Opin Pharmacother.* 2006;7:1571-1581.

170. Ginsberg MD. Adventures in the pathophysiology of brain ischemia: penumbra, gene expression, neuroprotection. *Stroke.* 2003;34:214.

171. Cheng YD, Al Khoury L, Zivin JA. Neuroprotection for ischemic stroke: two decades of success and failure. *NeuroRx.* 2004;1:36-45.

172. Albers GW, Clark WM, Atkinson RP, Madden K, Data JL, Whitehouse MJ. Dose escalation study of the NMDA glycine-site antagonist licostinel in acute ischemic stroke. *Stroke.* 1999;30:508-513.

173. Culmsee C, Junker V, Kremers W, Thal S, Plesnila N, Krieglstein J. Combination therapy in ischemic stroke: synergistic neuroprotective effects of memantine and clenbuterol. *Stroke.* 2004;35:1197-1202.

174. Piriyawat P, Labiche LA, Burgin WS, Aronowski JA, Grotta JC. Pilot dose-escalation study of caffeine plus ethanol (caffeinol) in acute ischemic stroke. *Stroke.* 2003;34:1242-1245.

175. Mehta SL, Manhas N, Raghubir R. Molecular targets in cerebral ischemia for developing novel therapeutics. *Brain Res Rev.* 2007;54:34-66. Green AR. Pharmacological approaches to acute ischaemic stroke: reperfusion certainly, neuroprotection possibly. *Br J Pharmacol.* 2008;153(S1):S325-S338.

176. Green AR, Shuaib A. Therapeutic strategies for the treatment of stroke. *Drug Discovery Today.* 2006;11:681-693.

177. Lees KR, Zivin JA, Ashwood T, et al. NXY-059 for acute ischemic stroke. *N Engl J Med.* 2006;354: 588-600.

178. Fisher M, Albers GW, Donnan GA, et al. Enhancing the development and approval of acute stroke therapies: Stroke Therapy Academic Industry roundtable. *Stroke.* 2005;36:1808-1813.

179. Shuaib A, Lees KR, Lyden P, et al. NXY-059 for the treatment of acute ischemic stroke. *N Engl J Med.* 2007;357:562-571.

180. Lees KR, Davalos A, Davis SM, et al. Additional outcomes and subgroup analyses of NXY-059 for acute ischemic stroke in the SAINT I trial. *Stroke.* 2006;37:2970-2978.

181. Diener HC, Lees KR, Lyden P, et al. NXY-059 for the treatment of acute stroke: pooled analysis of the SAINT I and II trials. *Stroke.* 2008;39:1751-1758.

182. O'Collins VE, Macleod MR, Donnan GA, Horky LL, van der Worp BH, Howells DW. 1,026 experimental treatments in acute stroke. *Ann Neurol.* 2006;59:467-477.

183. Lyden P, Wahlgren NG. Mechanism of action of neuroprotectants in stroke. *J Stroke Cerebrovasc Dis.* 2000;9:9-14.

184. Hoyte L, Kaur J, Buchan AM. Lost in translation: taking neuroprotection from animal model to clinical trials. *Exp Neurol.* 2004;188(2):200-204.

185. Jin K, Minami M, Xie L, et al. Ischemia-induced neurogenesis is preserved but reduced in the aged rodent brain. *Aging Cell.* 2004;3:373-377.

186. Dinapoli VA, Huber JD, Houser K, Li X, Rosen CL. Early disruptions of the blood-brain barrier may contribute to exacerbated neuronal damage and prolonged functional recovery following stroke in aged rats. *Neurobiol Aging.* 2008;29(5):753-764.

187. Tanne D, Yaari S, Goldbourt U. Risk profile and prediction of long-term ischemic stroke mortality: a 21-year follow-up in the Israeli Ischemic Heart Disease (IIHD) Project. *Circulation.* 1998;98: 1365-1371.

188. Sena E, van der worp HB, Howells D, Macleod M. How can we improve the pre-clinical development of drugs for drug? *Trend Neurosci.* 2007;30:433-439.

189. Mooradian AD. Effect of aging on the blood-brain barrier. *Neurobiol Aging.* 1988;9:31-39.

190. Spence JD, Donner A. Problems in design of stroke treatment trials. *Stroke.* 1982;13;94-99.

191. Wahlgren NG, Ahmed N. Neuroprotection in cerebral ischaemia: facts and fancies—the need for new approaches. *Cerebrovasc Dis.* 2004;17(Suppl 1):153-166.

192. Tymianski M. Can molecular and cellular neuroprotection be translated into therapies for patients?: yes, but not the way we tried it before. *Stroke.* 2010;41(10 Suppl):S87-S90.

193. Ginsberg MD, Hill MD, Palesch YY, Ryckborst KJ, Tamariz D. The ALIAS Pilot Trial: a dose-escalation and safety study of albumin therapy for acute ischemic stroke, I: physiological responses and safety results. *Stroke.* 2006;37:2100-2106.

194. Lampl Y, Boaz M, Gilad R, et al. Minocycline treatment in acute stroke. An open-label, evaluater-blinded study. *Neurology.* 2007;69;1404-1401.

195. Fagan SC, Waller JL, Nichols FT, et al. Minocycline to improve neurologic outcome in stroke (MINOS). A dose-finding study. *Stroke.* 2010;41:2283.

196. Saver JF, Kidwell C, Eckstein M, Starkman S, for the FAST-MAG Pilot Trial Investigators. Prehospital neuroprotective therapy for acute stroke. Results of the Field Administration of Stroke Therapy–Magnesium (FAST–MAG) Pilot Trial. *Stroke.* 2004;35:e106.

197. Amarenco P, Labreuche J, Lavallee P, Touboul PJ. Statins in stroke prevention and carotid atherosclerosis: systematic review and up-to-date meta-analysis. *Stroke.* 2004;35:2902-2909.

198. Cimino M, Gelosa P, Gianella A, Nobili E, Tremoli E, Sironi L. Statins: multiple mechanisms of action in the ischemic brain. *Neuroscientist.* 2007;13(3):208-213.

199. Bernard S. Therapeutic hypothermia after cardiac arrest: now a standard of care. *Crit Care Med.* 2006;34:923-924.

200. The Hypothermia After Cardiac Arrest Study Group. Mild therapeutic hypothermia to improve the neurological outcome after cardiac arrest. *N Engl J Med.* 2002;346:549-556.

201. Berger C, Schaibitz WR, Georgiadis D, et al. Effects of hypothermia on excitatory amino acids and metabolism in stroke patients: a microdialysis study. *Stroke.* 2002;33:519-524.

202. Globus MY, Alonso O, Dietrich WD, et al. Glutamate release and free radical production following brain injury: effects of post-traumatic hypothermia. *J Neurochem.* 1995;65:1704-1711.

203. Schwab S, Georgiadis D, Berrouschot J, Schellinger PD, Graffagnino C, Mayer SA. Feasibility and safety of moderate hypothermia after massive hemispheric infarction. *Stroke.* 2001;32:2033.

204. Lyden PD, Krieger D, Yenari M, Dietrich WD. Therapeutic hypothermia for acute stroke. *Int J Stroke.* 2006;1:9-19.

205. Hemmen TM, Lyden PD. Induced hypothermia for acute stroke. *Stroke.* 2007;38:794-799.

206. Krieger DW, De Georgia MA, Abou-Chebl A, et al. Cooling for Acute Ischemic Brain Damage (COOL AID): an open pilot study of induced hypothermia in acute ischemic stroke. *Stroke.* 2001;32:1847-1854.

207. De Georgia MA, Krieger DW, Abou-Chebl A, et al. Cooling for Acute Ischemic Brain Damage (COOL AID): a feasibility trial of endovascular cooling. *Neurology.* 2004;63:312-317.

208. Hemmen TM, Raman R, Gomez JA, et al. Intravenous thrombolysis plus hypothermia for acute treatment of ischemic stroke (ICTuS-l): final results. *Stroke.* 2010;41:e246.

209. Parker D, Rhoney DH, Liu-DeRyke X. Management of spontaneous nontraumatic intracranial hemorrhage. *J Pharm Pract.* 2010;23(5):398-407.

210. Mayer SA, Brun NC, Begtrup K, et al. Recombinant activated factor VII for acute intracerebral haemorrhage. *N Engl J Med.* 2005;352(8):777-785.

211. Almandoz JED, Yoo AJ, Stone MJ, et al. The Spot Sign Score in primary intracerebral hemorrhage identifies patients at highest risk of in-hospital mortality and poor outcome among survivors. *Stroke.* 2010;41:54-60.

212. Mayer SA, Brun NC, Begtrup K, et al. Efficacy and safety of recombinant activated factor VII for acute intracerebral haemorrhage. *N Engl J Med.* 2008;358(20):2127-2137.

213. Mayer SA, Davis SM, Skolnick BE, et al. Can a subset intracerebral haemorrhage patients benefit from haemostatic therapy with recombinant activated factor VII? *Stroke.* 2009;40(3):833-840.

214. Mendelow AD, Gregson BA, Fernandes HM, et al. Early surgery versus initial conservative treatment in patients with spontaneous supratentorial intracerebral haematomas in the International Surgical Trial in Intracerebral Haemorrhage (STICH): a randomised trial. *Lancet.* 2005;365:387-397.

215. Broderick J, Connolly S, Feldmann E, et al. Guidelines for the management of spontaneous intracerebral hemorrhage in adults: 2007 update: a guideline from the American Heart Association/American Stroke Association Stroke Council, High Blood Pressure Research Council, and the Quality of Care and Outcomes in Research Interdisciplinary Working Group. *Stroke.* 2007;38:2001-2023.

216. Prasad K, Mendelow AD, Gregson B. Surgery for primary supratentorial intracerbral haemorrhage (Review) In: *The Cochrane Library 2009.* Issue 1. Chichester, UK: John Wiley & Sons.

217. Morgan T, Zuccarello M, Nrayan R, et al. Preliminary findings of the minimally invasive surgery plus rtPA for intracerabral haemorrhage evacuation (MISTIE) clinical trial. *Acta Neurochir Suppl.* 2008;105:147-151.

218. Govan L, Weir CJ, Langhorne P; the Stroke Unit Trialists Collaboration. Organized inpatient (stroke unit) care for stroke. *Stroke.* 2008;39;2402-2403.

219. Alberts MJ, Felberg RA, Guterman LR, Levine SR, for Writing Group for Atherosclerotic Peripheral Vascular Disease Symposium II. Stroke intervention: state of the art. *Circulation.* 2008;118:2845-2850.

220. Garnett AR, Marsden DL, Parsons MW, et al. The rural Prehospital Acute Stroke Triage (PAST) trial protocol: a controlled trial for rapid facilitated transport of rural acute stroke patients to a regional stroke center. *Int J Stroke.* 2010;5(6):506-513.

221. Shuaib K, Khan K, Whittaker T, Amlani S, Crumley P. Introduction of portable computed tomography scanners, in the treatment of acute stroke patients via telemedicine in remote communities. *Int J Stroke.* 2010;5:62-66.

222. Walter S, Kostpopoulos P, Haass A, et al. Bringing the hospital to the patient: first treatment of stroke patients at the emergency site. *PloS One.* 2010;5(10);e13758.

223. Alberts MJ, Hademenos G, Latchaw RE, et al. Recommendations for the establishment of primary stroke centers: Brain Attack Coalition. *JAMA.* 2000;283:3102-3109.

224. Brainin M, Olsen TS, Chamorro A, et al. Organization of stroke care; education, referral, emergency management and imaging; stroke units and rehabilitation. *Cerebrovascular Dis.* 2004;17(Suppl 2);1-14.

225. Alberts MJ, Latchaw RE, Selman WR, et al. Recommendations for comprehensive stroke centers: a consensus statement from the Brain Attack Coalition. *Stroke.* 2005;36:1597-1616.

226. Stroke Unit Trialists' Collaboration. Organised inpatient (stroke unit) care for stroke. *Cochrane Database Syst Rev.* 1995;(2):CD000197.

227. Stroke Unit Trialists' Collaboration. Collaborative systematic review of the randomised trials of organised in-patient (stroke unit) care after stroke. *BMJ.* 1997;314:1151-1159.

228. Stroke Unit Trialists' Collaboration. Organised inpatient (stroke unit) care for stroke. *Cochrane Database Syst Rev.* 2002;(4).

229. Stroke Unit Trialists' Collaboration. Organised inpatient (stroke unit) care for stroke. *Cochrane Database Syst Rev.* 2007;(4):CD000197.

230. Govan L, Langhorne P, Weir CJ, for the Stroke Unit Trialists Collaboration. Does the prevention of complications explain the survival benefit of organized inpatient (stroke unit) care?: further analysis of a systematic review. *Stroke.* 2007;38(9):2536-2540.

231. CASPR (California Acute Stroke Pilot Registry) Investigators. The impact of standardized stroke orders on adherence to best practices. *Neurology.* 2005;65:360-365.

232. Forster A, Lambley R, Hardy J, et al. Rehabilitation for older people in long-term care. *Cochrane Database Syst Rev.* 2009;(1):CD004294.

233. Saposnik G, Hill MD, O'Donnell M, Fang J, Hachinski V, Kapral MK. Variables associated with 7-day, 30-day, and 1-yr fatality after ischemic stroke. *Stroke.* 2008;39;2318-2324.

234. Candelise L, Gattinoni M, Bersano A, et al. Stroke-unit care for acute stroke patients: an observational follow-up study. *Lancet.* 2007;369:299-305.

235. Saposnik G, Kapral MK, Coutts SB, et al. Do all age groups benefit from organized inpatient stroke care? *Stroke.* 2009;40:3321-3327.

236. The European Stroke Organization (ESO) Executive Committee and the ESO Writing Committee. Guidelines for management of ischaemic stroke and transient ischaemic attack 2008. *Cerebrovasc Dis.* 2008;25:457-507.

237. Kjellstrom T, Norrving B, Shatchkute A. Helsingborg Declaration 2006 on European stroke strategies. *Cerebrovasc Dis.* 2007;23;231-241.

Surgical Management of Acute Stroke

Alastair M. Buchan
J. David Spence
Joyce S. Balami

ISCHEMIC STROKE

In large hemispheric infarction with massive edema, death from increased intracranial pressure and uncal herniation ensues in approximately 72 hours, unless there is such atrophy that a large volume of swelling can be accommodated. The increased pressure in the compartment formed by the skull laterally, the relatively rigid falx medially, and the tentorium inferiorly causes progressive decline in cerebral blood flow, because cerebral blood flow is determined by arterial pressure, minus venous and tissue pressure. As the tissue pressure rises, cerebral blood flow to the ischemic but salvageable penumbra is progressively lost, and the infarction grows. This has been termed "malignant MCA infarction."

Malignant middle cerebral artery (MCA) infarction (Figure 17–1A and B) is a life-threatening condition, occurring in 10% to 15% of patients, with a mortality of up to 80% in untreated patients.[1] Younger patients are more prone to developing fatal malignant MCA syndrome than older patients, possibly because some degree of cerebral atrophy protects older people from developing space-occupying brain swelling.[2-4]

Therapies such as mannitol, glycerol, dexamethasone, and hyperventilation have little effect, but it is increasingly clear that hemicraniectomy markedly improves outcomes if done early enough. Hemicraniectomy can relieve increased intracranial pressure and prevent herniation and reduce mortality to about 5% to 27%,[5,6] unlike medical therapy where the mortality may be as high as 80%. This involves surgery to remove a large bone flap to permit the brain to swell, so that the swelling does not cause the infarction to grow progressively by strangulating its own blood supply (Figure 17–1C).

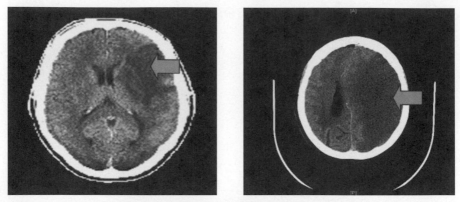

(A)   (B)

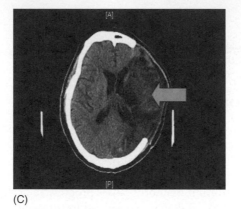

(C)

Figure 17–1. Unenhenced CT images. (A) Infarct in the middle cerebral artery territory with mild mass effect. (B) Subsequent extensive cerebral oedema with mass effect and mid-line shift (malignant MCA infarction) within 24 hours. (C) CT scan posthemicraniectomy following malignant MCA infarction.

It was difficult to show benefit of hemicraniectomy, perhaps mainly because neurosurgeons were reluctant to perform this procedure, fearing that they would save the patient's life only to suffer an outcome worse than death. Evidence of efficacy came from an imaginative, creative, and courageous approach: a combined analysis of three trials that were each having difficulty recruiting its planned sample size.

Although decompressive surgery was initially described in 1905,[7] it was not until early 1956 that it was reported as a potential treatment for large hemispheric infarction.[8] Since then, several case reports and case series have demonstrated the potential benefits of hemicraniectomy in relieving the mass effect associated with increased intracerebral pressure following malignant MCA.[5,6,9-11] Although these studies have reported improved survival with reduced mortality after hemicraniectomy, in patients with malignant MCA syndromes, no definitive conclusion was reached as to any benefit in functional outcomes after the procedure. Similarly, until recently, treatment of malignant MCA infarctions has been viewed with skepticism because of lack of evidence from randomized controlled trials (RCTs). However, results from the RCTs DECIMAL (Decompressive Craniectomy in Malignant Middle Cerebral Artery Infarct), DESTINY (Decompressive Surgery for the Treatment of Malignant Infarction of Middle Cerebral Artery), and HAMLET (Hemicraniectomy After Middle Cerebral Infarct With Life-Threatening Edema Trial) and their pooled analyses have provided evidence that hemicraniectomy undertaken within 48 hours of stroke onset improves survival and functional outcome in patients (<60 years) with malignant MCA infarction.[12-14]

This combined analysis,[15] presented to the International Stroke Conference in 2007 by Werner Hacke (whom we suspect was its chief architect), made it clear that early hemicraniectomy (within 48 hours) is remarkably efficacious. In the combined analysis data from DECIMAL, DESTINY, and HAMLET (excluding 34 patients in HAMLET, as at of the time of the analysis HAMLET was still ongoing), 51 patients received decompressive surgery and 42 had supportive therapy without decompression. Patients whose surgery was performed more than 45 hours after the onset of ischemia were excluded, as were patients with bilateral fixed dilated pupils or prestroke disability, with a modified Rankin Scale (mRS) score of 2 or greater.

Patients who had hemicraniectomy had significantly better survival (78% vs 29% [95% confidence interval {CI}, 33-67]), mRS score of 4 or less (75% vs 24%, 51% absolute risk reduction [34-69]), and mRS score of 3 or less (43% vs 21%; 23% absolute risk reduction [5-41]). Thus the number needed to treat was only two for survival or survival with mRS score of 4 or less, and four for mRS score of 3 or less.

Despite the increased favorable outcome in patients who have undergone decompressive surgery, it came at the expense of an increase in severe disability (mRS 4-5) at 12 months,[14] from 6% to 40%. The increase in severely disabled survivors after decompressive surgery has caused many to cast doubt about the effect of hemicraniectomy on long-term quality of life.

However, a medical decision analysis of surgical decompression versus medical management for space-occupying hemispheric swelling, based on data from the three randomized hemicraniectomy trials, suggests that over a one-year period, treatment of MMCA (Malignant MCA) infarctions with hemicraniectomy is associated with more quality-adjusted life-years (QALYs) than medical treatment alone.[16]

Notwithstanding the potential benefits of decompressive surgery with subsequent good functional outcome with acceptable quality of life (mRS ≤3), the results cannot be generalized to older stroke patients with malignant MCA infarction as none of the three randomized trials included patients above the age of 60 years. In light of this, DESTINY-2 is currently ongoing and may provide better evidence for hemicraniectomy in patients older than 60 years with space-occupying supratentorial infarctions. Hemicraniectomy is recommended in selected patients with marked brain ischemic swelling and life-threatening brain shifts.[17,18]

Space-occupying cerebellar infarctions can induce brainstem compression and obstructive hydrocephalus, and patients can often develop acute hydrocephalus.[19,20]

Rapid deterioration from cerebellar infarcts with swelling is common and may be associated with sudden apnea from brainstem compression and cardiac arrhythmias. Suboccipital decompressive craniectomy (SDC) is recommended as the treatment of choice to relieve both hydrocephalus and brainstem compression caused by large cerebellar infarctions.[21] Long-term outcome among survivors has been shown to be satisfactory, mostly in the absence of brainstem infarction.[21]

Hemicraniectomy is thus remarkably efficacious. The challenge at too many sites remains as that of convincing neurosurgeons to proceed early enough to decompression; to be most effective the procedure must be done before the swelling has caused progression of the stroke. Waiting until the patient has already shown signs of uncal herniation robs him or her of the huge potential benefit. Treating early enough requires courage that is all too often lacking.

Hypothermia Plus Hemicraniectomy

Nonrandomized studies suggest that moderate hypothermia between 32°C and 34°C may improve clinical outcome.[22] Several studies have shown a beneficial effect of hypothermia in malignant brain infarction by reducing the mortality to about 45%.[5,23,24] The first RCT that compared the safety and therapeutic benefit of hemicraniectomy combined with mild hypothermia therapy, with hemicraniectomy alone, enrolled 25 patients with malignant supratentorial infarctions: 13 to hemicraniectomy alone and 12 to combination therapy with hemicraniectomy and hypothermia of 35°C.[25] Although the trial demonstrated that mild hypothermia (35°C) in addition to decompressive surgery produced a trend toward a better clinical outcome than decompressive surgery alone at 6 months, as measured by the National Institutes of Health Stroke Scale (NIHSS) (10 ± 1 vs 11 ± 3; $P < .08$), there was no significant difference in the mortality rate between both groups. However, no recommendation is given regarding hypothermic therapy in patients with space-occupying infarction.[18]

HEMORRHAGIC STROKE

In contrast to ischemic stroke, the benefit of surgical treatment for spontaneous intracranial hemorrhage (ICH) has not been substantiated by evidence. The surgical procedures with varying degrees of evidence include conventional craniotomy, minimally invasive surgery, and decompressive craniectomy.

Conventional Craniotomy

Although open craniotomy could be beneficial in reducing hematoma volume and edema formation, and also lowering intracranial pressure with improved perfusion in the affected hemisphere, it may further damage the brain tissue around the hematoma.

The largest published trial of surgical management of ICH to date, the Surgical Trial in Intracerebral Hemorrhage (STICH) showed no overall benefit from early surgery compared with initial conservative treatment for patients (26% vs 24% favorable outcome, $P = .41$). However, a subgroup analysis found that patients with hematoma within a centimeter of the cortical surface showed a benefit for early surgery, although this did not reach statistical significance ($P = .41$).[26] Pending further data from STICH II, which is in progress and eagerly awaited, the current American Heart Association/American Stroke Association (AHA/ASA) guidelines suggest that craniotomy might be considered in patients with lobar clots greater than 30 mL and within 1 cm of the surface.[27,28]

A meta-analysis involving 10 trials of surgery for supratentorial ICH has demonstrated a benefit of surgery in primary supratentorial ICH in reducing the odds of an unfavorable outcome (death and dependence) at follow-up; however, the authors concluded that more trials were needed to make a definitive conclusion.[29]

Contrary to supratentorial ICH, there is much better evidence that patients with cerebellar hemorrhages exceeding 3 cm in diameter benefit from emergency surgical evacuation as brainstem compression and/or hydrocephalus from ventricular obstruction can lead to rapid deterioration within the first 24 hours of onset.[27,28]

Minimally Invasive Surgery

Minimally invasive surgery (MIS) is a promising option for removal of primary intracerebral hematomas with limited operative injury, as the techniques involve using endoscopic or stereotactic assistance to precisely locate the hematoma, thereby enabling minimal disturbance to the surrounding normal brain tissue during the surgical procedure. MIS has numerous advantages over conventional craniotomy such as shorter surgery time, reduced tissue damage, and the fact that the procedure could be performed under local anesthesia. The several methods of MIS include stereotactic guidance with aspiration and thrombolysis using recombinant human tissue-type plasminogen activator (rt-PA) or urokinase, endoscopic evacuation, and computed tomography (CT)-guided aspiration.

STEREOTACTIC ASPIRATION AND THROMBOLYSIS

The evidence for the potential beneficial effect of stereotactic infusion of urokinase for improving survival but not necessarily rebleeding has been provided by randomized trials.[30-33] The combination of frameless stereotactic aspiration and thrombolysis (FAST), in a phase 2 study of 28 patients with deep subcortical ICH found the procedure to be safe and associated with a reduction in ICH volume and early improvement in NIHSS with the potential to improve outcome.[34]

In another study of 15 patients who underwent FAST of the clot, there was demonstrable ICH reduction without perihematoma enlargement.[35] In the preliminary analysis of the Minimally Invasive Surgery plus T-PA for Intracerebral Hemorrhage Evacuation (MISTIE) trial, an ongoing open-label evacuation trial designed to determine the optimal dose of rt-PA and determine the safety of this approach, suggests that minimally invasive surgery plus rt-PA shows greater clot resolution than medical treatment.[36]

IMAGE-GUIDED STEREOTACTIC ENDOSCOPIC ASPIRATION

Numerous, small single-center randomized trials[37,38] and nonrandomized studies[39-43] have found the image-guided stereotactic endoscopic aspiration procedure to be effective in the immediate hematoma evacuation, with improved functional outcome and reduced mortality when compared to the best medical management. However, there is a need for further study to evaluate the real benefit of this minimally invasive procedure.

In view of the uncertainty of the effectiveness of MIS for hematoma evacuation and the need for further research, the application of MIS using either stereotactic or endoscopic aspiration with or without thrombolytic usage is not recommended for routine use by the AHA.[27,28]

DECOMPRESSIVE CRANIECTOMY

Although decompressive hemicraniectomy has been shown to be a life-saving procedure for malignant MCA infarction, no randomized controlled trial has been conducted in patients with ICH. The evidence for the potential beneficial effect of decompressive surgery comes from small case series. In one series of 12 patients with ICH treated with decompressive craniectomy, 11 (92%) patients survived at discharge, of which six (54%) had good function (mRS 0-3).[44] In another case series of 23 patients with autumnal hecatomb who underwent decompressive hemicraniectomy, 13 patients had a good outcome and 10 had a poor outcome (including 3 deaths) at 90 days.[45] Although decompressive hemicraniectomy may have a role in the management of ICH, there is a need for controlled trials to establish the benefit of such surgical decompression in patients with ICH.

REFERENCES

1. Huttner HB, Schwab S. Malignant middle cerebral artery infarction: clinical characteristics, treatment strategies, and future perspectives. *Lancet Neurol.* 2009;8:949-958.
2. Hacke W, Schwab S, Horn M, Spranger M, De Georgia M, von Kummer R. "Malignant" middle cerebral artery territory infarction: clinical course and prognostic signs. *Arch Neurol.* 1996;53:309-315.
3. Jaramillo A, Gongora-Rivera F, Labreuche J, Hauw JJ, Amarenco P. Predictors for malignant middle cerebral artery infarctions: a postmortem analysis. *Neurology.* 2006;66:815-820.
4. Chen RL, Balami J, Esiri M, Chen LH, Buchan AM. Stroke in ageing: an overview of evidence. *Nat Rev Neurology.* 2010;6:256-265.
5. Schwab S, Schwarz S, Spranger M, Keller E, Bertram M, Hacke W. Moderate hypothermia in the treatment of patients with severe middle cerebral artery infarction. *Stroke.* 1998;29:2461-2466.
6. Mori K, Nakao Y, Yamamoto T, Maeda M. Early external decompressive craniectomy with duroplasty improves functional recovery in patients with massive hemispheric embolic infarction: timing and indication of decompressive surgery for malignant cerebral infarction. *Surg Neurol.* 2004;62(5):420-429; discussion 429-430.
7. Cushing H. The establishment of cerebral hernia as a decompressive measure for inaccessible brain tumours; with the description of intramuscular methods of making the bone defect in temporal and occipital regions. *Surg Gynecol Obstet.* 1905;1297.
8. Scarcella G. Encephalomalacia simulating the clinical and radiological aspects of brain tumor: a report of six cases. *J Neurosurg.* 1956;13:366-380.
9. Walz B, Zimmermann C, Böttger S, Haberl RL. Prognosis of patients after hemicraniectomy in malignant middle cerebral artery infarction. *J Neurol.* 2002;249:1183-1190.
10. Leonhardt G, Wilhelm H, Doerfler A, et al. Clinical outcome and neuropsychological deficits after right decompressive hemicraniectomy in MCA infarction. *J Neurol.* 2002;249:1433-1440.
11. Gupta R, Connolly ES, Mayer S, Elkind MSV. Hemicraniectomy for massive middle cerebral artery territory infarction: a systematic review. *Stroke.* 2004;35:539-543.

12. Vahedi K, Vicaur E, Mateo J, et al, on behalf of the DECIMAL Investigators. Sequential-design, multicenter, randomized, controlled trial of early decompressive craniectomy in malignant middle cerebral artery infarction (DECIMAL). *Stroke.* 2007;38:2506-2517.

13. Juettler E, Schwab S, Schmiedek P, et al, for the DESTINY Study Group. Decompressive surgery for the treatment of malignant infarction of the middle cerebral artery (DESTINY): a randomized controlled trial. *Stroke.* 2007;38:2518-2525.

14. Hofmeijer J, Kappelle LJ, Algra A, Amelink GJ, van Gijn J, van der Worp HB, for the HAMLET Investigators. Surgical decompression for space-occupying cerebral infarction (the Hemicraniectomy after Middle Cerebral Artery infarction with Life-threatening Edema Trial (HAMLET). *Lancet.* 2009;8(4):326-333.

15. Vahedi K, Hofmeijer J, Juttler E, et al, for the DESTINY and HAMLET Investigators. Early decompressive surgery in malignant infarction of the middle cerebral artery: a pooled analysis of three randomised controlled trials. *Lancet Neurol.* 2007;6:215-222.

16. Kelly AG, Holloway RG. Health state preferences and decision-making after malignant middle cerebral artery infarctions. *Neurology.* 2010;75:682-687.

17. Adams HP Jr, del ZG, Alberts MJ, et al. Guidelines for the early management of adults with ischemic stroke: a guideline from the American Heart Association/American Stroke Association Stroke Council, Clinical Cardiology Council, Cardiovascular Radiology and Intervention Council, and the Atherosclerotic Peripheral Vascular Disease and Quality of Care Outcomes in Research Interdisciplinary Working Groups. *Stroke.* 2007;38;1655-1711.

18. The European Stroke Organization (ESO) Executive Committee and the ESO Writing Committee. Guidelines for management of ischaemic stroke and transient ischaemic attack 2008. *Cerebrovasc Dis.* 2008;25:457-507.

19. Jauss M, Krieger D, Homing C, et al. Surgical and medical management of patients with massive cerebellar infarctions: results of the German-Austrian Cerebellar Infarction Study. *J Neurol.* 1999;246:257-264.

20. Mathew P, Teasdale G, Bannan A, Oluoch-Olunya D. Neurosurgical management of cerebellar haematoma and infarct. *J Neurol Neurosurg Psychiatry.* 1995;59(3):287-292.

21. Pfefferkorn T, Eppinger U, Linn J, et al. Long-term outcome after suboccipital decompressive craniectomy for malignant cerebellar infarction. *Stroke.* 2009;40:3045-3050.

22. Steiner T, Friede T, Aschoff A, et al. Effect and feasibility of controlled rewarming after moderate hypothermia in acute stroke patients with malignant infarction of the middle cerebral artery. *Stroke.* 2001;32:2833-2835.

23. Schwab S, Georgiadis D, Berrouschot J, Schellinger PD, Graffangino C, Mayer SA. Feasibility and safety of moderate hypothermia after massive hemispheric infarction. *Stroke.* 2001;32:2033-2035.

24. Georgiadis D, Schwarz S, Aschoff A, Schwab S. Hemicraniectomy and moderate hypothermia in patients with severe ischemic stroke. *Stroke.* 2002;33(6):1584-1588.

25. Els T, Oehm E, Voigt S, Klisch J, Hetzel A, Kassubek J. Safety and therapeutical benefit of hemicraniectomy combined with mild hypothermia in comparison with hemicraniectomy alone in patients with malignant ischemic stroke. *Cerebrovasc Dis.* 2006;21:79-85.

26. Mendelow AD, Gregson BA, Fernandes HM, et al. Early surgery versus initial conservative treatment in patients with spontaneous supratentorial intracerebral haematomas in the International Surgical Trial in Intracerebral Haemorrhage (STICH): a randomised trial. *Lancet.* 2005;365:387-397.

27. Broderick J, Connolly S, Feldmann E, et al. Guidelines for the management of spontaneous intracerebral hemorrhage in adults: 2007 update: a guideline from the American Heart Association/American Stroke Association Stroke Council, High Blood Pressure Research Council, and the Quality of Care and Outcomes in Research Interdisciplinary Working Group. *Stroke.* 2007;38:2001-2023.

28. Morgenstern LB, Hemphill III JC, Anderson C, et al. Guidelines for the management of spontaneous intracerebral hemorrhage: a guideline for healthcare professionals from the American Heart Association/American Stroke Association. *Stroke.* 2010;41(9):2108-2129.

29. Prasad K, Mendelow AD, Gregson B. Surgery for primary supratentorial intracerbral haemorrhage (Review). In: *The Cochrane Library 2009.* Issue 1. Chichester, UK: John Wiley & Sons Ltd; 2009.

30. Zuccarello M, Brott T, Derex L, et al. Early surgical treatment for supratentorial intracerebral hemorrhage: a randomized feasibility study. *Stroke.* 1999;30:1833-1839.

31. Teernstra OPM, Evers SMAA, Lodder J. Stereotactic treatment of intracerebral hematoma by means of a plasminogen activator—a multicenter randomized controlled trial (SICHPA). *Stroke.* 2003;34(4):968-974.

32. Sun H, Liu H, Li D, Liu L, Yang J, Wang W. An effective treatment for cerebral hemorrhage: minimally invasive craniopuncture combined with urokinase infusion therapy. *Neurol Res.* 2010;32(4):371-377.

33. Zhou H, Zhang Y, Liu L, Huang Y, Tang Y, Su J. Minimally invasive stereotactic puncture and thrombolysis therapy improves long-term outcome after acute intracerebral hemorrhage. *J Neurol.* 2011;258(4):661-669.

34. Vespa P, McArthur D, Miller C, et al. Frameless stereotactic aspiration and thrombolysis of deep intracerebral hemorrhage is associated with reduction of hemorrhage volume and neurological improvement. *Neurocrit Care.* 2005;2(3):274-281.

35. Carhuapoma JR, Barrett RJ, Keyl PM, Hanley DF, Johnson RR. Stereotactic aspiration–thrombolysis of intracerebral hemorrhage and its impact on perihematoma brain edema. *Neurocrit Care.* 2008;8: 322-329.

36. Morgan T, Zuccarello M, Nrayan R, et al. Preliminary findings of the minimally invasive surgery plus rtPA for intracerabral haemorrhage evacuation (MISTIE) clinical trial. *Acta Neurochir Suppl.* 2008;105:147-151.

37. Auer LM, Ascher PW, Heppner F, et al. Does acute endoscopic evacuation improve the outcome of patients with spontaneous intracerebral hemorrhage? *Eur Neurol.* 1985;24:254-261.

38. Miller CM, Vespa P, Saver JL, et al. Image-guided endoscopic evacuation of spontaneous intracerebral hemorrhage. *Surg Neurol.* 2008;69(5):441-446; discussion 446.

39. Barlas O, Karadereler S, Bahar S, et al. Image-guided keyhole evacuation of spontaneous supratentorial intracerebral hemorrhage. *Minim Invasive Neurosurg.* 2009;52:62-68.

40. Chen CC, Lin HL, Cho DY. Endoscopic surgery for thalamic hemorrhage: a technical note. *Surg Neurol.* 2007;68:438-442.

41. Hsieh PC. Endoscopic removal of thalamic hematoma: a technical note. *Minim Invasive Neurosurg.* 2003;46:369-371.

42. Nishihara T, Nagata K, Tanaka S, et al. Newly developed endoscopic instruments for the removal of intracerebral hematoma. *Neurocrit Care.* 2005;2:67-74.

43. Nishihara T, Morita A, Teraoka A, Kirino T. Endoscopy-guided removal of spontaneous intracerebral hemorrhage: comparison with computer tomography-guided stereotactic evacuation. *Childs Nerv Syst.* 2007;23(6):677-683.

44. Murthy JM, Chowdary GV, Murthy TV, Bhasha PS, Naryanan TJ. Decompressive craniectomy with clot evacuation in large hemispheric hypertensive intracerebral hemorrhage. *Neurocrit Care.* 2005;2(3):258-262.

45. Ramnarayan R, Anto D, Anilkumar TV, Nayar R. Decompressive hemicraniectomy in large putaminal hematomas: an Indian experience. *J Stroke Cerebrovasc Dis.* 2009;18(1):1-10.

Stroke Rehabilitation

Robert Teasell

INTRODUCTION

Stroke rehabilitation is often required for those patients who are left with clinical deficits following an acute event. Stroke rehabilitation is undergoing a renaissance of sorts, sparked by increasing understanding of brain reorganization and neurological recovery, and a growing body of evidence (over 800 randomized controlled trials) that is helping us to unravel the "black box" of stroke rehabilitation. It has been estimated that over one-third of all stroke patients admitted to the hospital will require additional rehabilitation after the acute phase. This chapter focuses on brain reorganization and recovery poststroke, the key principles of stroke rehabilitation necessary to ensure best outcomes, specific interventions in stroke rehabilitation that will likely be of interest to the reader, and finally the importance and management of depression poststroke.

BRAIN REORGANIZATION AND RECOVERY FROM STROKE

Neurological Recovery

Neurological recovery is defined as recovery of neurological impairments and is often the result of brain recovery/reorganization; the latter has been increasingly recognized as being influenced by rehabilitation. Most neurological recovery occurs within the first 1 to 3 months, after which it may occur much more slowly for up to one year.[1] Reorganization of the brain after a stroke is dependent not only on the lesion site, but also on the surrounding brain tissue and on remote locations that have structural connections with the injured area. Following a stroke, brain reorganization has been best studied in relation to motor deficits (ie, hemiplegia or hemiparesis) and occurs in response to relearning motor activities, which involves primarily the contralateral (affected) hemisphere. Reorganization in response to training occurs along the cortical rim of the infarction with increased recruitment of secondary cortical areas such as the supplementary motor area and pre–motor cortex in the contralateral (affected) hemisphere. Ipsilateral cortical involvement is more prominent early on; however, persistence of ipsilateral cortical involvement is generally associated with larger strokes and a poorer recovery.

Functional Recovery

Functional recovery is defined as improvement in mobility and activities of daily living (ADLs); it has long been known that it is influenced by rehabilitation. Functional recovery is influenced by neurological recovery but is not entirely dependent on it. The two most powerful predictors of functional recovery are initial stroke severity and age.[2] Initial clinical assessment of stroke severity is the most predictive factor and correlates with the length of time to maximal neurological and functional recovery.

Stroke Rehabilitation Triage

Approximately 39% of patients will require inpatient rehabilitation services following stroke.[3] Although there is no set of universally accepted criteria for admission, patients who are admitted to a stroke rehabilitation unit must be (1) medically stable; (2) able to learn; and (3) have sufficient physical endurance to participate actively in therapeutic activities, as demonstrated by the ability to sit unsupported in a wheelchair for at least one hour at a time. Traditionally, stroke rehabilitation units have confined admissions to patients described as comprising the "middle band" of stroke severity. Patients recovering from milder stroke, with few or no disabilities, do not usually require the services of inpatient rehabilitation units and can be managed on an outpatient basis. The "lower band" patients, who present with profound disability, remain the most expensive to rehabilitate, as their progress is slow and the gains they make are more limited.[4] The benefit of rehabilitation for these patients may be more in the prevention of complications, a reduction in the length of hospital stay, and discharge planning.[5,6]

ORGANIZED STROKE CARE—INTERDISCIPLINARY CARE/TEAM

Efficacy of Stroke Rehabilitation

Many best practice guidelines now recommend that all patients who require inpatient rehabilitation services following stroke should be treated on a specialized rehabilitation unit.[7] Stroke rehabilitation programs are characterized by a collection of dedicated beds situated in a geographically defined area and staffed by an interdisciplinary team working cohesively and closely to provide a comprehensive rehabilitation program for each patient. These units are mainly found in stand-alone rehabilitation centers or large acute-care hospitals in urban areas. Another key feature of a well-functioning rehabilitation unit are weekly team conferences, which are held to establish or revise rehabilitation goals and plans, assess patient progress, identify barriers or complications, and develop a plan for discharge or transfer to another type of rehabilitation program. These programs may vary in terms of the types of therapies offered, as well as their intensity and duration. Stroke rehabilitation units organized in this fashion have been shown to improve functional outcomes, especially for patients recovering from moderately disabling strokes (modified Rankin Scale scores of 3-5),[5] and reduce mortality (especially in more severe strokes).[8] Although the mechanism by which specialized stroke care improves patient outcomes remains unclear, it is likely that the processes of care and the structures that support these processes contribute to their success. Specific interventions such as early mobilization and greater attention to medical complications have been suggested as factors. Staff specialization and greater education and involvement of caregivers may also contribute to their success.[9]

Although debate continues as to the optimal time to begin rehabilitation, there is evidence that the brain appears "primed" for recovery during the acute stage of the stroke, and delays may limit the patients' opportunity for recovery.[10] Admitting stroke patients earlier for inpatient rehabilitation has been shown to reduce the length of stay in acute hospital units and overall lengths of hospital stay, and improves functional outcome.[11,12]

Greater Intensity

When attempting to determine factors that contribute to the improved functional outcomes that are associated with specialized stroke rehabilitation, the intensity of rehabilitation therapies is often cited as an important element. Do patients who receive therapy for longer periods of time or at a higher level of intensity realize greater benefits compared to patients who receive conventional care? This hypothesis has been investigated extensively, although evidence suggests that there is only a weak correlation between intensity of rehabilitation therapies and functional recovery.[13-15] This weak association may be explained by differences in the time, duration, and composition of therapies provided and/or the characteristics of the stroke patients under study.

The optimal amount of therapy a given stroke patient should receive on a daily basis during inpatient rehabilitation remains unknown and is undoubtedly patient specific. In an effort to standardize care and to improve outcome following stroke, many national organizations have compiled some variation of a best practice guideline document intended for use by treating health care providers. Some of these guidelines, but not all, have included minimum standards of therapy provision, which range from 45 minutes to one hour, of occupational and physical therapy each day.[16-18]

Therapy Must Be Task Specific

The last few decades have been dominated by a debate among physiotherapists, and to a lesser extent occupational therapists, as to whether one should use a compensatory or a restorative therapeutic approach. The restorative approach focuses on traditional physical therapy exercises and neuromuscular facilitation, which involves sensorimotor stimulation, exercises, and resistance training designed to enhance motor recovery and maximize brain recovery of the neurological impairment.[19] This approach is facilitated by neurodevelopmental techniques (NDT) and is best known as the Bobath approach (one form of NDT) after its strongest and most popular proponent. The concepts of NDT emphasize that abnormal muscle patterns or muscle tone have to be inhibited, and that normal patterns should be used in order to facilitate functional and voluntary movements.[20]

In the compensatory approach, the goal is not motor recovery or reducing impairments but pragmatically learning an adaptive approach, one-handed if necessary. This approach is sometimes referred to as task-specific therapy; concerns are it may limit neurological recovery over the long term. It has been suggested that functional reorganization of brain cortex is greater when therapy is not only repetitive, but when focused on tasks that are important and meaningful to the patient. The use of Bobath and other NDT approaches are declining as evidence mounts that task-specific training results in short-term improvements in motor functioning and shorter lengths of hospital stay when compared to NDT.[21,22]

Early Supported Discharge

In recognition that patients may prefer to return home following a stroke and that inpatient interdisciplinary stroke rehabilitation may not always be necessary, early supported discharge (ESD) may be an option for some patients. Given that the goal of therapy is to establish skills that are applicable to the home environment, it has been suggested that there is no better place to learn such skills but in the home environment itself. Critics of ESD argue that most patients are already discharged as soon as it is feasible. Lincoln[23] maintained that rehabilitation on a stroke unit provides the best possible chance for recovery, due to the organized and highly specialized nature of the treatments provided, and argued that these key features could not be replicated in the community, while Young[24] argued that there is a definite place for rehabilitation in the home following stroke. Early supported discharge services provided by a well-resourced, coordinated, specialized interprofessional team can be an acceptable alternative to inpatient stroke rehabilitation unit care for some patients recovering from mild to moderate stroke. Patients appear to be more satisfied with ESD programs.[25] Additional benefits include reduced lengths of hospital stay, cost reduction,[26] and a greater likelihood of achieving independence in ADLs.[25]

SELECTED REHABILITATION ISSUES

Mobility and Lower Extremity

Treadmill training with partial body weight support (PWS) is a promising new approach that enables nonambulatory stroke survivors the repetitive practice of complex gait cycles rather than single-limb gait preparatory maneuvers. Patients are able to walk more symmetrically with less spasticity and improved cardiovascular efficiency, which the treadmill provides, when compared to floor walking.[27] Patient confidence is greater because of a reduced risk of falling while still engaging in the task. Body weight support can be gradually withdrawn as patients' posture, balance, and coordination improves. Although the weight of the evidence favors treadmill training with PWS, the treatment has not been widely adopted because it requires extensive equipment and is very labor (therapist) intensive.

Electrical stimulation has been used as a method to improve spasticity, muscle tone, sensory deficits, and pain reduction, which may lead to improvements in functional recovery. The application of an electrical current to the skin stimulates lower motor nerves and muscle fibers, resulting in improved contractility. Electrical stimulation is usually administered through two methods: functional electrical stimulation (FES) and transcutaneous electrical nerve stimulation (TENS).

TENS is a form of treatment that delivers electrical stimulation using a current intensity that it is beneath motor threshold, although capable of generating a "pins-and-needles sensation." Although TENS has been used most frequently as a means to reduce pain, it may also promote recovery of movement or functional ability following stroke. Similar to acupuncture or functional electrical stimulation, transcutaneous electrical stimulation is one method of achieving increased afferent stimulation.[28] TENS is also used to treat focal spasticity.

Functional electrical stimulation in the lower extremity has been used to enhance ankle dorsiflexion during the swing phase of gait. Weak ankle dorsiflexion with plantarflexion hypertonicity results in a drop foot, which is typically corrected by an ankle foot orthosis (AFO). FES of the common peroneal nerve during the swing phase of gait would appear to be a suitable alternative. Although not widely used or universally available, for highly motivated patients who are able to walk independently or with minimal assistance, there is growing evidence that treatment with FES can improve dropped foot, which in turn can improve gait. Both implantable and surface electrodes may be used. Although not widely used or available, there is growing evidence that FES combined with gait training improves hemiplegic gait.[29,30]

Upper Extremity

The hemiplegic upper extremity tends to recover more slowly and less completely than the lower extremity and tends to respond less well to treatment.[31] Over the last decade, a variety of new treatments have been examined as adjuncts to standard rehabilitation therapies.

The use of **mental imagery or mental practice** as a means to enhance performance following stroke was adapted from the field of sports psychology were the technique has been shown to improve athletic performance, when used in addition to standard training methods. The technique, as the name suggests, involves rehearsing a specific task or series of tasks, mentally. The most plausible mechanism to explain the success of the technique is that stored motor plans for executing movements can be accessed and reinforced during mental practice. Mental practice can be used to supplement conventional therapy at any stage of recovery and has been shown to improve motor function or ADL performance following stroke.[32,33]

Mirror therapy is a technique that uses visual feedback about motor performance to improve rehabilitation outcomes. It has been adapted from its original use for the treatment of phantom limb pain as a method to "retrain the brain" as a means to enhance upper-limb function following stroke and to reduce pain. In mirror therapy, patients place a mirror beside the unaffected limb, blocking their view of the affected limb, creating the illusion that both limbs are working normally. It is believed that by viewing the reflection of the unaffected arm in the mirror that it may act as a substitute for the decreased or absent proprioceptive input. To date, there have been only a small number of trials that have assessed its benefit. The results have not been convincing.

Constraint-induced movement therapy (CIMT) refers to a new set of rehabilitation techniques designed to reduce functional deficits in the more affected upper extremity of stroke survivors. The two key features of CIMT are restraint of the unaffected hand/arm and increased practice or use of the affected hand/arm.[34] Because stroke survivors may experience "learned non-use" of the upper extremity within a short period of time, CIMT is designed to overcome learned non-use by promoting cortical reorganization.[35] Although the biological mechanism(s) responsible for the benefit are unknown, and the contribution from intense practice is difficult to disassociate from the contribution of constraining the good limb, this form of treatment shows promise, especially for survivors with moderate disability following stroke. The results from the largest and most rigorously conducted trial, the *Extremity Constraint Induced Therapy Evaluation (EXCITE)*, may provide the strongest evidence of a benefit of CIMT treatment to date.[36] The study recruited 222 subjects with moderate disability three to nine months following stroke over three years from seven institutions in the United States. Treatment was provided for up to six hours a day, five days a week, for two weeks. Patients were reassessed up to 24 months following treatment. At 12 months, compared with the subjects in the control group who received usual care, subjects in the treatment group had significantly higher scores on sections of the Wolf Motor Function test and the Motor Activity Log, which were maintained at 24 months. Although these results are encouraging, the number of patients for whom this treatment may be suitable for remains uncertain. In the EXCITE trial, only 6.3% of patients screened were eligible. Although estimates of 20% to 25% have been suggested, it remains uncertain if subjects with greater disability would benefit from treatment.

Traditional CIMT is delivered over a two-week period, consisting of restraint of the unaffected upper extremity during waking hours for 14 days coupled with six hours of "shaping" practice in using the impaired upper extremity over 10 of the treatment days. Because such an intensive program is not practical or feasible in most clinical settings, modifications have been proposed. They include a less intense, modified CIMT (mCIMT) that combines structured functional practice sessions of a half-hour to two hours each day, in addition to restraint of the unaffected arm and hand.

The optimal timing of treatment remains uncertain. Although there is evidence that patients treated in the acute phase of stroke may benefit preferentially,[37] there is also evidence that it may, in fact, be harmful.[38,39] The greatest benefit is likely to be conferred during the chronic stages.

FUNCTIONAL ELECTRICAL STIMULATION (FES) IN HEMIPARETIC UPPER EXTREMITY

Neuromuscular electrical stimulation (NMES) can be used to improve motor recovery, reduce pain and spasticity, strengthen muscles, and increase range of motion following stroke. Functional electrical stimulation (FES) refers to the application of NMES to help achieve a functional task. Three forms of NMES are available: (1) cyclic NMES, which contracts paretic muscles on a preset schedule and does not require participation on the part of the patient; (2) electromyogram (EMG)-triggered NMES, which may be used for patients who are able to partially activate a paretic muscle and may have a greater therapeutic effect; (3) neuroprosthetic applications of NMES, which can ultimately improve or restore the grasp and manipulation functions required for typical ADLs.[40] FES has been well studied and found to be an effective treatment in both acute stroke (less than six months) and chronic stroke (more than six months).

SPASTICITY POSTSTROKE

Spasticity is usually seen days to weeks post–ischemic stroke and is characterized by velocity-dependent resistance to passive movement of affected muscles at rest. Spasticity can be painful, interfere with functional recovery in the upper extremity, and hinder rehabilitation efforts. The incidence of spasticity in the upper extremity is reported to be approximately 20%.[41]

One treatment for localized spasticity in stroke patients is botulinum toxin injections. Botulinum toxin works by weakening spastic muscles by blocking the neuromuscular junction for up to six months. Botulinum toxin has been shown to reduce spasticity in the upper extremity. However, it has not been shown to necessarily improve function, likely because underlying weakness more than spasticity results in the limitation of function. Modest improvements in the dressing, grooming, and eating on the Barthel Index score have been reported following botulinum toxin injections (Table 18–1 and Figure 18–1).

Table 18–1. Common Indications for the Use of Botulinum Toxin in the Spastic Upper Extremity

- Adducted/internally rotated shoulder (subscapularis/pectoralis major) to improve on adduction and internally rotated shoulder tightness/contracture and pain
- Flexed elbow (brachioradialis/biceps/brachialis) to make ADLs and hygiene easier as well as improve cosmesis
- Pronated forearm (pronator quadratus/pronator teres) to improve hand orientation
- Flexed wrist (flexor carpi radialis/brevis/ulnaris/extrinsic finger flexors) to improve ADLs and reduce pain
- Clenched fist (flexor digitorum profundus/sublimis) to improve hygiene
- Thumb in palm deformity (adductor pollicis/flexor pollicis longus/thenar group) to improve thumb for key grasp

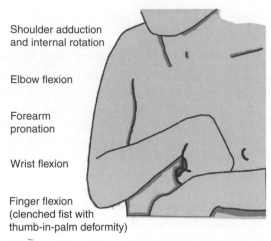

Shoulder adduction
and internal rotation

Elbow flexion

Forearm
pronation

Wrist flexion

Finger flexion
(clenched fist with
thumb-in-palm deformity)

Figure 18–1. The typical hemiplegic upper extremity posturing. (Reprinted by permission of Robert Teasell.)

Brashear et al[42] in a landmark study conducted a randomized, double-blinded, placebo-controlled multicenter trial investigating the efficiency and safety of one-time injections of BTx-A in 126 subjects with increased flexor tone in the wrist and fingers after a stroke. Modified Ashworth Scale scores for the wrist and fingers were significantly different between groups ($P < .001$) at 4, 6, and 12 weeks follow-up. Overall, there is strong evidence that treatment with botulinum toxin either alone or in combination with therapy significantly decreases spasticity in the upper extremity in stroke survivors. However, it is not clear that the improvements are sustained, nor is there strong evidence that they are associated with improved function and quality of life.

VISUAL-SPATIAL PERCEPTUAL DEFICITS

Visual-spatial perceptual deficits are characteristic of right hemispheric parietal strokes and may be defined as deficits in the ability to process, organize, interpret, and act on, in an appropriate fashion, incoming visual or tactile-kinesthetic information, or both.[43] There are two main approaches to the treatment of perceptual disorders: a transfer of training approach and the functional approach.[44] The transfer of training approach assumes that practice on a particular perceptual task will improve performance on similar perceptual tasks. The functional approach strives to promote functional independence through the repetitive practice of particular tasks, usually ADLs. When occupational therapists treat stroke patients having cognitive impairments, they often use a functional approach in ADL retraining to reduce the consequences of cognitive-perceptual impairments such as visual-spatial neglect.[45]

Unilateral spatial neglect (USN) is defined as a failure to report, respond, or orient to sensory stimuli presented to the side contralateral to the stroke lesion.[46] Neglect, in itself, is not a disorder, but rather a complex combination of symptoms

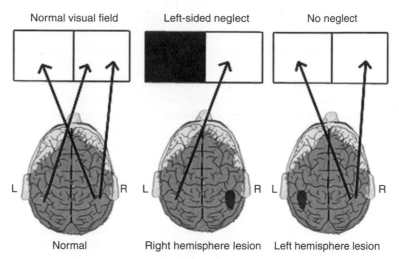

Normal visual field   Left-sided neglect   No neglect

L   R   L   R   L   R

Normal   Right hemisphere lesion   Left hemisphere lesion

Figure 18–2. Why is left-sided neglect more common than right-sided neglect? The right hemisphere regulates attention more than the left hemisphere. The left hemisphere is responsible for modulating attention and arousal for the right visual field only, and the right hemisphere is responsible for controlling these processes in both the right and left hemispheres. Hence the right hemisphere is more able to compensate for the left hemisphere when it suffers a stroke, and the left hemisphere is not able to compensate for the right hemisphere if it is injured in a stroke. (Reprinted by permission of Robert Teasell.)

that differ from patient to patient. USN occurs in approximately 23% of individuals following stroke[47,48] and is more common in patients with right-sided lesions than left (Figure 18–2).[48,49] In many cases, conspicuous manifestations of USN resolve spontaneously with the first four weeks of a stroke event.[50] In the case of persistent neglect, further recovery may continue at a less significant rate than seen during the acute phase poststroke.[50,51] The presence of USN may be associated with poorer functional outcomes, reduced mobility, longer length of stay in rehabilitation, and a greater chance of institutionalization upon discharge.[52,53]

Clinicians have the responsibility to systematically screen all clients for cognitive impairments and disabilities poststroke, including USN, using standardized assessment tools and stroke scales.[7,54,55] A recent literature review reported that there are currently 61 standardized and nonstandardized assessment tools available to assess USN in each of the hemispaces at both impairment and disability levels.[56] Common screening tests include the line bisection test, the single-letter cancellation test, and the behavior inattention test.

In general, rehabilitation interventions to improve neglect may be classified into **two major rehabilitation types**: (1) those that attempt **to increase the stroke patient's awareness of or attention** to the neglected space and (2) those that focus on the **remediation of deficits of position sense or body orientation**.[57,58] Examples of interventions that attempt to improve awareness of or attention to the neglected space include the use of visual scanning retraining, arousal or activation strategies, and feedback to increase awareness of neglect behaviors.[57] Interventions that attempt to improve neglect by targeting deficits associated with position sense and spatial representation include the use of prisms, eye patching and hemispatial glasses, caloric stimulation, optokinetic stimulation, TENS, and neck vibration.

The most common type of intervention designed to increase attention to the neglected space is **visual scanning retraining**. Typically, patients with neglect do not visually scan their whole environment, often paying no attention to their left hemispace.[59,60] Visual scanning involves teaching patients to look to their left side in a consistent manner, whether by retraining specific scanning behavior or through the remediation of functional activities that require spatial ability. In general, interventions utilizing enhanced visual scanning techniques have produced a positive effect on neglect when assessed either in isolation or in combination with other strategies including training of functional tasks requiring spatial ability.[61,62] In addition, improvements in USN derived from visual scanning interventions have been associated with significant functional gains.[59,63]

The most common treatments for the remediation of deficits in position sense or body orientation include the use of **prisms** and **eye patching**. Prisms affect spatial representation by causing an optical deviation of the visual field to either the left or the right, usually by 5 to 10 degrees, on average. One of the most common low-vision interventions for stroke-induced hemianopia is the incorporation of binocular sector prisms in the person's habitual spectacle lenses. These may be Fresnel membrane lenses or prisms that are cemented onto the lens surface. The prism is located so that it remains outside the residual field of view when the person is looking straight ahead. When gaze is shifted in the direction of the non-seeing hemifield, the prismatic effect gives a more peripheral view to the affected side than would otherwise be possible without a larger magnitude eye movement. Although prism adaptation appears to be effective in improving various aspects of perceptual performance and may be used in the treatment of both acute and chronic neglect,[64-68] improvements in visuospatial neglect following prism treatment have not been demonstrated to be associated with improvements in ADL function[68] or motor recovery.[69]

Shulman[70] noted that in healthy subjects, **eye patches** should increase eye movements toward the contralateral space. Thus eye patching of the eye ipsilateral to the lesion causes patients to look toward the contralateral space by either moving their eye or by movement of the head. The use of hemispatial patching, in which right half-field patches are used over both eyes, has shown promising results on assessments of visual neglect.[71-73] However, studies have provided conflicting reports regarding the generalizability of such improvements to functional ability.[71,73]

VASCULAR COGNITIVE IMPAIRMENT

According to O'Brien et al,[74] the term vascular cognitive impairment refers to all forms of cognitive impairment caused by cerebrovascular disease. The authors noted that vascular dementia, vascular cognitive impairment without dementia, and vascular mild cognitive impairment all fall within this definition (Table 18–2). Stroke

Table 18–2. Vascular Versus Alzheimer Dementia

Characteristic	Vascular Dementia	Alzheimer Disease
Onset	Sudden or gradual	Gradual
Progression	Slow, stepwise fluctuation	Constant insidious decline
Neurological findings	Evidence of focal deficits	Subtle or absent
Memory	Mildly affected	Early and severe deficit
Executive function	Early and severe	Late
Dementia type	Subcortical	Cortical
Neuroimaging	Infarcts or white matter lesions	Normal; hippocampal atrophy
Gait	Often disturbed early	Usually normal
Cardiovascular history	TIAs, strokes, vascular risk factors	Less common

From Salter K, Teasell R, Bhogal S, Zettler L, Foley N. Aphasia. In: Teasell R, Foley N, Salter K, Bhogal SK, Jutai J, Speechley M, eds. *Evidence-Based Review of Stroke Rehabilitation*. 13th ed. London, Ontario: 2010.

survivors with vascular cognitive impairment but no dementia exhibit impairments of attention and executive function, but have preservation of memory and orientation when compared to those who have vascular dementia.[75,76] Progression to dementia may be predicted by the relative severity of memory impairment.[76,77] Reported prevalence rates of vascular cognitive impairment have varied substantially from 15% to 20% in various clinical settings to 39%, 35%, 30%, and 32% at three months, one year, two years, and three years poststroke, respectively, as reported by Patel et al.[78] Although not all individuals with cognitive impairment have or will develop dementia, poststroke cognitive impairment is associated with a twofold greater risk for dementia.[79] All stroke patients entering rehabilitation should be screened for cognitive impairment using a validated screening tool. The Montreal Cognitive Assessment may be a more accurate screening tool than the Mini Mental Status Exam for detecting milder forms of vascular cognitive impairment in individuals with stroke.[80]

Cognitive rehabilitation refers to a systematic intervention or series of interventions or activities that are based on the evaluation and understanding of an individual's deficits and is oriented toward function.[61] Various interventions aim to (1) reinforce, strengthen, or reestablish previously learned patterns of behavior; (2) establish new patterns of cognitive activity through compensatory cognitive mechanisms for impaired neurological systems; (3) establish new patterns of activity through external compensatory mechanisms such as personal orthoses or environmental structuring and support; and (4) enable persons to adapt to their cognitive disability. A meta-analysis of the reviews conducted by Cicerone et al[61,81] reported that overall, cognitive rehabilitation interventions are associated with small but significant treatment effects. Effectiveness of treatment may be moderated by variables such as treatment domain, etiology of injury (eg, traumatic brain injury [TBI] vs stroke), and time since injury. It should be noted, however, that studies of individuals with stroke included in the analyses were primarily in the areas of language and visuospatial interventions only. Studies of attention or executive function, memory, or comprehensive cognitive function have focused more often on individuals with TBI or other brain injury. Specific interventions used to address aspects of cognition, such as attention, memory, and executive function, include imagery-based training; the use of assistive, electronic devices; and training in problem solving. In these areas, the development of compensatory strategies rather than the restoration or remediation of function may be the most effective approach to rehabilitation.[81]

Various **pharmacotherapeutic approaches** to the management of vascular cognitive impairment have been evaluated. Acetylsalicylic acid (ASA), for example, is a common antithrombotic therapy used in the treatment of vascular dementia that may be effective in stabilizing cognitive deficit.[82,83] Other medications that have been investigated include donezepil, memantine, hydergine, pentoxifylline, propentofylline, piracetam, nimodipine, and ginkgo biloba. Most of these have all shown only modest and/or clinically irrelevant effects.[84] Chui[84] also notes that therapeutic effects are usually very similar in patients with Alzheimer disease and vascular dementia, suggesting that the these two types of dementia may share a common or similar pharmacodynamic basis. (See Chapter 14 for further discussion of prospects for preventing dementia.)

APHASIA

Aphasia is one of the most common consequences of stroke in both the acute and chronic phases. A recent report based on data from the Ontario Stroke Audit (Ontario, Canada) estimated that 35% of individuals with stroke have symptoms of aphasia at the time of discharge from inpatient care.[85] Aphasia is generally described as an impairment of language as a result of focal brain damage to the language-dominant cerebral hemisphere. This serves to distinguish it from language and cognitive-communication problems associated with non–language dominant hemisphere damage, dementia, and TBI.[86] The Boston classification system is used frequently by researchers and clinicians to classify types of aphasia on the basis of fluency (Table 18–3 and Figure 18–3). Type of aphasia (eg, Broca

Table 18–3. Boston Classification System—Characteristic Features of Aphasia

Type	Fluency	Comprehension	Repetition
Broca's	Nonfluent	Good	Poor
Transcortical motor	Nonfluent	Good	Good
Global	Nonfluent	Poor	Poor
Wernicke's	Fluent	Poor	Poor
Transcortical sensory	Fluent	Poor	Good
Anomic	Fluent	Good	Good
Conduction	Fluent	Good	Poor

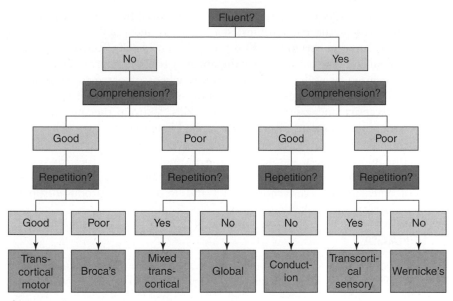

Figure 18–3. Assessment of aphasia.

aphasia) is determined, primarily, by lesion location (see Figure 18–4).[87] For many, aphasia improves during the first year following the stroke event. A review by Ferro et al[50] reported that approximately 40% of acutely aphasic patients experience complete or almost complete recovery by one year poststroke. Pedersen et al[88] reported that during these first 12 months, aphasia of all types (even global aphasia) tended to evolve to a less severe form. Nonfluent aphasias evolved to fluent aphasias, although the reverse was not observed. Although 61% of aphasic patients in the Copenhagen Aphasia Study still experienced aphasia at 1 year poststroke, it was usually of a milder form.[88]

The presence of aphasia has an adverse effect on mood, functional, and social outcomes as well as overall quality of life.[50,89,90] Conversation is important in social

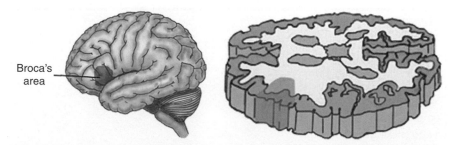

Figure 18–4. Broca aphasia. Posterior-inferior frontal lobe stroke characterized by non-fluent, effortful speech with preserved comprehension and poor repetition. (Reprinted by permission of Robert Teasell.)

participation and plays an important role in many social functions such as establishing and maintaining relationships, sharing ideas and opinions, and making plans. Speech language therapy (SLT) is generally considered effective in the treatment of aphasia poststroke.[91] Intensive therapy may result in improved written and receptive language, as well as in overall severity when compared to conventional therapy.[13,91] Social support and communication stimulation is also associated with improved receptive and expressive language skills.[91] Group therapy for aphasic patients is a potential means to maximize limited language therapy resources and encourage social interactions. Training conversation or communication partners within the aphasic's social setting may also promote opportunities for restored access to conversation.[92] In addition, volunteer-facilitated therapy appears to produce outcomes similar to conventional SLT and, in one study, produced superior results on measures of spoken repetition.[91]

DYSPHAGIA

Dysphagia is defined as difficulty with swallowing and is a common complication of stroke (Table 18–4). The incidence rates are reported to be 29% to 67% in the acute stage of stroke.[93] The presence of dysphagia in stroke survivors has been associated with increased mortality and morbidities such as malnutrition, dehydration, and pulmonary compromise.[94-96] Evidence indicates that detecting and managing dysphagia in acute stroke survivors improves outcomes such as reduced risk of pneumonia, length of hospital stay, and overall health care expenditures.[94]

Aspiration following stroke, the most clinically significant symptom of dysphagia, has long been associated with pneumonia, sepsis, and death. Silver et al[97] and Bounds et al[98] reported that pneumonia was the second most common cause of death during the acute phase of a stroke, with up to 20% of individuals with stroke-related dysphagia dying during the first year poststroke from aspiration pneumonia.[99] Detection of aspiration, both silent and audible, and subsequent adaptive management strategies are regarded as important in the prevention of pneumonia.[100-102] Management of dysphagia largely focuses on strategies to avoid

Table 18–4. Signs and Symptoms of Dysphagia

- Choking on food
- Coughing during meals
- Drooling or loss of food from mouth
- Pocketing of food in cheeks
- Slow, effortful eating
- Difficulty swallowing pills
- Avoiding foods or fluids

Complaining of

- Food sticking in throat
- Problems swallowing
- Reflux or heartburn

Table 18–5. Factors Associated With Aspiration Poststroke

- Brainstem stroke
- Difficulty swallowing oral secretions
- Coughing/throat clearing, choking, or wet, gurgly voice quality after swallowing water
- Weak voice and cough
- Recurrent lower respiratory infections
- Aspiration or pharyngeal delay on VMBS
- Immunologically compromised or chronic lung disease
- Poor oral hygiene

aspiration following stroke. Factors associated with aspiration poststroke are listed in Table 18–5.

Assessment

Following a stroke, patients should have their swallowing ability evaluated using a simple, valid, reliable bedside screening test before initiating oral intake of medications, fluids, or food. Most of these screening tests are comprised of two (or more) components. Typically, there is some form of swallowing trial, which is preceded by a questionnaire or preliminary examination. Patients who pass the screening are unlikely to have significant swallowing difficulties and have a minimal risk of dysphagic complications. Patients who fail the screen should be assessed by a speech-language pathologist. Several forms of clinical or bedside swallowing evaluations have been described. Some of these methods target specific functions or tasks, and others evaluate swallowing ability using a more comprehensive approach.

When aspiration is suspected, the **videofluoroscopic modified barium swallow (VMBS) study** is often considered the "gold standard" in confirming the diagnosis.[103] A VMBS study examines the oral and pharyngeal phases of swallowing. The patient must have sufficient cognitive and physical skills to undergo testing.[104] Radio-opaque materials of various consistencies are tested: barium-impregnated thin and thick liquids, pudding, bread, and cookies are routinely used. Various aspects of oral, laryngeal, and pharyngeal involvement are noted during the radiographic examination. The VMBS study is then followed by a chest x-ray to document any barium that may have been aspirated into the tracheobronchial tree.

The VMBS assessment not only establishes the presence and extent of aspiration but may also reveal the mechanism of the swallowing disorder. Aspiration most often results from a functional disturbance in the pharyngeal phase of swallowing related to reduced laryngeal closure or pharyngeal paresis. A VMBS study is recommended in those cases where the patient is experiencing obvious problems maintaining adequate hydration/nutrition, where concern is expressed regarding frequent choking while eating, or in the case of recurrent respiratory infections. A definitive criterion to determine if a VMBS study is required has yet to be determined in a systematic and scientific manner. Repeat VMBS studies are usually conducted at the discretion of the SLP/MD based on the progress and prognosis of the individual patient. No standard schedule for reassessment exists.

Treatment

Modified-texture diets are usually the first step in the management of dysphagia. They serve three purposes: (1) to decrease the risk of aspiration, (2) to provide adequate nutrients and fluids, and (3) to provide a progressive approach to feeding based on improvement or deterioration of swallowing function.[104] No single dysphagia diet exists. Dysphagia diets include modified food and liquid textures. Five different consistencies of food—thin and thick fluids, pureed, minced, and solids—are used, usually in conjunction with thickened fluids. Dysphagia soft diet eliminates all hard, small, and stringy food particles. Although **dietary modifications** are a commonly used strategy, evidence that their use reduces the risk of aspiration pneumonia has not been yet well established.

Nonoral feedings are a well-established practice for those patients who cannot handle oral feeds and increasingly are implemented early, within three to four days of the stroke. In the short term, a nasogastric feeding tube is the most commonly used device. If dysphagia is severe (ie, still aspirating) and the patient is expected to remain unsafe with oral intake for more than six weeks, a gastrostomy or jejunostomy tube is indicated. Enteral feeding tubes have been shown to deliver adequate nutrition and hydration to stroke survivors, and can improve indicators of nutritional status.[105,106] Although enteral feeding tubes are often used with the aim of preventing aspiration pneumonia, their use has been identified as both protective and a risk factor for pneumonia.[107-109]

POSTSTROKE DEPRESSION (PSD)

Incidence of Poststroke Depression

Depression is a common complication of stroke. In a systematic review of prospective, observational studies of PSD, Hackett et al[110] reported that 33% of stroke survivors exhibit depressive symptoms at some time following stroke (acute, medium-term, or long-term follow-up). This is likely to be an underestimation attributable to under-reporting of unusual mood, difficulties in the assessment of depression in neurologically impaired individuals, and variability in the methods used to assess and define depression within the literature.[110] The highest rates of incident depression have been reported in the first month following stroke,[111-113] and although the incidence of major depression poststroke may decrease over the first 24 months following stroke,[114,115] minor depression tends to persist or increase over the same time period.[115,116] Risk factors associated with PSD include female sex, past history of depression or psychiatric illness, and severity of functional limitations.[117,118] In addition, the association between the brain lesion as a result of stroke and PSD has been the topic of much research. However, there remains a wide diversity of findings in studies looking at the relationships between stroke location and depression. Not all studies have confirmed the hypothesized relationship, and meta-analyses have failed to establish a definitive relationship between the site of the brain lesion and depression.[119-121]

Impact of Depression Poststroke

PSD is associated with reduced functional ability and may have a negative impact on recovery. Although patients with PSD may experience significant recovery over time, functional ability will remain at a lower level than nondepressed patients, despite rehabilitation interventions.[122-124] Goodwin and Devanand[125] demonstrated that co-occurrence of stroke and depression is associated with greater physical limitations than either condition on its own. Physical impairment and PSD appear to act upon each other, and each influences the recovery of the other. PSD has also been associated with reduced frequency and satisfaction with social contacts (family and friends),[126] increased cognitive impairment (referred to as the dementia of depression),[127] and increased risk for mortality.[128-130]

Treatment of Poststroke Depression

Treatment of PSD usually involves the use of medications, with or without the addition of psychosocial therapies. Drug therapy for depression is based on the notion that depression is associated with an imbalance and underactivity of the cerebral noradrenergic and serotonergic systems. The use of pharmacotherapy has been associated with significant positive treatment effects,[131,132] particularly as the duration of treatment increases.[131] There are two classes of drugs used most frequently in the treatment of PSD: heterocyclic antidepressants (eg, nortriptyline, imipramine) and selective serotonin reuptake inhibitors (SSRIs; eg, fluoxetine, citalopram, sertraline). Although heterocyclic antidepressants may be an effective treatment for PSD,[133] the relatively high incidence of side effects associated with their use, especially in elderly patients, must be taken into account.[134-136] SSRIs may be as effective as heterocyclic antidepressants,[16,137,138] but response to treatment may be quicker and side effects fewer and less severe than those associated with heterocyclic drugs.[138] Successful treatment of PSD has been associated with improved functional recovery[139] and increased survival.[140] Because depression is a treatable condition, with significant consequences, it should be taken into account in the evaluation and treatment of all stroke patients.

There are several sets of current rehabilitation guidelines that make recommendations for the assessment and treatment of mood disorders following stroke.[7,14,141] In general, all acknowledge the importance of the identification and diagnosis of depression. All recommend the use of standardized assessment, and most indicate that a clinical interview conducted by an appropriate mental health care professional is required for diagnosis. Treatment, in the form of antidepressant medication (usually an SSRI), is recommended, although the details and possible duration of treatment are not clearly stated. The possible role of psychotherapy is acknowledged, although there is little evidence of its effectiveness within this population.

SUMMARY

Once a stroke occurs, stroke rehabilitation offers the best opportunity to maximize recovery and obtain best outcomes. Stroke rehabilitation units, characterized by dedicated beds grouped within a geographically defined space and staffed by a stroke specialized interdisciplinary team, is important to ensuring best outcomes. However, it is not enough to just have a specialized stroke rehabilitation unit; processes of care such as early admission to rehabilitation, intensity of rehabilitation therapy, task-specific therapies, and accessibility to outpatient therapies have been shown to be as important if not more important. Evidence is building for a number of specific rehabilitation interventions: treadmill training with partial body weight support, functional electrical stimulation, mental imagery, constraint-induced movement therapy, and botulinum toxin injections, as well as group and volunteer-driven aphasia therapy. Depression has the potential to derail or limit the impact of rehabilitation, and its assessment and treatment is increasingly recognized as being as important as physical rehabilitation.

REFERENCES

1. Dombovy ML. Stroke: clinical course and neurophysiologic mechanisms of recovery. *Phys Med Rehabil.* 1991;2(2):171-188.

2. Alexander MP. Stroke rehabilitation outcome. A potential use of predictive variables to establish levels of care. *Stroke.* 1994;25(1):128-134.

3. Hall R, O'Callaghan C, Bayley M, et al. *Ontario Stroke Evaluation Report 2010: Technical Report.* Toronto: Institute for Clinical Evaluative Sciences; 2010.

4. Garraway WM, Akhtar AJ, Smith DL, Smith ME. The triage of stroke rehabilitation. *J Epidemiol Community Health.* 1981;35(1):39-44.

5. Kalra L, Dale P, Crome P. Improving stroke rehabilitation. A controlled study [see comments]. *Stroke.* 1993;24(10):1462-1467.

6. Teasell RW, Foley NC, Bhogal SK, Chakravertty R, Bluvol A. A rehabilitation program for patients recovering from severe stroke. *Can J Neurol Sci.* 2005;32(4):512-517.

7. Lindsay MP, Gubitz G, Bayley M, et al. Canadian Best Practice Recommendations for Stroke Care (Update 2010). On behalf of the Canadian Stroke Strategy Best Practices and Standards Writing Group. 2010; Ottawa, Ontario Canada: Canadian Stroke Network. http://www.strokebestpractices.ca (accessed accessed January 14, 2012).

8. Langhorne P, Duncan P. Does the organization of postacute stroke care really matter? *Stroke.* 2001;32(1):268-274.

9. Langhorne P, Pollock A. What are the components of effective stroke unit care? *Age Ageing.* 2002;31(5):365-371.

10. Schallert T, Fleming SM, Woodlee MT. Should the injured and intact hemispheres be treated differently during the early phases of physical restorative therapy in experimental stroke or parkinsonism? *Phys Med Rehabil Clin N Am.* 2003;14(1 Suppl):S27-S46.

11. Maulden SA, Gassaway J, Horn SD, Smout RJ, DeJong G. Timing of initiation of rehabilitation after stroke. *Arch Phys Med Rehabil.* 2005;86(12 Suppl 2):S34-S40.

12. Salter K, Jutai J, Hartley M, et al. Impact of early vs delayed admission to rehabilitation on functional outcomes in persons with stroke. *J Rehabil Med.* 2006;38(2):113-117.

13. Bhogal SK, Teasell R, Speechley M. Intensity of aphasia therapy, impact on recovery. *Stroke.* 2003;34(4):987-993.

14. Duncan PW, Zorowitz R, Bates B, et al. Management of adult stroke rehabilitation care: a clinical practice guideline. *Stroke.* 2005;36(9):e100-e143.

15. Kwakkel G, van PR, Wagenaar RC, et al. Effects of augmented exercise therapy time after stroke: a meta-analysis. *Stroke.* 2004;35(11):2529-2539.

16. Andersen G, Vestergaard K, Lauritzen L. Effective treatment of poststroke depression with the selective serotonin reuptake inhibitor citalopram [see comments]. *Stroke.* 1994;25(6):1099-1104.

17. *Clinical Guidelines for Stroke Management.* Melborne, Australia: National Stroke Foundation; 2010.

18. Intercollegiate Stroke WP. *National Clinical Guideline for Stroke.* 3rd ed. London: Royal College of Physicians; 2008.

19. Gresham G, Duncan P, Adams H, et al. *Post-Stroke Rehabilitation.* Clinical Practice Guidelilne No. 16, CAHCPR Publication No. 95-0662. Rockville, MD: Department of Health and Human Services, Public Health Service, Agency for Health Care Policy and Research; 1995.

20. Bobath B. *Adult Hemiplegia: Evaluation and Assessment.* 3rd ed. London: Heinemann; 1990.

21. Langhammer B, Stanghelle JK. Bobath or motor relearning programme? A comparison of two different approaches of physiotherapy in stroke rehabilitation: a randomized controlled study. *Clin Rehabil.* 2000;14(4):361-369.

22. Langhammer B, Stanghelle JK. Bobath or motor relearning programme? A follow-up one and four years post stroke. *Clin Rehabil.* 2003;17(7):731-734.

23. Lincoln NB. Is stroke better managed in the community? Only hospitals can provide the required skills. *BMJ.* 1994;309(6965):1357-1358.

24. Young J. Is stroke better managed in the community? Community care allows patients to reach their full potential. *BMJ.* 1994;309(6965):1356-1357.

25. Langhorne P, Holmqvist LW. Early supported discharge after stroke. *J Rehabil Med.* 2007;39(2): 103-108.

26. Teng J, Mayo NE, Latimer E, et al. Costs and caregiver consequences of early supported discharge for stroke patients. *Stroke.* 2003;34(2):528-536.

27. Hesse S, Werner C, vonFrankenberg S, Bardelben S. Treadmill training with partial body weight support after stroke. *Phys Med Rehab Clin N Am.* 2003;14(1 Suppl):S111-S123.

28. Sonde L, Gip C, Fernaeus SE, Nilsson CG, Viitanen M. Stimulation with low frequency (1.7 Hz) transcutaneous electric nerve stimulation (low-tens) increases motor function of the post-stroke paretic arm. *Scand J Rehabil Med.* 1998;30(2):95-99.

29. Kottink AI, Oostendorp LJ, Buurke JH, Nene AV, Hermens HJ, IJzerman MJ. The orthotic effect of functional electrical stimulation on the improvement of walking in stroke patients with a dropped foot: a systematic review. *Artif Organs.* 2004;28(6):577-586.

30. Robbins SM, Houghton PE, Woodbury MG, Brown JL. The therapeutic effect of functional and transcutaneous electric stimulation on improving gait speed in stroke patients: a meta-analysis. *Arch Phys Med Rehabil.* 2006;87(6):853-859.

31. Hiraoka K. Rehabilitation effort to improve upper extremity function in post-stroke patients: a meta-analysis. *J Phys Ther Sci.* 2005;13:5-9.

32. Page SJ, Levine P, Sisto SA, Johnston MV. Mental practice combined with physical practice for upper-limb motor deficit in subacute stroke. *Phys Ther.* 2001;81(8):1455-1462.

33. Page SJ, Levine P, Leonard A. Mental practice in chronic stroke: results of a randomized, placebo-controlled trial. *Stroke.* 2007;38(4):1293-1297.

34. Fritz SL, Light KE, Patterson TS, Behrman AL, Davis SB. Active finger extension predicts outcomes after constraint-induced movement therapy for individuals with hemiparesis after stroke. *Stroke.* 2005;36(6):1172-1177.

35. Taub E, Uswatte G, Pidikiti R. Constraint-induced movement therapy: a new family of techniques with broad application to physical rehabilitation—a clinical review. *J Rehabil Res Dev.* 1999;36(3): 237-251.

36. Wolf SL, Thompson PA, Morris DM, et al. The EXCITE trial: attributes of the Wolf Motor Function Test in patients with subacute stroke. *Neurorehabil Neural Repair.* 2005;19(3):194-205.

37. Taub E, Morris DM. Constraint-induced movement therapy to enhance recovery after stroke. *Curr Atheroscler Rep.* 2001;3(4):279-286.

38. Dromerick AW, Lang CE, Birkenmeier RL, et al. Very early constraint-induced movement during stroke rehabilitation (VECTORS): a single-center RCT. *Neurology.* 2009;73(3):195-201.

39. Grotta JC, Noser EA, Ro T, et al. Constraint-induced movement therapy. *Stroke.* 2004;35(11 Suppl 1):2699-2701.

40. Popovic MR, Popovic DB, Keller T. Neuroprostheses for grasping. *Neurol Res.* 2002;24(5):443-452.

41. Sommerfeld DK, Eek EU, Svensson AK, Holmqvist LW, von Arbin MH. Spasticity after stroke: its occurrence and association with motor impairments and activity limitations. *Stroke.* 2004;35(1): 134-139.

42. Brashear A, Gordon MF, Elovic E, et al. Intramuscular injection of botulinum toxin for the treatment of wrist and finger spasticity after a stroke. *N Engl J Med.* 2002;347(6):395-400.

43. Titus MN, Gall NG, Yerxa EJ, Roberson TA, Mack W. Correlation of perceptual performance and activities of daily living in stroke patients. *Am J Occup Ther.* 1991;45(5):410-418.

44. Edmans JA, Webster J, Lincoln NB. A comparison of two approaches in the treatment of perceptual problems after stroke. *Clin Rehabil.* 2000;14(3):230-243.

45. Steultjens EM, Dekker J, Bouter LM, van de Nes JCM, Cup EHC, van den Ende CHM. Occupational therapy for stroke patients. A systematic review. *Stroke.* 2003;34:676-687.

46. Heilman KM, Watson RT, Valenstein E. Neglect and related disorders. In: Heilman KM, Valenstein E, eds. *Clinical Neurospychology.* New York: Oxford Press; 1985:243-293.

47. Appelros P, Karlsson GM, Seiger A, Nydevik I. Neglect and anosognosia after first-ever stroke: incidence and relationship to disability. *J Rehabil Med.* 2002;34:215-220.

48. Pedersen PM, Jorgensen HS, Nakayama H, Raaschou HO, Olsen TS. Hemineglect in acute stroke—incidence and prognostic implications: the Copenhagen Stroke Study. *Am J Phys Med Rehabil.* 1997;76(2):122-127.

49. Ringman JM, Saver JL, Woolson RF, Clarke WR, Adams HP. Frequency, risk factors, anatomy, and course of unilateral neglect in an acute stroke cohort. *Neurology.* 2004;63(3):468-474.

50. Ferro JM, Mariano G, Madureira S. Recovery from aphasia and neglect. *Cerebrovasc Dis.* 1999; 9(Suppl 5):6-22.

51. Appelros P, Nydevik I, Karlsson GM, Thorwalls A, Seiger A. Recovery from unilateral neglect after right-hemisphere stroke. *Disabil Rehabil.* 2004;26(8):471-477.

52. Paolucci S, Antonucci G, Grasso MG, Pizzamiglio L. The role of unilateral spatial neglect in rehabilitation of right brain-damaged ischemic stroke patients: a matched comparison. *Arch Phys Med Rehabil.* 2001;82:743-749.

53. Gillen R, Tennen H, McKee T. Unilateral spatial neglect: relation to rehabilitation outcomes in patients with right hemisphere stroke. *Arch Phys Med Rehabil.* 2005;86(4):763-767.

54. Royal College of Physicians (RCP) London. National Clinical Guidelines for Stroke. 2002. http://bookshop.rcplondon.ac.uk.

55. Kelly-Hayes M, Robertson JT, Broderick JP, et al. The American Heart Association Stroke Outcome Classification. *Stroke.* 1998;29(6):1274-1280.

56. Menon A, Korner-Bitensky N. Evaluating unilateral spatial neglect post stroke: working your way through the maze of assessment choices. *Top Stroke Rehabil.* 2004;11(3):41-66.

57. Butter CM, Kirsch NL, Regev I. The effect of lateralized dynamic stimuli on unilateral spatial neglect following right hemisphere lesions. *Restor Neurol Neurosci.* 1990;2:39-46.

58. Pierce SR, Buxbaum LJ. Treatments of unilateral neglect: a review. *Arch Phys Med Rehabil.* 2002; 83(2):256-268.

59. Weinberg J, Diller L, Gordon WA, et al. Visual scanning training effect on reading-related tasks in acquired right brain damage. *Arch Phys Med Rehabil.* 1977;58(11):479-486.

60. Ladavas E, Menghini G, Umilta C. A rehabilitation study of hemispatial neglect. *Cogn Neuropsychol.* 1994;11(1):75-95.

61. Cicerone KD, Dahlberg C, Kalmar K, et al. Evidence-based cognitive rehabilitation: recommendations for clinical practice. *Arch Phys Med Rehabil.* 2000;81(12):1596-1615.

62. Cappa SF, Benke T, Clarke S, Rossi B, Stemmer B, van Heugten CM. EFNS guidelines on cognitive rehabilitation: report of an EFNS task force. *Eur J Neurol.* 2005;12(9):665-680.

63. Weinberg J, Diller L, Gordon WA, et al. Training sensory awareness and spatial organization in people with right brain damage. *Arch Phys Med Rehabil.* 1979;60(11):491-496.

64. Rossetti Y, Rode G, Pisella L, et al. Prism adaptation to a rightward optical deviation rehabilitates left hemispatial neglect. *Nature.* 1998;395(6698):166-169.

65. Farne A, Rossetti Y, Toniolo S, Ladavas E. Ameliorating neglect with prism adaptation: visuo-manual and visuo-verbal measures. *Neuropsychologia.* 2002;40:718-729.

66. Frassinetti F, Angeli V, Meneghello F, Avanzi S, Ladavas E. Long-lasting amelioration of visuospatial neglect by prism adaptation. *Brain.* 2002;(125):608-623.

67. Rode G, Pisella L, Rossetti Y, Farne A, Boisson D. Bottom-up transfer of sensory-motor plasticity to recovery os spatial cognition: visuomotor adaptation and spatial neglect. *Prog Brain Res.* 2003;142: 273-287.

68. Shiraishi H, Yamakawa Y, Itou A, Muraki T, Asada T. Long-term effects of prism adaptation on chronic neglect after stroke. *NeuroRehabilitation.* 2008;23(2):137-151.

69. Maravita A, McNeil J, Malhotra P, Greenwood R, Husain M, Driver J. Prism adaptation can improve contralesional tactile perception in neglect. *Neurology.* 2003;60:1829-1831.

70. Shulman GL. An asymmetry in the control of eye movements and shifts of attention. *Acta Psychol (Amst).* 1984;55(1):53-69.

71. Beis JM, Andre JM, Baumgarten A, Challier B. Eye patching in unilateral spatial neglect: efficacy of two methods. *Arch Phys Med Rehabil.* 1999;80(1):71-76.

72. Zeloni G, Farne A, Baccini M. Viewing less to see better. *J Neurol Neurosurg Psychiatry.* 2002;73(2): 195-198.

73. Tsang MH, Sze KH, Fong KN. Occupational therapy treatment with right half-field eye-patching for patients with subacute stroke and unilateral neglect: a randomised controlled trial. *Disabil Rehabil.* 2009;31(8):630-637.

74. O'Brien JT, Erkinjuntti T, Reisberg B, et al. Vascular cognitive impairment. *Lancet Neurol.* 2003; 2(2):89-98.

75. Ballard C, Stephens S, McLaren A, et al. Neuropsychological deficits in older stroke patients. *Ann N Y Acad Sci.* 2002;977:179-182.

76. Stephens S, Kenny RA, Rowan E, et al. Neuropsychological characteristics of mild vascular cognitive impairment and dementia after stroke. *Int J Geriatr Psychiatry.* 2004;19:1053-1057.

77. Ingles JL, Wentzel C, Fisk JD, Rockwood K. Neuropsychological predictors of incident dementia in patients with vascular cognitive impairment, without dementia. *Stroke.* 2002;33(8):1999-2002.

78. Patel M, Coshall C, Rudd AG, Wolfe CDA. Natural history of cognitive impairment after stroke and factors associated with its recovery. *Clin Rehabil.* 2003;17:158-166.

79. Ivan CS, Seshadri S, Beiser A, et al. Dementia after stroke: the Framingham Study. *Stroke.* 2004; 35(6):1264-1268.

80. Pendlebury ST, Cuthbertson FC, Welch SJ, Mehta Z, Rothwell PM. Underestimation of cognitive impairment by Mini-Mental State Examination versus the Montreal Cognitive Assessment in patients with transient ischemic attack and stroke: a population-based study. *Stroke.* 2010;41(6):1290-1293.

81. Cicerone KD, Dahlberg C, Malec JF, et al. Evidence-based cognitive rehabilitation: updated review of the literature from 1998 through 2002. *Arch Phys Med Rehabil.* 2005;86(8):1681-1692.

82. Meyer JS, Rogers RL, McClintic K, Mortel KF, Lotfi J. Randomized clinical trial of daily aspirin therapy in multi-infarct dementia. A pilot study. *J Am Geriatr Soc.* 1989;37(6):549-555.

83. Rands G, Orrel M, Spector A, Williams P. Aspirin for vascular dementia. *Cochrane Database Sys Rev.* 2000;(4):CD001296.

84. Chui H. Vascular dementia, a new beginning, shifting focus from clinical phenotype to ischemic brain injury. *Neurol Clin.* 2000;18:951-978.

85. Dickey L, Kagan A, Lindsay MP, Fang J, Rowland A, Black S. Incidence and profile of inpatient stroke-induced aphasia in Ontario, Canada. *Arch Phys Med Rehabil.* 2010;91(2):196-202.

86. Orange JB, Kertesz A. Efficacy of language therapy for aphasia. *Phys Med Rehabil.* 1998;12(3): 501-517.

87. Godefroy O, Dubois C, Debachy B, Leclerc M, Kreisler A. Vascular aphasias: main characteristics of patients hospitalized in acute stroke units. *Stroke.* 2002;33(3):702-705.

88. Pedersen PM, Vinter K, Olsen TS. Aphasia after stroke: type, severity and prognosis. The Copenhagen aphasia study. *Cerebrovasc Dis.* 2004;17(1):35-43.

89. Davidson B, Howe T, Worrall L, Hickson L, Togher L. Social participation for older people with aphasia: the impact of communication disability on friendships. *Top Stroke Rehabil.* 2008;15(4): 325-340.

90. Wade DT, Hewer RL, David RM, Enderby PM. Aphasia after stroke: natural history and associated deficits. *J Neurol Neurosurg Psychiatry.* 1986;49(1):11-16.

91. Kelly H, Brady MC, Enderby P. Speech and language therapy for aphasia following stroke. *Cochrane Database Syst Rev.* 2010;5:CD000425.

92. Kagan A, Black SE, Duchan FJ, Simmons-Mackie N, Square P. Training volunteers as conversation partners using "Supported Conversation for Adults with Aphasia" (SCA): a controlled trial. *J Speech Lang Hear Res.* 2001;44(3):624-638.

93. Martino R, Foley N, Bhogal S, Diamant N, Speechley M, Teasell R. Dysphagia after stroke: incidence, diagnosis, and pulmonary complications. *Stroke.* 2005;36(12):2756-2763.

94. Smithard DG, O'Neill PA, Parks C, Morris J. Complications and outcome after acute stroke. Does dysphagia matter? *Stroke.* 1996;27(7):1200-1204.

95. Gordon C, Hewer RL, Wade DT. Dysphagia in acute stroke. *Br Med J (Clin Res Ed).* 1987; 295(6595):411-414.

96. Barer DH. The natural history and functional consequences of dysphagia after hemispheric stroke. *J Neurol Neurosurg Psychiatry.* 1989;52(2):236-241.

97. Silver FL, Norris JW, Lewis AJ, Hachinski VC. Early mortality following stroke: a prospective review. *Stroke.* 1984;15(3):492-496.

98. Bounds JV, Wiebers DO, Whisnant JP, Okazaki H. Mechanisms and timing of deaths from cerebral infarction. *Stroke.* 1981;12(4):474-477.

99. Scmidt EV, Smirnov VE, Ryabova VS. Results of the seven-year prospective study of stroke patients. *Stroke.* 1988;19(8):942-949.

100. Horner J, Massey EW. Silent aspiration following stroke. *Neurology.* 1988;38(2):317-319.

101. Horner J, Massey EW, Riski JE, Lathrop DL, Chase KN. Aspiration following stroke: clinical correlates and outcome. *Neurology.* 1988;38(9):1359-1362.

102. Teasell RW, McRae M, Marchuk Y, Finestone HM. Pneumonia associated with aspiration following stroke. *Arch Phys Med Rehabil.* 1996;77(7):707-709.

103. Splaingard ML, Hutchins B, Sulton LD, Chaudhuri G. Aspiration in rehabilitation patients: videofluoroscopy vs bedside clinical assessment. *Arch Phys Med Rehabil.* 1988;69(8):637-640.

104. Bach DB, Pouget S, Belle K, et al. An integrated team approach to the management of patients with oropharyngeal dysphagia. *J Allied Health.* 1989;18(5):459-468.

105. Finestone HM, Greene-Finestone LS, Wilson ES, Teasell RW. Malnutrition in stroke patients on the rehabilitation service and at follow-up: prevalence and predictors. *Arch Phys Med Rehabil.* 1995;76(4):310-316.

106. Norton B, McLean KA, Holmes GK. Outcome in patients who require a gastrostomy after stroke. *Age Ageing.* 1996;25(6):493.

107. Finucane TE, Bynum JP. Use of tube feeding to prevent aspiration pneumonia. *Lancet.* 1996; 348(9039):1421-1424.

108. Dziewas R, Ritter M, Schilling M, et al. Pneumonia in acute stroke patients fed by nasogastric tube. *J Neurol Neurosurg Psychiatry.* 2004;75(6):852-856.

109. Nakajoh K, Nakagawa T, Sekizawa K, Matsui T, Arai H, Sasaki H. Relation between incidence of pneumonia and protective reflexes in post-stroke patients with oral or tube feeding. *J Intern Med.* 2000;247(1):39-42.

110. Hackett ML, Yapa C, Parag V, Anderson CS. Frequency of depression after stroke: a systematic review of observational studies. *Stroke.* 2005;36(6):1330-1340.

111. Morrison V, Pollard B, Johnston M, Macwalter R. Anxiety and depression 3 years following stroke: demographic, clinical, and psychological predictors. *J Psychosom Res.* 2005;59(4): 209-213.

112. Aben I, Lodder J, Honig A, Lousberg R, Boreas A, Verhey F. Focal or generalized vascular brain damage and vulnerability to depression after stroke: a 1-year prospective follow-up study. *Int Psychogeriatr.* 2006;18(1):19-35.

113. Bour A, Rasquin S, Aben I, Boreas A, Limburg M, Verhey F. A one-year follow-up study into the course of depression after stroke. *J Nutr Health Aging.* 2010;14(6):488-493.

114. Astrom M, Adolfsson R, Asplund K. Major depression in stroke patients. A 3-year longitudinal study. *Stroke.* 1993;24(7):976-982.

115. Verdelho A, Henon H, Lebert F, Pasquier F, Leys D. Depressive symptoms after stroke and relationship with dementia. A three-year follow-up study. *Neurology.* 2004;62:905-911.

116. Berg A, Palomaki H, Lehtihalmes M, Lonnqvist J, Kaste M. Poststroke depression: an 18-month follow-up. *Stroke.* 2003;34(1):138-143.

117. Paolucci S, Gandolfo C, Provinciali L, Torta R, Sommacal S, Toso V. Quantification of the risk of post stroke depression: the Italian multicenter observational study DESTRO. *Acta Psychiatr Scand.* 2005;112(4):272-278.

118. Hackett ML, Anderson CS. Frequency, management, and predictors of abnormal mood after stroke: the Auckland Regional Community Stroke (ARCOS. study, 2002 to 2003). *Stroke.* 2006;37(8): 2123-2128.

119. Singh A, Herrmann N, Black SE. The importance of lesion location in poststroke depression: a critical review. *Can J Psychiatry.* 1998;43(9):921-927.

120. Carson AJ, MacHale S, Allen K, et al. Depression after stroke and lesion location: a systematic review. *Lancet.* 2000;356(9224):122-126.

121. Bhogal SK, Teasell R, Foley N, Speechley M. Lesion location and poststroke depression: systematic review of the methodological limitations in the literature. *Stroke.* 2004;35(3):794-802.

122. Nannetti L, Paci M, Pasquini J, Lombardi B, Taiti PG. Motor and functional recovery in patients with post-stroke depression. *Disabil Rehabil.* 2005;27(4):170-175.

123. Paolucci S, Gandolfo C, Provinciali L, Torta R, Toso V. The Italian multicenter observational study on post-stroke depression (DESTRO). *J Neurol.* 2006;253(5):556-562.

124. Saxena SK, Ng TP, Koh G, Yong D, Fong NP. Is improvement in impaired cognition and depressive symptoms in post-stroke patients associated with recovery in activities of daily living? *Acta Neurol Scand.* 2007;115(5):339-346.

125. Goodwin RD, Devanand DP. Stroke, depression, and functional health outcomes among adults in the community. *J Geriatr Psychiatry Neurol.* 2008;21(1):41-46.

126. Sienkiewicz-Jarosz H, Milewska D, Bochynska A, et al. Predictors of depressive symptoms in patients with stroke—a three-month follow-up. *Neurol Neurochir Pol.* 2010;44(1):13-20.

127. Murata Y, Kimura M, Robinson RG. Does cognitive impairment cause post-stroke depression? *Am J Geriatr Psychiatry.* 2000;8(4):310-317.

128. Williams LS, Ghose SS, Swindle RW. Depression and other mental health diagnoses increase mortality risk after ischemic stroke. *Am J Psychiatry.* 2004;161(6):1090-1095.

129. Peters R, Pinto E, Beckett N, et al. Association of depression with subsequent mortality, cardiovascular morbidity and incident dementia in people aged 80 and over and suffering from hypertension. Data from the Hypertension in the Very Elderly Trial (HYVET). *Age Ageing.* 2010;39(4): 439-445.

130. Ellis C, Zhao Y, Egede LE. Depression and increased risk of death in adults with stroke. *J Psychosom Res.* 2010;68(6):545-551.

131. Chen Y, Guo JJ, Zhan S, Patel NC. Treatment effects of antidepressants in patients with post-stroke depression: a meta-analysis. *Ann Pharmacother.* 2006;40(12):2115-2122.

132. Hackett ML, Anderson CS, House A, Xia J. Interventions for treating depression after stroke. *Cochrane Database Sys Rev.* 2008;(4):Art.

133. Robinson RG, Schultz SK, Castillo C, et al. Nortriptyline versus fluoxetine in the treatment of depression and in short-term recovery after stroke: a placebo-controlled, double-blind study. *Am J Psychiatry.* 2000;157(3):351-359.

134. Lauritzen L, Bendsen BB, Vilmar T, Bendsen EB, Lunde M, Bech P. Post-stroke depression: combined treatment with imipramine or desipramine and mianserin. A controlled clinical study. *Psychopharmacology (Berl).* 1994;114(1):119-122.

135. Kumar V. Post-stroke depression and treatment strategies including Aniracetam. *Int J Geriatr Psychopharmacol.* 1999;2:40-46.

136. Steffens DC, Chung H, Krishnan KR, Longstreth WT Jr, Carlson M, Burke GL. Antidepressant treatment and worsening white matter on serial cranial magnetic resonance imaging in the elderly: the Cardiovascular Health Study. *Stroke.* 2008;39(3):857-862.

137. Wiart L, Petit H, Joseph PA, Mazaux JM, Barat M. Fluoxetine in early poststroke depression: a double-blind placebo-controlled study. *Stroke.* 2000;31(8):1829-1832.

138. Fruehwald S, Gatterbauer E, Rehak P, Baumhackl U. Early fluoxetine treatment of post-stroke depression—a three-month double-blind placebo-controlled study with an open-label long-term follow up. *J Neurol.* 2003;250(3):347-351.

139. Narushima K, Kosier JT, Robinson RG. Preventing poststroke depression: a 12-week double-blind randomized treatment trial and 21-month follow-up. *J Nerv Ment Dis.* 2002;190(5):296-303.

140. Jorge RE, Robinson RG, Arndt S, Starkstein S. Mortality and poststroke depression: a placebo-controlled trial of antidepressants. *Am J Psychiatry.* 2003;160:1823-1829.

141. Turner-Stokes L, Macwalter R. Use of antidepressant medication following acquired brain injury: concise guidance. *Clin Med.* 2005;5(3):268-274.

Index

NOTE: Page numbers followed by *f* and *t* denotes figures and tables, respectively.